DRUGS AND PHARMACY
IN THE
LIFE OF GEORGIA
1733-1959

DRUGS AND PHARMACY

IN THE

LIFE OF GEORGIA

1733-1959

By

ROBERT CUMMING WILSON

Dean Emeritus
School of Pharmacy
University of Georgia
Athens, Georgia

© 1959 by Robert Cumming Wilson
Paperback edition published in 2010 by
The University of Georgia Press
Athens, Georgia 30602
www.ugapress.org
All rights reserved
Printed digitally in the United States of America

The Library of Congress has cataloged the hardcover edition
of this book as follows:
Library of Congress Cataloging-in-Publication Data
LCCN Permalink: http://lccn.loc.gov/59014611

Wilson, Robert Cumming, 1878–
Drugs and pharmacy in the life of Georgia, 1733–1959.
ix, 443 p. illus. 25 cm.
Bibliography: p. 439–443.
1. Pharmacy—Georgia. 2. Medicine—Georgia. I. Title.
RS67.U7 G4
615.09758   59-14611

Paperback ISBN-13: 978-0-8203-3556-8
ISBN-10: 0-8203-3556-8

DEDICATED TO
MY FORMER STUDENTS
AND THOSE PHARMACISTS OF GEORGIA, PAST AND PRESENT,
WITH WHOM CLOSE ASSOCIATION AND COOPERATION
HAVE EXISTED THROUGH THE YEARS

CONTENTS

	Preface	ix
I	Reasons for the Establishment of the Colony of Georgia—The Search for Drugs a Prominent Factor	1
II	The Founding Fathers of the Profession of Pharmacy and Medicine in Georgia	16
III	Disease and Drug Problems Confronting the Colony	38
IV	Self-Diagnosis and Treatment of Ordinary and Epidemic Diseases Became a Necessity in the Life of the Colony and of the State, 1733-1807	58
V	With the Appearance of Newspapers in Georgia in 1763, the Value of Advertising Is Discovered and Is Promptly Adopted by Those Having Medicinal Products or Medical Services to Offer the Public, 1763-1820	97
VI	Public Health, Organization, Medical and Pharmaceutical Education, and Legislation Begin a Slow But Definite Process of Evolution, 1760-1828-1959	124
VII	The Retail Drug Store in Georgia— Past and Present	163

CONTENTS

VIII   Specialized Fields of Pharmacy—Wholesale and Manufacturing, the Professional Store (The Apothecary Shop), Hospital Pharmacy, Education, and Research 181

IX   The Soda Fountain—Soda Water: At First a Medicinal Agent, Becomes a Beverage . . . 203

X   Ether Anaesthesia, 1842, and Coca-Cola, 1886: Born in Georgia Drug Stores. A Story Whereby Coca-Cola Becomes the Complement of Ether Anaesthesia 217

XI   Drugs in the Modern Era 233

Supplement A: Medical Education 255

Supplement B: Pharmaceutical Education . . 267

Supplement C: Laws Governing the Practice of Medicine and Pharmacy, 1825-1958 279

Supplement D: The Georgia Pharmaceutical Association and the Women's Auxiliary . . . 317

Appendix 1: Glossary of Terms and Formulas of the Period, 1733-1800 423

Appendix 2: Some Drugs Used by the American Indians 428

Appendix 3: List of Drugs for Filling Medicine Chests or Boxes 430

Appendix 4: Diseases Transmittable from Certain Domestic Animals to Man 433

Appendix 5: Members of the Georgia State Board of Pharmacy, 1881-1958 436

Appendix 6: A Medical Fee Bill of Vintage 1865 438

Bibliography 439

PREFACE

IF WE would properly interpret the present and chart a new course for the future, we must of necessity look at the past. Recognizing this fact, Cicero in 50 B.C. pointed out to us that "If we fail to make use of the knowledge and labors of past ages, we will forever remain in the infancy of knowledge." He might also have said: We are what we are, and what we hope to become, because of what has been.

If we would understand the evolutionary processes by or through which pharmacy, as we know it today, has evolved, we must consider the history of drugs and the part they have played in the building of our civilization.

Whether operating under the name of apothecary, pharmacist, druggist, or drug dealer, these individuals, throughout the ages, have been charged with the responsibility of discovering, testing, preserving, manufacturing, standardizing, distributing, and dispensing medicinal agents whether for the treatment or prevention of diseases of man, animals, fowls, or plants.

Briefly, but solemnly stated, it is the function of pharmacy to supply the tools with which the physician treats disease, it being the function of the physician to supply the know-how of the use of these tools. This teamwork on the part of pharmacy and medicine is responsible for the progress being made in the treatment and/or prevention of disease. Therefore, the history of drugs becomes the history of pharmacy.

The vast amount of research and clerical work involved in the preparation of the manuscript for this volume could not have been possible but for the financial assistance and encouragement of that great friend and benefactor of Georgia pharmacy, Robert W. Woodruff of The Coca-Cola Company.

THE AUTHOR

CHAPTER I

REASONS FOR THE ESTABLISHMENT OF THE COLONY OF GEORGIA — THE SEARCH FOR DRUGS A PROMINENT FACTOR

FOR four thousand years and more, prior to the settlement of Georgia, the people of the earth had for all time depended upon drugs in the treatment or prevention of disease. Except perhaps for the Arctic Regions, native peoples, even though primitive in character, have relied upon the vegetable kingdom for their drugs. Their knowledge of the medicinal properties of plants and their ability to identify the particular plant and distinguish it from all others have been passed down to them from generation to generation from the beginning of time. This was certainly true of the American Indians, and we are told that they were a hardy, healthy race of people. And the same is true today wherever primitive peoples are found, whether in the isolated sections of America, the South Sea Islands, or the heart of Africa. They know how to identify and to use their native vegetable drugs in the prevention and treatment of disease.

There are some grounds for the belief on the part of some religious sects, and others, that the growing and the use of vegetable drugs began in the Garden of Eden as the first of the thousands of botanical gardens the world was to know thereafter. The theory was advanced by these religious sects, and others, that disease was produced by sin and that following the Fall of Man in the Garden of Eden there were provided for him various vegetable drugs there in the Garden which were considered to be sufficient for the treatment of any disease that flesh might be heir to. They believed further that the seeds, or other reproducing organs of these plants, were distributed to all sections of the world by way of the winds or the waters of the earth. This theory is not far removed from what John Wesley, the famous creator of Methodism, pronounced. During his stay in Georgia, and his contact with the American Indians, Wesley, impressed with their health and hardiness, began the observation and study of drugs, and later on began the practice of medicine and pharmacy following his return to England. Several years after his return to England, he wrote a textbook on the subject of medicine which was entitled, "Primitive Physick, or An Easy Way To Treat Any Ordinary Disease." This little booklet went through twenty-three editions and reprintings prior to his death and nine reprintings after his death, as the most popular of the many books he authored, even though it was frowned upon by practitioners of pharmacy and medicine.[1]

The preface in Wesley's book places the blame for illness on sin and divine retribution. He states that in the beginning "as man knew no sin, so he knew no pain, no sickness, no weakness or bodily disorders." Later, however, he declares, "The seeds of wickedness and pain, of sickness and death, are lodged in our inmost substance, whence a thousand disorders continually spring, even without the aid of external violence." The particular drugs mentioned in Wesley's book, and which were prescribed and dispensed by him, were some of those Indian vegetable drugs which he learned about during his stay in America, and which he gave one at a time, never using a mixture of them.

Accept or reject this theory as you will, but the fact remains as recorded by history that vegetable drugs have been in use longer than any other type of drug, and even today constitute an important factor in the prevention and treatment of many of our common diseases; though, throughout the centuries, Man, while continuing his exploration of the vegetable kingdom for new and better drugs, has also probed the animal and the mineral kingdoms for medicinal agents. In addition to this, in recent years, thousands of new medicinal products have come into existence as a result of the expansion of our knowledge through the practice of synthetic pharmaceutical chemistry.

The use of vegetable drugs, however, came on down through the centuries. Hippocrates, Aristotle, Asclepiades, Dioscorides, Galen and others were practicing medicine and pharmacy, and were exploring the vegetable kingdom constantly for new and better medicinal agents.

1. M. B. Gordon, *Aesculapius Comes to the Colonies,* p. 497.

℞ DRUGS IN THE COLONY

It is now revealed that the possibility of finding valuable vegetable drugs growing on the new Continent was a prominent factor in the mind of Oglethorpe and the apothecaries, physicians, botanists and surgeons of England who were instrumental in helping the English Government to arrive at the decision to begin the settlement of the Colony of Georgia.

In the settlement of the Colony of Virginia in 1607, the London Company promoted the settlement of the Colony by arguing the possibility of finding or growing drugs and other botanicals as one of the feasible means of financing the Colony. It was therefore logical that the Apothecaries Company should, 127 years later, use the same argument in promoting the colonization of Georgia.

In order to interpret the meaning of the various moves of the Spanish Government and the English Government in the latter part of the 15th century and the early part of the 16th century in so far as the American Continent is concerned, it is interesting to consider here some dates: in 1494 Columbus returns to this Continent and conquers Cuba; in 1513 Ponce de Leon discovers Florida and claims the entire Continent for the Spanish Government, though he did not settle in Florida at that time; in 1520 Mexico was conquered and settled by the Spaniards; in 1531 Peru in South America was conquered by the Spaniards; in 1540 De Soto explored Georgia, but established no settlement there; in 1565 and 1566 some Spanish missions were settled on the coast of Florida and of Georgia and Carolina; in 1607 the English settled Jamestown; and in 1670-1680 Charles Town, South Carolina, was settled by the English. The movement of the English southward and of the Spaniards northward along the coast set the stage for an eventual clash between them which culminated in the Battle of Bloody Marsh in 1742.

Landing in Mexico, the Spaniards began the exploration of that country for gold, and other minerals perhaps, but also in the hope of finding further commercial products growing there in the vegetation of that region. Among the valuable discoveries that were made was the Cochineal insect, which was growing on various plants of the Cactus family. The Cochineal insect, when killed and dried, came to be the source of most of the red dye that was available in the world at that time and for many years thereafter (especially as a food coloring), and therefore became a valuable commercial product.

Along with the Cochineal, the Spaniards found the natives

using a number of the native vegetable products as medicinal agents, some of which they adopted upon finding them of value, and promptly began the introduction of them on the European Continent, thereby promoting a monopoly not only in Cochineal, but also of the vegetable drugs they had found. In their effort to protect their monopolies in Mexico, they began the exploration of South America, and conquered Peru in 1531. Living among the natives there, they found them using the leaves of a plant which proved to be a remarkable stimulant, enabling them to do larger quantities of work without tiring. These leaves proved to be those of the Coca plant.

They also found the natives using some plant we now know as Ipecac, which is used as an expectorant in cough remedies, as a specific in the treatment of amoebic dysentery, in fevers, and also as an emetic.

But the drug they found which was to become world-wide in importance and significance was the bark of a tree. They found the natives using the bark in the treatment of fevers which were common to that particular area, (whether malarial fever no one knows). The legend is to the effect that the Countess Chinchon was cured of what may have been malarial fever, and the drug was given the name "Cinchona" in her honor.[2] The drug was introduced on the European Continent in 1640 as a secret remedy, and it was 100 years later before the source of the bark was known in Europe. From that date 1640 until after the war between England and Spain in 1742, in which war Spain was destroyed as a world power, the South American countries where Cinchona was grown were ruled by Spain, thus giving that country a complete monopoly so long as it could be protected. Years after the value of the bark was established, the active principle was isolated and given the name "Quinine." Quinine gave Spain and her armies a degree of protection not available to other countries when they were living and fighting in malaria-infested countries, for Quinine was recognized as the only remedy then known to be of value in the treatment of malaria. Before the Cinchona plant had received its botanical name and classification, it was called by various names: first, as "The Bark," Peruvian Bark, Calisaya Bark, Red Bark, Yellow Bark, Countess' Powder, or Jesuit's Bark. It was called Jesuit's Bark due to the fact that the Jesuits had introduced the drug in Europe in the treatment

---

2. The error in spelling is attributed to the botanist Linné. The name "Chinchona," if it were to honor the Countess Chinchon, should have prevailed.

of fever, and the Spanish Government had given these priests somewhat of a monopoly in its use and sale. It was for many years used as a secret remedy, and exorbitant prices charged for it. But for a number of years very little of the Bark was allowed to be exported to other countries of the world, particularly to England, which was a natural competitor of Spain for world power. A writer has well said that "What the discovery of gunpowder did for warfare, the discovery of Quinine has done in the fight against malaria."

Whether it is a coincidence or not is worth considering, but bear in mind that Cinchona had been introduced on the European Continent in 1640, and its value was being recognized more and more as the only drug which made it possible for armies to fight in malarial areas of the world. It seems significant that just a few years later the Spaniards should begin to expand the settlement of the Atlantic coast of the Continent of North America, which they had begun in 1565.

Their settlements were extended on up the Florida and Georgia coasts as far as Carolina. What their motives were in establishing those settlements may be somewhat speculative, but it is natural to suppose that they were thinking perhaps that these medicinal and coloring products which they had discovered in Mexico and in South America might by chance be growing in Georgia and Florida; and therefore, to protect their valuable monopolies in these products, they had moved in and begun the settlement of those areas.

The Spanish merchantmen, as well as the English merchantmen, had been coming into the Georgia Coast for some years and exporting therefrom the drug Sassafras, which was bought in large quantities, and the business developed to such an extent that an island off the coast of Georgia was named Sassafras.[3]

Some of the older physicians of that era gave Sassafras credit for being a cure-all. Whether or not it had anything to do with Ponce de Leon's dream of the Fountain of Youth in the Florida or the Georgia area, the legend is to the effect that the Sassafras tea that was drunk, having ascribed to it such extravagant powers as a medicinal agent, may have had some connection with the Fountain of Youth. At any rate, the drug Sassafras, which is the root of the plant, was the first product of which there is any record as far as we can find, to be exported from Georgia. Sassa-

---

3. *Georgia Historical Quarterly*, Vol. XXII-XXIII (March 1938-December 1939), p. 369.

fras tea is still a popular drink, at least with our Southern people. Many adult readers will recall that, in the spring of the year, Sassafras tea was deemed necessary as a blood purifier and was routine practice in most households. Along with many others of the older vegetable drugs, this product might, in the public interest, be re-surveyed in the light of present-day research.

As early as 1700 the British Government and its professional people, including physicians, surgeons, apothecaries and botanists, were recognizing the importance of the drugs the Spanish Government had discovered in Mexico and South America, and over which they held a strict monopoly. These included Cinchona Bark, Ipecac, Jalap, Coca, Cochineal, and various other drugs, many of which are in extensive use today. The matter was discussed over a period of years, but no concrete steps were taken until 1730-31 when the Apothecaries Company of England, a subsidiary of the Society of Apothecaries of London, encouraged by the Trustees of the Colony of Georgia, was formed for the purpose of exploring the various colonies of England to determine whether or not these drugs might be growing there; or, if they were not growing there, whether they might be grown. They also hoped to find drugs which might be used as substitutes or which might be perhaps even better than the original drug.

On the basis of previous reports from Jamaica and Madeira as to the possibility of finding drugs, the Company felt justified in searching for a botanist with a broad background of character, judgment, and experience. They chose for the purpose Dr. William Houstoun. The Trustees of the Colony agreed to aid the Apothecaries Company in the venture and to administer the funds contributed for that purpose.

On August 23, 1732 the Trustees ordered that a book be prepared for the taking of subscriptions in money and materials for the promotion of the Colony of Georgia under the following heads.[4]

Item:

1—For the establishing of the Colony
2—For encouraging and improving the Botany and Agriculture of the Colony
3—For religious purposes

It was agreed that all contributions of money and/or materials were to be handled by the Trustees of the Colony.

---

4. *Colonial Records of Georgia*, Vol. I, p. 72.

℞   DRUGS IN THE COLONY   7

For Item Number 2 above, various subscriptions in cash are recorded in varying amounts.[5] Among these cash contributors were the following individuals, who agreed to pay yearly for three years towards the botanist's salary:

His Grace, the Duke of Richmond   Charles DuBois, Esq.
The Rt. Hon. Earl of Derby   George Heathcoate, Esq.
Sir Hans Sloane   James Oglethorpe
Company of Apothecaries

In addition to those making cash contributions, other persons made contribution of materials:[6]

Christopher Tower   2 gallons Lucerne Seed
Richard Martyn   1 box Tellicherry Bark
Phillip Millar of Chelsea   White Mulberry Seed
   ”   ”   ”   ”   2 papers Egyptian Kali
   ”   ”   ”   ”   1 paper Cotton Seed
Thomas Hyan   10 Olive Trees
Solomon Merrett   1 bag Basilla Seed
Samuel Skinner   4 large tubs Bamboo Plants
Henry L'Apostre   1 bottle of Salistrum Seed

The Trustees of the Colony received a publication entitled, *Reasons For Establishing The Colony Of Georgia.* Impressed with the arguments advanced in this publication, the Trustees ordered 600 copies to be printed in book form to be distributed to all members of the House of Lords and the House of Commons, to all institutions and individuals interested in promoting or opposing the establishment of the Colony.

Since drugs are mentioned as a possible source of revenue as one of the reasons for the establishment of the Colony, there appears herewith a photostat of the cover page of this book, and in succeeding pages will be found a number of quotes from this publication.

Excerpts from *Reasons For Establishing the Colony of Georgia* are as follows:

It is undoubtedly a self-evident maxim that the wealth of a nation consists in the number of her people. But this holds true only insofar as employment can be found for them; if there be any poor who cannot, or do not, add to the riches of their country by labor, they must lie a dead weight

---

5. *Egmont Manuscripts* of the Phillipps Collection, p. 64 (185), University of Georgia Library.
6. *Colonial Records of Georgia*, Vol. II, p. 54, June 15, 1733.

REASONS

For Establishing the

COLONY of GEORGIA,

With Regard to the

TRADE of GREAT BRITAIN,

THE

Increase of our People, and the Employment and Support it will afford to great Numbers of our own Poor, as well as foreign persecuted PROTESTANTS.

With some Account of the COUNTRY, and the Design of the TRUSTEES.

By BENJAMIN MARTYN, Esq;

Hoc Natura præscribit, ut homo homini, quicunque sit, ob eam ipsam Causam tamen, quod is homo sit, consultum velit.
CICERO De Officiis, Lib. III.

The SECOND EDITION.

LONDON:

Printed for W. MEADOWS, at the *Angel* in *Cornhill*. MDCCXXXIII.

on the public; and, as every wise government, like the bees, should not suffer any drones in the state, these poor should be situated in such places where they might be easy themselves and useful to the commonwealth.

If this can be done by transplanting such as are necessitous and starving here, and consequently unnecessary, it is encumbent on us at this time more particularly to promote and enlarge our settlements abroad, with unusual industry, when the attention of almost all the powers in Europe is turned towards the improvement of theirs. The French are continually undermining us, both in the East and West Indies. The Emperor is attempting the same: Portugal owes her riches chiefly to her plantations: Sweden, Denmark, and Germany find themselves poor because they have none at present, though they abound with laborious men. The Colonies of Spain supply the want of industry in her natives, and trade in her towns.

It is at all times our interest to naturalize as much as we can the products of other countries; especially such as we purchase of foreigners with ready money, or otherwise to our disadvantage such as are necessary or useful to support or carry on our manufactures: such as we have a great demand for: and such as we can raise ourselves as good in kind as any other country can furnish us with. Because by so doing we not only gain a new position for our poor, and an increase of our people by increasing their employment; but by raising such materials ourselves, our manufacture comes cheaper to us whereby we are enabled to cope with other nations in foreign markets and at the same time prevent our home consumption of them being a luxury too prejudicial to us.

I hope in the following tract to make these evidently appear, and show the advantages that must accrue to our trade by establishing the Colony of Georgia. I shall give some account of the country and the proceedings of the Trustees, and with candour take notice of the objections that are made to this design, and endeavour to answer them in the clearest and fullest manner I can. I think it may be proved that we have many who are and will be useless at home, and that the settling such a Colony with these, and the foreign persecuted Protestants, is consistent with the interest and reputation of Great Britain.

Then comes a discussion of Silk, Flax, Hemp and Potashes as products which may be produced in commercial quantities in Georgia:

Though these articles are so very considerable, and enough to justify the settling of such a Colony of Georgia; they are not the only ones in which she will be advantageous to us. She can supply us with *Indigo, Cochineal, Olives, Dyeing Woods, and Drugs of various kinds* [this item being also stressed by General Oglethorpe himself, as recorded in a biography by Ettinger], *and many others which are needless to enumerate.** One

---

* The italics are the author's.

article more I shall mention; namely, wine, of which, as she is about the same latitude as Madeira, she may raise, with proper application and care, sufficient quantities not only for part of our consumption at home, but also for the supply of our other plantations (colonies) instead of our going to Madeira for it. The country abounds with varieties of grapes, and the Madeira vines are known to thrive there extremely well. A gentleman of great experience in botany, who has his salary from the Trustees by a particular contribution of some noblemen and gentlemen for that purpose, sailed from hence almost five months ago to procure the seeds and roots of all useful plants. He has already, I hear, sent from Madeira a great number of Malmsey and other vines to Charles Town for the use of Georgia, with proper instructions for cultivating the vines and making the wine.

Two chief objections to the establishment of the Colony of Georgia were being raised, as follows:

Objection 1. Our Colonies may in time grow too great for us and throw off their dependency.

Objection 2. The planting of our Colony may take off our people who are wanted to cultivate our lands at home.

Mr. Martyn answers to his satisfaction and to the satisfaction of the Trustees of the Colony each of these objections to its establishment, and concludes his arguments with these three statements:

Of all public-spirited actions, perhaps none can claim a preference to the settling of colonies, as none are, in the end, more useful.

Whoever then is a lover of liberty will be pleased with an attempt to recover his fellow subjects from a state of misery and oppression, and stake them in happiness and freedom. Whoever is a lover of his country will approve of a method for the employment of her poor, and the increase of her people, and trade. Whoever is a lover of mankind will join his wishes to the success of a design so plainly calculated for their good, undertaken and conducted with so much disinterestedness.

Few arguments surely are requisite to incite the generous to exert themselves on this occasion. To consult the welfare of mankind regardless of any private views is the perfection of virtue, as the accomplishing and consciousness of it is the perfection of happiness.

Sentiment having thus been created for establishing the Colony of Georgia with assurances of proper governmental support, moral and financial, the Trustees of the Colony, acting for and in cooperation with the Apothecaries Company, contracted with Dr. William Houstoun, a botanist of note and an employee of the Apothecaries Company, at a salary of £ 200 per year to go to Jamaica, where he was to set up headquarters for operations in the Caribbean area in a search for medicinal or other plants which might be grown in Georgia, as witnessed by the contract between the Trustees and Dr. Houstoun, dated the 4th of October, 1732:[7]

To all whom it may concern Know Ye That I William Houstoun Doctor of Physick of the University of St. Andrews Do Covenant and Agree that in Consideration of the yearly salary of £ 200 to be paid unto me on my Order in the manner following Viz. £ 100 at the Feast of St. Michael and £ 100 on the 25th of March, That I will serve the Trustees for establishing the Colony of Georgia in America in the following manner Viz. That I will forthwith embark on board a Ship bound for the Madeiras and will from thence proceed to America and will for the Space of Two Years at my own Charge and Expense travel to such Parts thereof as the Trustees shall think proper in order to collect all such Plants as shall be contained in my Instructions from the said Trustees and that I will carry or cause them to be carried to Georgia and that I will constantly correspond with and from time to time transmit to the said Trustees all such Observations as I shall apprehend may be useful to the said Colony of Georgia at my own Charge and Expence and use my utmost Endeavours there for the preserving and propagating of the said Plants and follow such Orders therein as I shall receive from the said Trustees.

(Signed) William Houstoun.

The copy of instructions mentioned above was issued to Dr. Houstoun dated October 12, 1732. They read as follows:

Sir: You are ordered by the Common Council of the Trustees for establishing the Colony of Georgia in America to go on board the Ship Amelia Captn. Brooks Commander now lying in the River Thames and bound for Madeira and Jamaica. When you arrive at Madeira you are ordered to inform your self of the manner of cultivating the Vines and making the Wines there, and to carry with you to Jamaica Cuttings of their best Sorts of Vines, and Seeds, Roots or Cuttings of any other useful Plants you shall meet with on that Island wch. are wanting in the British Colonies, but particularly the Cinnamon Tree. And if you can find any vessel going from thence to South Carolina, you must also send some of each of the above-mentioned things directly there addressed to Mr. St. Julian at Charles Town.

From Jamaica you are ordered to go to the several Spanish settlements at Carthagena, Puerto Bello, Campechy and Vera Cruz, as soon as you can have the opportunity of any Vessel's going to the said Places; and if you can you are to cross the Country to Panama.

7. *Egmont Manuscripts* of the Phillipps Collection. Letters to Georgia, Vol. 14207, pp. 1-4 (33-38).

At all these Places you are to use your utmost Diligence to procure Seeds, Roots of all useful Plants, such as Ipecac, Jalap, Contrayerva, Sarsaparilla, and Jesuits Bark, the Trees which yield Peruvian and Capivi Balsam, the Gum Elemi, etc., the Cockineal Plant with the Animals upon it, and all other things you shall judge may be of use to the Colony of Georgia.

When you return from any of the said Places to Jamaica you are to leave the things you shall have brought over with the person you shall find most capable and willing to take care of them, while you go to the other Spanish Ports in search of others; but if you can have the opportunity of a ship going to Charles Town, you are still to send some of each kind to Mr. St. Julian there.

When you have visited each of the aforesaid Places and collected from them all that shall be in your Power, you are to expect our further Orders to be sent you to Jamaica directing you how to proceed in transporting your self and them to Georgia, where you are to spend the remaining part of the Three years in taking Care of the Culture of what you shall carry with you.

You are particularly desired to inform your self of the Nature and Culture of the White Mulberry Tree, which is most proper for the Nourishment of Silkworms.

As like wise all Sorts of Logwood and other Woods and Barks of use in Dyeing, in order to the Propagating of them in Georgia.[8]

Dr. Houstoun accepted the contract for this mission for the Trustees, and after serving six months, sent back some plants to Charles Town. In a letter from Mr. Martyn to Mr. Oglethorpe, dated March 31, 1733, he says that he has had "two letters from Dr. Houstoun, the first dated November 9, 1732," and stating that Houstoun had shipped two tubs of cuttings and vines to Mr. St. Julian, of Charles Town, and in the second letter, dated December 31, 1732, said "There is but one Cinnamon Tree in Madeira."[9]

In another letter from Mr. Martyn to Mr. Oglethorpe, September 22, 1733, there is found this paragraph: "As the Trustees are desirous of producing Raisins and Currants if possible, some are sent by this Ship to be sowed there. As likewise, the Cubebs and Cardamums (Cardamons), and the Gourd Seeds. The Shells of these (Gourds) may serve for Bottles."[10]

In the final paragraph of a letter from Mr. Martyn to Mr. Oglethorpe, dated November 22, 1733, the statement is made:

8. *Ibid.,* pp. 2-4 (34-38).
9. *Ibid.,* p. 44 (134).
10. *Ibid.,* p. 44 (134).

℞ DRUGS IN THE COLONY

"They have sent by this Ship some of the seeds of Egyptian Kali that produces a Plant that makes the best Potashes. This Seed is to be tried in all the different kinds of Land."[11]

But Dr. Houstoun died after six months' service, and Robert Millar, the brother of Phillip Millar, the chief gardener at Chelsea, London, and Assistant Botanist to Houstoun, was chosen to carry on the work of Dr. Houstoun. Millar's orders and instructions were almost identical with those of Houstoun.

In the meanwhile, Oglethorpe had landed in Savannah in 1733 with the first settlers; the town site was laid out; plans were put into operation for the development of the agricultural industries which were the objectives of the Trustees, these to include the growing of Silk, Hemp, Flax, Indigo, Drugs, Cochineal, Fruits and Vegetables.

The stage was all set then for the shipments of botanical products from Millar, who, following his shipments of "Potash Seed," Cotton Seed, Mulberry Plants, Burgundy Vines, Lucerne Seed, Caper Plants, and Madder Roots, wrote that, in addition, he had Ipecac, Balsam of Capivi and Tolu Plants, and that he would try to get Jalap, Sarsaparilla, and Cochineal, as well as the Cinchona or Jesuit Plant.[12]

Through some political maneuvering, permission was granted for Millar to go into Mexico, where he hoped to learn something of the Cochineal industry and whether it might be practical to grow the insects in Georgia. He was also instructed to learn as much about such drugs as have been mentioned as a possible source of revenue for the Colony and which had been known to exist in Mexico and other countries controlled by the Spanish government. But at Vera Cruz he was restrained on board his ship from entering the country by order of the Governor, who put him under arrest, and ordered him sent back to Jamaica. Millar then sought the privilege of entering Florida to explore that area for medicinal plants, but here again the Spanish Government turned him down.[13]

Thus there was no getting Jesuits Bark, and Millar's activities of necessity ended with the Declaration of War with Spain in 1740. The Company which Millar headed never produced any great amount of suggestions for improvement of the medicinal

---

11. *Ibid.,* p. 58 (170).
12. *Georgia Historical Quarterly,* Vol. XX, p. 328. Article by Dr. Joseph Krafka, "Medicine in Colonial Georgia."
13. *Ibid.,* p. 329.

plant situation in Georgia, and there is no record of the Company's further attempting to introduce herbs into the Colony.[14]

In view of the importance of vegetable drugs, it was customary at that time that both physicians and apothecaries should be trained in botany, so that they might be able to identify medicinal plants wherever they might be located, and to note particularly those which might be poisonous in character. For many years, up until the comparatively recent past, botany was required in every pharmaceutical and medical curriculum for the reason indicated above.

There came with Oglethorpe, or shortly after he arrived in Georgia, a number of scientifically trained people, some of whom were listed as surgeons, some as medicos, some as apothecaries, some as nurses, and some as botanists. Some, however, were listed as apothecaries *and* surgeons, or as surgeons *and* apothecaries. The number of these botanists, physicians, or apothecaries, whatever their classification, seemed to be all out of proportion to the number of people whom they were to serve. It therefore seems a good guess that many of them came specifically for the purpose of looking for vegetable drugs. They did find some drugs, and every boat returning to England carried its consignment of "Bear's Oyl, Snake-root, Rattlesnake-root, Sea-rod, China Root, Sassafras, and Shumack (Sumac)."[15]

The proposed Trustees' Garden in Savannah, to be used as an experimental plant for growing vegetable drugs and other products, was located on a ten-acre tract on the banks of the Savannah River, and a number of items were planted there. But, due to the fact that the Apothecaries Company was not able to locate the seed or plants of the medicinal products with which they were most concerned, they had ceased their operations in 1739. The Garden, therefore, was in time abandoned. However, a number of individuals and institutions later on carried out the idea of experimental botanical gardens, not only for medicinal products, but for spices and other products which might be industrialized.

Oglethorpe, writing to the Trustees as late as October, 1739, describes in detail conditions in the Province of Georgia. He mentions the following trees: "Pine, Walnut, Oak and Beech; Laurel, Cedar, Cypress, Bays and Live Oaks."[16] He writes

14. *Ibid.*
15. *Colonial Records of Georgia,* Vol. III, p. 97.
16. *Egmont Manuscripts,* Phillipps Collection, Vol. 14204, pp. 32-36.

further: "In this Province which but seven years ago was all Forests, are four towns. It is well watered, every part of it fit for Pasture, a great deal stock'd with Cattle; great part of it very rich land fit for Agriculture, and what is cultivated produces Vines, Mulberrys, Orange and Olive Trees, Peaches, Figs and most kinds of Fruits, that grow in Europe and Asia; Potatoes, Cabbage, Carrots and all Pulse, Roots and Grain that grow in Europe; Cotton, Indigo, Cochineal, Aloes, true Aloes, Sassafras, Snake-root, Sumac, Myrtle and many other Drugs that will not grow in England."[17]

The Trustees did not abandon hope that something might be done in the apothecary line. The dreams of the Apothecaries Company and of the Trustees may even yet be realized when, and if, we turn the light of present-day research on this potentially fabulous opportunity. The "Acres of Diamonds," referred to by those who were describing DeSoto's travels through Georgia, may yet reveal themselves in the light of research. Those who trusted in the efficacy of vegetable drugs for thousands of years could not all be wrong.

17. *Ibid.*, p. 34.

Chapter II

THE FOUNDING FATHERS OF THE PROFESSIONS OF PHARMACY AND MEDICINE IN GEORGIA

IT MUST be borne in mind that the use of the terms surgeon, medico, apothecary, pharmacist, nurse, midwife, were all broad terms in the Colonial Period. And, as a matter of fact, in many instances it seems that all of these terms might apply to any one individual, as witnessed by the fact that some were called upon to render service in all of these fields. At the time of the settlement of the Colony the term "apothecary" in England was described as follows: "In England the licensed apothecary is a small shopkeeper or dealer in drugs and druggist's articles, and a chemist and pharmacist, within the necessities of his business, and, as a special requirement, before he can proclaim himself an apothecary, he must receive a license as a person competent to prescribe medicines and practice surgery to a limited extent."[1]

It must be further borne in mind that there was not enough business in the Colony in any one of these fields to justify specialization, and that income necessary for maintenance had to be reinforced by any number of activities outside the professional field, including agriculture, merchandising, governmental and military service, and so on. It must be further borne in mind that under the preceptorship system it was possible for any person to qualify himself in a short period of time for activities in any or all of these fields.

Among the professionally trained people who came from Europe in the period from 1733 to 1740, here is an incomplete list of those who came as apothecary or surgeon, or as both apothecary and surgeon: William Bowler, Isaac King Clarke,

---

1. *Proceedings of the American Pharmaceutical Association,* 1868, p. 289.

William Cox, William Elphinston, Loyd Gibbons, Patrick Graham, Thomas Hawkins, Patrick Hunter, Henry Lascelles, Richard Lobb, John Ludowick Meyer, Samuel Nunez, Samuel Pensyre, John Regnier, Joseph Smith, George Symes, Patrick Tailfer, Christian Thilo, William Watkins, and Johann Zwiffler.[2]

In addition, there is added a short list of reported professional midwives: Lucy Mouse, public mid-wife; Elizabeth Stanley, aged 38, public mid-wife, returned to England to "ly in" in October, 1736; Mrs. Harrison, who was paid five pounds for officiating as mid-wife at Frederica; and Jane Leak, school mistress and midwife.[3]

In addition to those who came to the Colony of Georgia from Europe during the early days from 1733 to 1740, there is an incomplete list of surgeons, apothecaries, M. D.'s, physicians and apothecaries, and drug dealers who came into prominence during the period from 1740 to 1800, among whom were Dr. Lyman Hall, a practicing physician and pharmacist, and Button Gwinnett, who was a merchant dealing in drugs and medicines. These two men were to play an important part not only in the health of the community but in public life. They were active in promoting the spirit of liberty which resulted in Georgia's becoming one of the thirteen Colonies to throw off the yoke of England, and in 1775 were signers of the Declaration of Independence from Georgia, the third signer being George Walton. Biographical data on these two prominent Georgians appear at the end of this chapter.

The list of those who came in this period 1740 to 1800 who were physicians or apothecaries, or were physicians *and* apothecaries, or who came as dealers in drugs, as gleaned from the newspapers of Savannah and Augusta for this period, were the following: Dr. Henry Lewis Bourquoin, Dr. James Cuthbert, Dr. David Brydie, Dr. Andrew Johnston, Dr. Lyman Hall, Dr. Irvine, Dr. White, Edmond Dillon, Dr. George Harral, Johnson & Wylly, James Furse, John and Alexander MacIver, Adam Austin, William Belcher, Kollock & Parker, Carpenter & Havens, Samuel Brown, Dr. Nathan Brownson, Edward & Clement Stebbins, Dr. Cornelius Dysart, Dr. Payne, Dr. Henry Todd, Dr. William Wyatt Bibb, Dr. Burke, Dr. John Murray, Dr. Smelt, Dr. Hull, Dr. Cocke, Harper & Maher, Montgomery & Bird,

---

2. Coulter and Saye, eds., *A List of the Early Settlers of Georgia.* Athens, Georgia: 1949.
3. *Ibid.*

James O. Prentiss, Dr. Watkins, Collin Reed & Company, Dr. Thomas I. Wray, Dr. H. M. Fendall, Dr. Harris, Dr. Childers, Dr. Benjamin Gantt, and Dr. Poisson.

Those who came as drug dealers—who apparently were neither physicians nor apothecaries—as gleaned from early Georgia newspaper notices and advertisements, were the following: Button Gwinnett, Alexander Fyffe & Company; Sawyer, Morel & Blogg; Maquere, Lerray & Company; John Willson & Company; Joseph Chouler & Company; The Venet & Company; William H. Jack; J. & F. D. L'Homaca; and Alexander Habersham.

Following is a biographical sketch of each of those men who came during the early days from 1733 to 1740:

William Bowler, a surgeon, came to Charleston in July, 1741, and presented a memorial claiming that he went over to Georgia in May, 1738, and was stationed at St. Andrews on the Island of Cumberland, to attend two companies of General Oglethorpe's regiment there, where a party of Highlanders (mostly servants of the Trustees) had hitherto kept guard under the command of Ensign Hugh Mackay with a surgeon to attend them, all supported by an establishment from the Trustees. That about July 20, 1738, those Highland servants with their officer were sent from St. Andrews to Amelia to settle a plantation and guard the Inland Passage between that Island and the Main, continuing there until some time in January, 1739, when they were all recalled and sent to Darien. That from the fore-mentioned 20 July, 1738 till their removal to Darien he (Bowler) solely attended them, making journeys to visit them at all calls from St. Andrews to Amelia. That he never received any consideration for his trouble. That he also attended 80 women and children belonging to the soldiers and some of them at Mackays Town. That he also did business for scout boat people at the Amelia Station without receiving any gratuity before the Highland servants were sent there.[4]

Isaac King Clarke, apothecary, embarked 11 September 1733; arrived 16 December 1733; lot number 123 in Savannah. He went away to Carolina, quitting the Colony in 1738.

William Cox, aged 41, is listed as a surgeon. In England in November, 1732, the Palace Court reported that "Mr. [Dr.]

---

4. Journal of the Earl of Egmont, *Colonial Records of Georgia,* Vol. V, pp. 523-524.

Cox, the Surgeon attending, agreed to give his attendance to the sick and wounded in Georgia the first year without any fee or reward, except that his house should be built and the land tilled like the others by joint labor." The Court also agreed to allow him a case of instruments and bedding.[5]

In 1733 William Cox arrived. But he died of consumption within six months after his arrival here. He had been granted a lot in Savannah, on which his widow and son made a claim in 1735.

William Elphinston, apothecary, arrived 14 January, 1734, but died 27 January, 1734, leaving his wife Anne. Prior to leaving England he contributed 20 pounds for a collection for religious inhabitants of the Parish of St. Mary's.[6]

Henry Garret, M. D., was given Lot Number 127 in Savannah in May, 1737, but in 1738 he "flung it up." During the year he practiced "physick" in Savannah. Mr. John Wesley represented him a "direct Deist" 17 June, 1737.[7]

On the first of August, 1740, he addressed a letter to the "Rt. Honble Matthew Lord Ducie" in which he said: "Tho' my profession is physick, as no body can pay for services done in that way, we are obliged to do everything we can to get a livelyhood, and was imployed by the Magistrates here in behalf of the Honble the Trustees to bring up their long Neglected Orphans Accts., about which they kept me as an Assistant 16 Months imployed."[8]

In a letter dated the first of August, 1740, and addressed to the "Rt. Honble George Lord Carpenter," Garret says, "I am the Unfortunate Chymist of Brooks Street who by too Close a Conjunction with that very bad Man Slingsby Cressy Sustained the Loss of above £ 2000 from his Extravagance."[9]

Loyd Gibbons, apothecary, arrived in Savannah 12 March, 1734, and died 27 September, 1734, leaving wife Frances, who married Henry Molton 7 September, 1736.[10]

Dr. Patrick Graham came to the Colony in 1733 as apothecary and surgeon to the Trustees. He had a grant of 100 acres

5. *Colonial Records of Georgia,* Vol. I, p. 82.
6. *Colonial Records of Georgia,* Vol. III, p. 32.
7. Coulter and Saye, *Early Settlers of Georgia,* No. 424.
8. *Col. Recs. of Ga.,* Vol. XXII, pp. 393-396. Part II.
9. *Ibid.,* p. 399.
10. Coulter and Saye, *op. cit.*

from the Trustees and upon petition was given Lot Number 44 in Georgetown. Each lot measured 120 by 80 feet. In March of 1740 it is recorded that he had made very considerable improvement in building on his lot, as well as having been "a constant planter for two or three years past." "Having Ann Cuthbert, sister to the late Captain Cuthbert for his Patient, dangerously ill in a Fever and at that time a Lodger in his House; the Doctor took the Opportunity of prescribing Matrimony to her, as a Specifick which he was sure should Compleat her cure; and on consenting to take his Advice in it, they were married at her late Brother's Plantation; Mr. Jones and I [Mr. Stephens] were pressingly invited to the wedding; which we complied with. We rowed up to Joseph Town this Forenoon, but the ceremony of the wedding was over, the Marriage performed yesterday by Mr. Norris."[11]

On November 21, 1741, "the said Commissioners having sent over Patrick Graham's account with the Trust for November 30, 1737, to October 4, 1739, for Physick administered at Savannah whereon the Balance due to him appeared to be 40 pounds, 17 shillings and 6 pence, the Committee finds that said account includes the sums for Medicines for Soldiers left sick at Savannah —Part of the first Detachment of Gen'l Oglethorpe's Regiment —and the said Patrick Graham having duly administered Medicines to the sick at Savannah, the Committee are of the Opinion the sum reported due to him should be paid."[12]

A later record shows that Graham came from his plantation up the river (formerly Mr. Cuthbert's) when Colonel Cochran first arrived with part of the Regiment who were sickly and "who had been attended by Mr. [Dr.] Graham in his Profession as an Apothecary."[13]

He was reported in Stephens' Journal as being a very successful grower of mulberry plants, and he sold a lot of these plants for the people at Frederica for 25 pounds. His price for the plants was one penny per plant.

In 1745 Graham was Assistant to Mr. William Stephens, President, along with Henry Parker, William Spencer and Samuel Mercer. In 1748 he was appointed Co-Adjutor to Mr. Stephens to aid in distributing presents from the English Government to the Indians. In 1751, he and "Mr. James Habersham,

11. *Stephens Journal,* 1737-1740.
12. *Ibid.*
13. *Col. Recs. of Ga.,* Vol. V, p. 564.

THE FOUNDING FATHERS

Noble Jones, Pickering Robinson and Francis Harris, or any two of them, were appointed as Commissioners, for meeting, conferring and treating with the Nations of the Creek Indians for the purchasing of the Lands from Pipemakers Bluff to Savannah, and the three islands of St. Catherine, Ossabaw and Sapelo for the Use and Benefit of the Trustees; and for them or any two of them to Subscribe and Affix any Seal to the said Treaty as they shall see proper, and likewise to do and perform all further Acts and Requisites Which the Cause may require."[14]

Dr. Graham in his official capacity addressed the following letter "to our Friends and loving Brothers the Chickasaws: We send you as a Token of our Love by your Traders Ten Bags of Powder and twenty Bags of Bullets and some Paint, Flints and Knives to be distributed among you."[15]

On the second day of June, 1755, the Minutes of the Board (the Common Council) record that "the Honorable Patrick Graham, Esquire, the first named member of this Board, dyed [died] the 30th Ult. and was interred yesterday."[16]

Graham was President of the Common Council when the first Royal Governor John Reynolds was appointed. He was elected to the first Legislature under Governor Reynolds.

Dr. James Cuthbert, the son of the Widow Cuthbert, served as an apprentice under Dr. Graham as his preceptor, and in 1763 we find him operating a place of business in Savannah under the name Cuthbert & Brydie, in which business he and his partner David Brydie advertised a parcel of family medicines for sale and offered to buy pinkroot and Virginia snakeroot from the settlers and/or Indians.

Thomas Hawkins came as Apothecary and Surgeon to Oglethorpe in 1736. He was Oglethorpe's personal physician as well as Regimental Surgeon to the Army. He was the first bailiff in Frederica, due to the fact that he was one of the few people there who could read. He was given Lot Number 28 in Frederica.

Dr. Hawkins reports in a letter to the Trustees on 28 February, 1736, that "by God's Divine Providence we enjoy a great Share of health, the people in general are hearty and strong, which in great Measure is owing to our Temperance. We have 'Burred' (buried) no People Since my last Account but Mrs.

---

14. *Col. Recs. of Ga.*, Vol. I, p. 561, June 1, 1751.
15. *Col. Recs. of Ga.*, Vol. VI, p. 450.
16. *Col. Recs. of Ga.*, Vol. VII, p. 181.

Loope a person of 60 years and a child of four months so that Since our Inbarkation (Embarkation) no people have been favour'd with the like Success."[17]

In January, 1737, he requests an "Invoice of Drugs necessary for the Settlement" and repeats this request from time to time. On the same date in another letter to the Trustees, he reports "no Loss by Death except one Infant and Mrs. Humble, a woman aged upwards of 60 who died of old age rather than any Illness."

Hawkins also reported in this same letter some events of the trip over by boat from England: "The chief Illness that happen'd was a Cow's during our Passage, the most Complaints of the people were of Coughs and Colds Occasion'd by the Change of Weather and Living due in part to want of Exercise. On our Arrival here Some few had pains in their Limbs and Rheumatic Disorders, Inflammations on their Feet, and Leggs, most of which were Cured by Strong Purgatives. As yet (January 1737) Fluxes have not proved so obstinate as we could reasonably expect. I vomited them with the Ipecac in the Evening; the next Morning if necessary I gave them a Purge, and in the Evening a small Draught of Burnt Rice Liquor, or the white Drink of Burnt Hartshorn with 20 Drops of Laudanum; with which Treatment several have recovered. Their Drink was chiefly of the same Liquor and the following Electuary, viz. Conserve of Roses and Lusceallhus Balsam, of each an Ounce, Bole and Spermaceti, of each 2 drams, made into an Electuary with a sufficient Quantity of Diacodium of which the patient took a small Quantity 5 times a day. A little burnt Claret relieved them when weak and languid; Fevers yielded to Bleeding, etc."[18]

On the 24th of June, 1737, Hawkins reported to General Oglethorpe that, "We have lost no people Since my last at either Settlement, and have but few people Ill at Present, most of which are on the Recovery. Dr. Lascelles' Son was Drown'd being in the River with many other Boys he was found the 14th and Buried by his Father. There is about 4 pounds and 10 shillings lodged in my hands which shall be remitted his Brother or defray the Charges of the Funeral as your Hon'r shall Advise."[19]

Dr. Hawkins complained: "The Acct of the Public Building is so Bad that I dread mentioning it to you there not having been a Brick made since your Departure from Savannah or a Board

17. *Col. Recs. of Ga.*, Vol. XXI, pp. 331-332.
18. M. B. Gordon, *Aesculapius Comes to the Colonies.*
19. *Ibid.*

saw'd. My House is yet unfinish'd but hope in a month's time to do it on My own Expence if they don't proceed.

"We have a good Sortment of Druggs remaining in the Chest and have Occasion only for the enclosed Catalogue to Mr. Verelst. There is and has been for near 2 Months since a great Want of Provisions and great Complainings among the People."

Dr. Hawkins rendered a bill to the Trustees for 50 pounds for the cost of boats and men being kept to pass from Frederica to Darien to visit patients there. The Trustees argued that this bill should be reduced to about 16 pounds. And on October 21, 1740 he wrote to the Trustees "that the Trustees use me Ill," and if the balance of the account with them was not paid, that he would "fling up" his office.

In May, 1741, Captain William Thompson had delivered a package of drugs and medicines to Dr. Hawkins in the amount of £ 29, s. 9, d. 6, "part whereof being to replace Medicines taken out of the King's Chest for the Trust Service."[20]

On November 5, 1742, Hawkins complains that "I continue the care of the sick Widows and Servants and Indians and Objects of Charity, as well as the Bailiffship, but cannot get regular Payment for either, even tho' I delivered 50 Babies in Frederica alone in 1740."

Dr. Hawkins was in the Battle of Bloody Marsh, where he served as Surgeon for as many as fifty patients per day, most of whom required surgery, as indicated by the fact that in one day he "paid one shilling to Richard Hughes for sharpening [his] surgical saws."[21]

Patrick Hunter, apothecary, is recorded as an inmate at Savannah in 1738, on Lot Number 18.

The Reverend George Whitefield, returning to Georgia on his second voyage in 1740, opened the Town House of the Moravians as a hospital and free clinic. This was the first hospital and the first free clinic in the Colony of Georgia.[22] He also organized an orphanage, later to be known as Bethesda Orphanage, to house 70 children. The hospital and clinic was turned over to Patrick Hunter, who was then reported to have been apothecary and surgeon who had come to Georgia out of devotion to the Reverend George Whitefield. The surgeon was supplied with all

20. *Col. Recs. of Ga.*, Vol. II, p. 373.
21. *Ibid.*
22. M. B. Gordon, *op. cit.*

needed apparatus at Whitefield's own expense, and drugs for use in the hospital were manufactured by the apothecary (Hunter).

There was some excitement in the Colony in 1740 due to the charge that two ministers were preaching false doctrines, and Patrick Hunter was one of the witnesses who testified. It is also recorded that Hunter was a witness at the marriage of James Habersham (one of Whitefield's trustworthy agents in his absence).

In 1742 at a meeting of the Presidents and Assistants for the County of Savannah, it was represented to this Board by Dr. Hunter that "Landry and his Wife at Highgate are both dead in the last Sickness, leaving a Family of five Children behind them," (children who no doubt would be inmates at the Orphanage under Dr. Hunter). Following the statement from Dr. Hunter, the Board "ordered two Shillings and six Pence be weekly laid out."[23]

At a similar meeting of the Presidents and Assistants in October, 1742, the following resolution was presented: "Whereas Application was formerly made by numbers of the Inhabitants after their Return to Savannah from their Places of Retreat during the late Commotions, when a grievous Sickness (Smallpox) began to spread among'em, that they were destitute of all Help, for Want of proper Medicines being applied (there being none in the Stores); whereupon we did then engage Dr. Hunter —Surgeon & Apothecary belonging to the Orphan House to visit and relieve such Persons, (he giving at the same Time an Account to this Board of their respective Names, whereby we might judge of their Necessity, or Ability to help themselves); and said Dr. Hunter now delivered sundry Bills containing the Expence of Medicines and his Care thereon, amounting in the Whole to £ 43 s.17 d.0, which there being no Objection to, the Same was ordered to be paid."[24]

In March, 1743 at a subsequent meeting of the Presidents and Assistants of Savannah, the following account: "Information being given us by Mr. Hunter (Dr. Hunter), who visited the poor lad that had his Limbs broken, that during the present Extremities he lay under 'twas needful some extraordinary Care should be taken that he might not want proper Assistance to move him on Occasion, and be frequently helpful otherwise; which was more than his Father or Mother could do, without

---

23. *Col. Recs. of Ga.*, Vol. VI, Sept., 1742.
24. *Ibid.*, October, 1742.

giving up their Plantation work, to their future irrevocable Loss; It is judg'd thereupon reasonable that ten Shillings a Week be allow'd."[25]

A letter from Mr. John Dobell to "the Honble the Trustees for Establishing the Colony of Georgia":

"Just now an Unlucky Accident happen'd. William Ryley an Orphan, but lives with Joseph (Patrick) Hunter an Apothecary in this Town, being in the Woods a Hunting, as also happen'd to be John Seillier; the latter shot at the former, mistaking him for some wild beast, and lodg'd about 20 Shots in his Body at which said Seillier is exceedingly Griev'd. Tis supposed that the Lad is not dangerously wounded. I have since been to the House of Mr. (Dr.) Hunter to see the Boy but he was laid to sleep. Mr. (Dr.) Hunter tells he is dangerously wounded and thinks he will not recover."[26]

One of Mr. Stephens' letters to Mr. Secretary Martyn from Savannah:[27]

"Mr. (Dr.) Graham is a Man generally well esteem'd among us All; but from the Time of his Marriage several Years since to the late Mr. Cuthbert's Sister, whereby he came possess'd of that Tract of Land (good part whereof was well cultivated) he gave up all his Practice as an Apothecary entirely and left the Town wholly destitute; which gave Room for another (one Joseph (Patrick) Hunter who came out of England with Mr. Whitefield) to come to the Orphan House and settle with his Family in Savannah, where a while after he made Purchase of a very good Lot, that formerly was Mr. West, whose Son sold it to Hunter. He has practised with very great Success, which has render'd him much esteem'd by the whole Town and many miles around; and on that Occasion I proposed it to him several times to accept the £ 20 design'd by the Trust, together with the Use of their Medicines; but he still declin'd it, and the Reason indeed was evident; for communibus Annis his Bills have amounted to near double, tho we have allow'd none to be charg'd to the Trust, excepting only such as the Parties by Reason of their Poverty were in no wise able to discharge, and we hear of no Complaint against him for extravagant Bills, but on the Contrary he is look'd on very modest in all his Demands, as well in Physick as broken Bones and . . ."

(Signed, William Stephens)

Henry Lascelles, surgeon, arrived in the Colony in February, 1736.

In a letter from A. Anderson to Mr. Verelst at the Georgia

---

25. *Ibid.,* March, 1743.
26. *Col. Recs. of Ga.,* Vol XXIV, Oct. 31, 1743.
27. *Ibid.,* August 31, 1745.

Office in Old Palace Yard, Westminster: "Poor Lascelles, the Bonesetter, received with great thankfulness Mr. Tower's generous Instance of his great Humanity, and the Money Mr. Oglethorpe directed to be given him, but he was not able to set out for Gravesend 'till Tuesday last, which makes me fear he came too late."[28]

Richard Lobb, apothecary, arrived February 15, 1734. He was given Lot Number 90 in Savannah.

He was "fyn'd double the value for killing a chicken May 18, 1734." He was also "fyn'd for Defamation three Shillings and four Pence on the 26th of May, 1735."

John Ludowick Meyer, surgeon, aged 30, Saltzburger, arrived in the Colony December 2, 1741, with his wife Elizabeth, aged 38.

The Reverend Mr. Bolzius in a letter to Mr. Martyn in August, 1747,[29] stated from Ebenezer that "our Surgeon Mr. (Dr.) Meyer is a very well qualified person, and beloved in our whole settlement on account of his prudent behavior and usefulness to our Inhabitants in several respects. Mr. Von Munch and the Reverend Mr. Senior Urlsperger have placed a great deal of confidence in him, being very sensible of his fine natural Parts and great unfeign'd inclination to serve our Settlement and Colony."

Rev. Bolzius is asking the Council that they "graciously please to take the burden of the secular affairs and of a Conservator of Peace from me and put it upon his (Dr. Meyer's) shoulders, which he is willing to take upon him, if the Province of God and the Pleasure of their Honours order it so." He states that he will be glad to act as Meyer's Assistant and Adviser in anything, and that without his (Bolzius') or Mr. Lemke's concurrence Dr. Meyer will do nothing. Further, Rev. Bolzius says, "We live all three in intimate conjunction of heart, and have nothing else in our view, but the true happiness of our and other people. Dr. Meyer (as a German) is not yet fully acquainted with the English tongue to speak and to write: till he has made better improvements I'll write according to my weak capacity anything for him, and Mr. Habersham will be our Agent at Savannah, if we have Matters to lay before the Council there, or if the Council have anything or Orders for us: till Mr. (Dr.) Meyer is better used to the language, Customs and other necessary Qualifications,

---

28. *Col. Recs. of Ga.,* Vol. XXI, Oct. 23, 1735.
29. *Col. Recs. of Ga.,* Vol. XXV, August, 1747.

Mr. Habersham will do all for nothing merely out of love to us and our people; but Mr. (Dr.) Meyer has nothing to live from, if he spend his time for the common Good, and if their Honours could not allow him something for his subsistence, till we come in the way by God's assistance to get ourselves more ability to pay him a Salary. He undertakes likewise the sale of our boards, and I hope, the time will come that shipping is no more attended with so many expences and dangers."

Again in September, 1747, Rev. Mr. Bolzius pleads in a letter to Mr. Verelst that the Council appoint Mr. (Dr.) Meyer "Conservator of the Peace and Manager of the secular Affairs at our Place" for his relief. On March 9, 1748 Dr. Meyer was appointed a Conservator of the Peace at Ebenezer.[30]

On October 8, 1748, Rev. Mr. Bolzius reports to the Council that he wants to know when Dr. Meyer's salary commences and what Mr. Martyn means in his letter when he says "The Trustees have resolved to grant to Dr. Meyer the sum of £ 20 sterling within one year to enable him to go between Savannah and Ebenezer as agent for the affairs of our settlement."

Later in 1748, Bolzius writes to Mr. Verelst: "The Trustees have constituted Dr. Meyer Constable of Peace with an Allowance of £ 20 Sterling. He is a well qualified person tho subject to many bodily Infirmities and much esteem'd in our and the neighboring settlements for his skill, honesty and good conduct, and upon that account their Honors have not only enabled him to subsist comfortably among us but have thereby promoted peoples joy and contentment, and have made my burden a great deal easier for the better performance of my ministerial office."[31]

On December 3, 1750, the Colonial Records show, Dr. Meyer wrote that the box of some "necessary glasses for stilling and with some medicines" had arrived safely, and nothing was broken. It seems also that Dr. Meyer was in charge of the store warehouse where various goods or merchandise including medicines were kept for the convenience of the people.

In addition to his other duties as physician, surgeon, Conservator of the Peace, and storekeeper, Dr. Meyer was made Justice of the Peace for Ebenezer and Cowpens in August, 1756.[32]

In December, 1756, the Council of the Colony granted 125 acres in the District of Ebenezer to Dr. Meyer and others in

30. *Ibid.*
31. *Ibid.,* Oct. 26, 1748.
32. *Col. Recs. of Ga.,* Vol. VII, 1756.

trust for a mill at Ebenezer. In February, 1757, he petitioned for 100 additional acres on Mill Island opposite to the other land and stated that he now had a wife and three children.

Finally, in the *Georgia Gazette,* the early Savannah newspaper, for 23 February, 1764, there is a public notice to this effect:

To be sold on Monday the fifth of November at three o'clock in the afternoon at the house of the late Dr. Meyer: all the medicines, medical books, and chyrurgical instruments of the said deceased. The condition of the sale to be ready money. The medicines may be viewed before the sale. (Signed)
Barbar Meyer, Executrix
J. Zubly, Executor.

The story of *Dr. Samuel Riberio Nunez* must be mentioned in any account of pharmacy and medicine in Colonial Georgia. The following information has been given by M. M. Noah, Esquire: "Dr. Samuel (Riberio) Nunez of Lisbon was one of the foremost practitioners in that city at a time when the Jews were already being persecuted under the Inquisition. Colleagues, begrudging the good man his well-earned success, denounced him to the Tribunal of the Inquisition, and he and his family were arrested and thrown into the dungeon as heretics. This was one of the many sad epochs in Jewish history. Dr. Nunez, a man of fine personality and proven medical skill, became physician to the Grand Inquisitor himself. The Grand Inquisitor did his best to ameliorate the sufferings of the doctor's family. Nonetheless, his kinswoman Abby de Lyon, who passed away in Savannah, carried to her grave the impression left by ropes on her wrists when put to the question."[33]

Dr. Nunez and his family escaped to England, and came to Georgia with a party who arrived July 11, 1733, and he was given Lot Number 43 in Savannah. In 1734, Dr. Nunez delivered the first two white babies born in the Colony, the male child being Philip Minis, who came to be a prominent financial influence in Georgia during the Revolution,[34] and whose grandson Philip Minis came to be a prominent physician in Savannah in the 1800's.

Dr. Nunez set up the first apothecary shop in Savannah.[35]

33. Gordon, *Aesculapius Comes to the Colonies,* p. 491.
34. "The Minis Family," in *Georgia Historical Quarterly,* Vol. I, p. 45ff.
35. Gordon, *op. cit.,* p. 492.

Indicating that there must have been some close relationship between Dr. Nunez and the Wesleys, there are two small towns to be found just a few miles apart in Emanuel County, Georgia, — one named for Dr. Nunez and the other named for John or Charles Wesley (or both).

Samuel Pensyre said of himself in a letter dated, Savannah, January 18, 1735: "I have visited ye sick ever since I been ye." He also spoke of buying medicines and distilling herbs.[36]

John Regnier was a Swiss nurse who came with the Moravian Colony to Georgia in 1733 and gave medical aid to the general population.[37] His knowledge and art were of a high type. His scientific curiosity led him to perform the first autopsy in this settlement, at which he was assisted by John Wesley.[38] In 1739 he left the Colony, along with the Moravians, just prior to the War with Spain.

Joseph Smith, apothecary and surgeon in England, was awarded Lot Number 33 in Frederica in 1734, but he did not embark for Georgia until 1735. He is said to have been one of a group of church wardens and members of the Vestry of the Parish of St. Margaret's who received money from the Trustees for establishing the Colony. It is recorded that in 1735 "Twenty-five pounds was appropriated to pay the freight of Joseph Smith, his wife and daughter, and also his manservant John Jones," all of whom came to Georgia on the *Prince of Wales,* being recommended by Dr. Hales and Oglethorpe.[39]

George Symes, aged 55, apothecary, arrived February 1, 1733 and was given Lot Number 21 in Savannah. He married Elizabeth Gray, servant to Jo Baillie.

In November, 1732, back in England, the *Colonial Records* show that Mr. Oglethorpe is directed "to set out 300 acres of land in America for the use of the church in the Town of Savannah and a site for the church and the Minister's House in Town and likewise a burial place at the proper distance from the Town, and George Symes is appointed Conservator to keep the Peace in Town, replacing Peter Gordon."

36. *Col. Recs. of Ga.*
37. *Georgia Historical Quarterly,* Vol. XX, p. 335. Article by Dr. Joseph Krafka.
38. Gordon, *op. cit.,* p. 496.
39. *Col. Recs. of Ga.,* Vol. II, p. 6.

Patrick Tailfer, surgeon and apothecary, arrived in August, 1734. He settled first on the River Nece, but quitted to practice surgery in Savannah. Prior to his embarking for America, he had a grant of 500 acres dated October, 1733.

He was a proud, saucy fellow and ringleader for allowance of Negroes and change of tenure. He finally went away to Carolina for fear of the Spaniards on August 31, 1740.

Before coming to Georgia, Patrick Tailfer had been a practicing physician in Edinburgh, Scotland. Upon reaching the Colony, he evidently became dissatisfied with its agricultural and industrial prospects, for he immediately decided to resume his medical practice and hire out his servants to other planters.

The scheme to change land tenure and to introduce slave labor into the Colony was headed by Robert Williams, Patrick Tailfer, Patrick Mackay, Andrew Grant and others.

Williams and his brother-in-law, Dr. Patrick Tailfer, became sellers of rum and dispensers of physick, for which by August, 1739, they "had almost all of the Town of Savannah indebted to them."

It appears that, altogether, Patrick Tailfer and his brother-in-law Williams were a disturbing element in the community, and precipitated much criticism of Oglethorpe and the conduct of the Colony by Stephens.

Just prior to evidence that war with Spain was approaching, Dr. Tailfer and his associates began sending off their goods and luggage, and selling off their property. Late in 1740, Tailfer left the Colony in disgrace, never to return. He settled in Charles Town, South Carolina, and practiced there.

Christian Thilo (Thielo), Surgeon to the Saltzburgers, arrived January 16, 1738. He settled at Ebenezer, and it was agreed to grant his passage, three years' allowance, and a servant.

It appears that Dr. Thilo was being brought to the Colony to succeed Dr. Zwiffler (see later biographical data on Dr. Zwiffler) at Ebenezer, where Dr. Zwiffler had been Apothecary and Surgeon to the Saltzburgers. Dr. Thilo brought with him letters of recommendation which certified that he was a man equally skilled in medical science and noted for sincere piety. He was further recommended as having had as tutor on the Continent the physician in charge of an Orphan House there, a Doctor Professor Juncker, a most worthy man, and, from his medical writing, most famous. Juncker gave Dr. Thilo diligent work for some years in the hospital, from which it happened that Thilo was trained not only in school and doctrine, but also in practice and experience; not simply in medicine and pharmacy, but in surgical practice as well. He laid solid foundations for securing the "honor of doctrine" and of extending his medical art in Germany, so that he was by no means deficient or inferior. While all else being considered least important, he resolved to devote his time and talents to the "poor exiles of Christ."

Some drugs from the pharmacy department in the Orphanage in Germany were sent to be used by Dr. Thilo in case of need.

In a letter from the Reverend Mr. Bolzius to Mr. Henry Newman in June, 1740, he requested that some small salary be appropriated Dr. Thilo, physician at Ebenezer, whose contract for residing with the Saltzburgers for three years was nearly expired. It was later agreed to give Dr. Thilo a 50-acre lot of land, together with a servant, to be maintained one year at the Trustees' expense, and he was to have the proper tools, a cow, a calf, and a hog.

It seems that inhabitants of the Northern District of Savannah petitioned the Council after some time to procure for them a physician, there being at that time in the District neither physician, apothecary, nor surgeon to attend them in sickness. They pointed out that there was at the Orphan's House one Hunter, and there was also one Thilo, a Saltzburger at Ebenezer, who had been four years in the Colony and by now was supposed to have learned some English, and who was reported to be a useful man to the Saltzburgers and might be also to the English. It was provided that in the event Dr. Thilo would come to Savannah to attend all of the sick of the Northern District who should want his assistance, an allowance of £ 50 and chest of medicines might every year be sent to him, the value of which for 600 persons would approximate £ 75.

William Watkins, surgeon, aged 44, arrived on December 16, 1733. The first reports of Dr. Watkins are not very flattering, for it is reported that he was given 100 lashes for marrying a second wife, his first wife still living, and to give security to return to Abercorn, his settlement. He was finally convicted of adultery and sentenced to imprisonment December, 1736, for two years. But he ran away in 1737.

In 1734, Isaac King Clarke, previously referred to in this chapter, requested that Dr. Watkins of Abercorn should not be allowed to practice in Savannah, so that he (Clarke) might be able to reap such small advantages as might accrue by those persons who came to the Colony on their own account.

(Author's note: A distinction was made between those people who came on their own account and those who came at the expense of the government. Those who came at the expense of the government were provided with free medical services, so that Dr. Clarke's practice was drawn strictly from those who came "on their own account" and who were able to pay for medical services.)

J. Andrew Zwiffler, M. D., came on March 12, 1734, as apothecary and medico, with the first transport for Ebenezer. He was a Saltzburger and settled at Ebenezer and was made Constable there in 1736. A summary from the Saltzburgers' tracts says that Johann Andreas Zwiffler came as "apothecarian and medico." On the 14th day of May, 1734, during the ocean voyage, he "learned barbering and bleeding and gave service as a medico." Shortly after his arrival, he was lost for 12 days, when Indians were sent out to find him. They brought him safely home, and he was reported well.

Rev. Bolzius in a letter to Oglethorpe stated that he was to "spend some money for buildings at old Ebenezer and in this new settlement."[40] "The school master," he stated, "and likewise Mr. [Dr.] Zwiffler, are disable to pay for huts and garden fences."

Mr. John Vat in a letter to Mr. Newman on February 15, 1735, said, "I could hardly stand on my legs, which weakness continued for several weeks, but upon taking proper medicines of Dr. Zwiffler, am recovering."

Late in 1736 Zwiffler refused a position as medico in Frederica and resolved to return to Germany, where he considered the climate better and healthier. By March of 1737 he had left, and the Colony received Dr. Thilo as his replacement at Ebenezer.

In addition to these early surgeons and apothecaries, there are given below some sketches concerning some of the men who came into prominence in Georgia during the period from 1740 to 1800, and who were to play various roles in the health life of the Colony and State, and also in promoting the spirit of liberty which stirred the people to independence from England.

---

40. *Col. Recs. of Ga.,* Vol. XXI.

One of the signers of the Declaration of Independence from Georgia, Lyman Hall, was born in Wallingford, Connecticut, in 1724. He graduated from Yale in 1747, and under the direction of his uncle, the Reverend Samuel Hall, he entered upon the study of theology. (One writer says that Lyman Hall actually entered the ministry, and left the ministry on account of some misunderstanding or unpleasantness).[41] He soon abandoned preaching, however, apprenticed himself to a local physician, and adopted medicine as his profession, in which he became very proficient.

About this time Hall married Mary Osborne. In the twenty-eighth year of his age, he removed from Connecticut to Dorchester, South Carolina, and cast his lot among the Puritan colonists who had moved to that place from Massachusetts a few years before, and who were prospering greatly in their new home. Here he was warmly welcomed, and for some years he ministered to the health needs of these sturdy people. Owing to the unhealthfulness of this locality and the impoverished condition of the lands, many of these settlers removed to the Midway District of what is now Liberty County, Georgia. Along with the secondary stream of this immigration came Dr. Hall, who purchased a small plantation a few miles north of Midway Meeting-House. Owing to the swampy condition of the adjacent country, much sickness prevailed in the new settlement, and Dr. Hall found ample opportunity for the exercise of his professional skill. After some time, he removed to Sunbury, where many of the settlers had summer homes, and soon became the leading physician of the town and country around.

From the Colonial Records comes the following petition dated 1760, from Sunbury, Georgia: "Governor and Council, February 5, 1760. Petition of Lyman Hall and Samuel Miller. Desirous of becoming inhabitants of this Province, the petitioner Hall had a wife. Prayed 250 acres in joint tenancy on a swamp, the north branch of Newport River, near Robert Smallwood. Petition granted."[42]

Notice is found in the *South Carolina Gazette,* July 24, 1764, published at Charleston, South Carolina:

"The subscriber, practitioner in physic and surgery, having removed to Pon Pon, solicits friends and others for their practice; also family medi-

---

41. Gordon, *op. cit.,* p. 509.
42. *Col. Recs. of Ga.,* Vol. VIII, p. 242.

cines, perfumed waters, and cosmetics, which may also be had of Mr. John Milner in Church Street, Charleston."

(Signed) Lyman Hall.

St. Bart's Parish, Colleton County, South Carolina, *1769 Court Records* (Conveyances 1769-1771) pages 15 and 17, show: "Deed to Dr. Lyman Hall, 2000 acres of estate of Dr. John Lupton on Midway Swamp, St. John's Parish."

St. John's Parish, Georgia: Deed dated September 19, 1769. "Lyman Hall, of St. John's Parish, practitioner of physic, and wife Mary, and Samuel Miller of said parish, who is a merchant, and wife Mary, to Robert Smallwood of same parish, planter, consideration of £ 30, conveys 30 acres St. John's Parish, D. and B. S-E Robert Smallwood, other sides vacant when surveyed."

The *Revolutionary Records of Georgia,* St. John's Parish, 1774, show the following: "Committee in charge of the Meeting of Protest, August, 1774: Joseph Clay, Lyman Hall, Samuel Farley, George Walton, William Gibbons, Benjamin Andrew, John Wynn, John Stirk, E. Powell, D. Zubly, Eliza Butler, William Baker, Parmenas Way, John Baker, John Mann, John Stacey."

Dr. Hall represented Georgia in the Continental Congress and was one of the signers of the Declaration of Independence from Georgia. He was elected Governor of Georgia in 1783. He died in Burke County, Georgia, in October, 1790.

Button Gwinnett. Though not a pharmacist, unless perchance he may have been so designated under a preceptorship system, Button Gwinnett did own and operate a store handling drug items in the year 1765, as witnessed by the following advertisement in the *Georgia Gazette,* dated September 12, 1765:

"Just imported
To be sold on the most reasonable terms
by
BUTTON GWINNETT
At the store lately occupied by Messrs. Johnson & Wylly
The following Goods, Viz.
Rhubarb, Turlington's Balsam of Life, Dr. James's Powders for Fever, Flake Manna, Glauber Salts, Florence Oil, Mustard, Tin Ware . . . ."

"Button Gwinnett was born in England in the year 1732. He became a merchant in Bristol, a city in the West of England, which, more perhaps than any other English city, owes its growth and prosperity to commerce with the vast Western world. He was doubtless drawn to consider coming to the American Continent by reason of the wealth gained through trade."[43]

The *Colonial Records* of 1766 show: "The Governor and Council on December 3, 1766, heard a petition of Button Gwinnett. He was settled in the Province and had made a large purchase of land, and being concerned in the shipping industry, prayed on purpose for 1000 acres of pineland on Sapelo River for cutting. This was granted."[44]

A year later, the following: "The Governor and Council, May 5, 1767, Petition of Button Gwinnett. He purchased the Island of St. Catherine whereon he was now settled. Opposite to the said Island are some small hammocks lying on Newport Marshes; of little value, but might be injurious to petitioner if granted to another. Supposed to contain not more than 1000 acres. Prayed grant for same, and it was granted."[45]

And this item comes from White's *Historical Collections,* pages 38 to 41: "Button Gwinnett, Justice of the Peace for St. John's Parish, took the oath of Allegiance and Supremacy."

By 1769 this notice comes from the *Journal* of the Commons House, dated St. John's Parish, November 14, 1769: "Button Gwinnett, Esquire, one of the representatives for Midway and the Parish of St. John, excused for his absence through sickness. Qualified and took his seat."[46]

An advertisement in the *Georgia Gazette,* Savannah, for September 3, 1766, reads, "All persons whatever are hereby prohibited from hunting and shooting upon the Island of Saint Catherine's. I do hereby offer a reward of £ 20 Sterling to any person or persons reporting the name of any trespasser." (Signed) "Button Gwinett."

Button Gwinnett was chosen as one of the signers of the Declaration of Independence from Georgia, and in 1777 he was Governor of Georgia for a few months. His career ended on May 19, 1777, when he was killed in a duel with General Lachlan McIntosh. Lyman Hall was executor of Gwinnett's estate.

In view of the fact that most, or all, of those who practiced medicine in Georgia prior to 1800 were also practicing pharmacy

43. *The Atlanta Journal,* July 10, 1927.
44. *Col. Recs. of Ga.,* Vol. X, p. 163.
45. *Col. Recs. of Ga.,* Vol. IX, p. 699.
46. *Col. Recs. of Ga.,* Vol. XV, p. 43.

and were advertising and dispensing their own drugs, it is reasonable to include this further list of early practitioners:

Dr. Nathan Brownson, of Liberty County, who served as Governor; Dr. William Barnett, a Representative to the United States Congress from Elbert County; Dr. William Wyatt Bibb, from Petersburg, Elbert County, who served in the United States Congress and in the United States Senate.

Dr. Noble Wymberly Jones, a Revolutionary patriot, was born in England in 1724, coming to Georgia in the early days of the Colony. He was a protege of General Oglethorpe, and was made a Cadet in Oglethorpe's regiment and later promoted to Lieutenant, but he was too young to participate in Oglethorpe's attack on Saint Augustine in 1740. He studied medicine and practiced in Savannah. In 1755 he served in the Commons House of Assembly, and in 1768 was made Speaker of that body. He was active in the Revolutionary War, even though his father Noble Jones, remained loyal to the Crown. Leaving Savannah prior to its capture by the English, he went to Charleston; and when that city was captured, he was taken prisoner but was later exchanged and found himself in Philadelphia, where he practiced medicine until the War was over. But during his stay in Philadelphia he served as Representative from Georgia in the Continental Congress; in 1795 was elected President of the State Constitutional Convention; and in 1803 was elected President of the Medical Society.

Dr. George Jones, son of Dr. Noble Wymberly Jones, of Savannah, studied medicine under his father, and later served in the United States Senate for a time.

The names of Dr. William Terrell, of Hancock County, and Dr. Joel Abbot, of Wilkes County, are associated together because of the fact that they served in the United States Congress at the same time and, while serving in the Congress, represented Georgia in the organization of the First Pharmacopoeial Convention, held in Washington, D. C., in 1820. It is interesting also to note that both Dr. Terrell and Dr. Abbot served as Trustees of the University of Georgia, and that Dr. Terrell gave to the University a sum of money for the establishment of a Chair of Agricultural Chemistry.

Of the early physicians, apothecaries, surgeons, or drug dealers in Georgia, several served in governmental positions.

Serving Georgia as Governor were Nathan Brownson, Button Gwinnett, and Lyman Hall.

Serving in the United States Senate: Lyman Hall, Homer Virgil Miller, W. W. Bibb, and George Jones.

Serving in the House of Representatives: W. W. Bibb, William Terrell, Joel Abbot, Charles E. Haynes, and William Barnett.

Serving in the First Provincial Assembly of Georgia were Patrick Graham and Noble Wymberly Jones, the latter being elected Speaker of the House.

This group of scientifically trained people, in addition to those who were to come after them, were among the relatively few educated people coming into the Colony in its early days, and they were called upon to serve not only in the professional capacity in which they were trained, but also in various governmental and military capacities. They were to set up, in the Colony, a system of preceptorship training—as botanists, as apothecaries, as surgeons, or as medicos—which would have to serve in an educational capacity for a period of one hundred to one hundred fifty years, since it was at least that long before a system of basic education could be established, and many more years were to elapse before professional education could be contemplated.

There must have been some wonderful teaching on the part of many of the preceptors of those years. But, naturally, as in all educational processes, there was some poor teaching, which left us with educational and professional problems from which we have never been completely divorced.

Chapter III

DISEASE AND DRUG PROBLEMS CONFRONTING THE COLONY.

HEALTH conditions in the area of Savannah in 1733 must have been excellent, for the American Indians are reported to have been a healthy, hardy race of people. The health picture in the Colony was to change rapidly with the appearance of settlers from England and the European Continent, who brought with them into the Colony the diseases incident to the region or country from which they came. The health problems were still further multiplied with the appearance of the African slaves, who brought with them the infectious and contagious diseases then, and perhaps long, existing on the African Continent.

The physicians, surgeons and apothecaries of the Colonial period were inexperienced in the treatment of these (to them) new diseases. This condition necessitated much experimentation with the drugs with which they were familiar and with locally growing drugs, the end result being that large numbers of the early settlers were lost by death and many others left the Colony when confronted with the various epidemics which visited the Colony from time to time.

The population in the Colony in 1733 was 114, but by 1740 the all-white population was reported to have been approximately 2,000. Shortly thereafter, this number was materially decreased due to the fact that many died from an epidemic of smallpox and others fled the Colony. Prior to and during the early days of the War with Spain, others left the Colony.

A chart, indicating the population changes in the Colony and the State between the years of 1751 and 1850, is shown on the following page.

PROBLEMS CONFRONTING THE COLONY

Population Changes in the Colony and State[1]

Date	White	Negro	Total
1751	1,700	400	2,100
1760	6,000	3,000	9,000
1773	18,000	15,000	33,000
1800	102,261	60,425	162,686
1850	521,572	384,613	906,185

This relatively rapid increase in the population of the Colony meant that the settled area in the Colony was expanding rapidly and widely. Many of these new settlers were probing into the wilderness farther and farther, and were settling there, most of them in isolated areas, since the only areas which could be considered urban in character were Savannah, Frederica, Ebenezer, Augusta, and the environs of these communities. This condition placed upon the government and the surgeons and apothecaries the responsibility of safeguarding not only the health of these settlers but their physical safety as well, particularly in view of the fact that the War with Spain was imminent, and the Revolutionary War was in the offing. The disease problems, including their treatment and prevention, were multiplying rapidly, particularly those conditions which came in epidemic form,—including hookworm, smallpox, dysentery, malaria, typhus and typhoid fever, and yellow fever, and the supply of drugs for their treatment was limited in quantity and quality.

The cause of these contagious diseases was not known at that time, nor were diagnostic or preventive measures, nor corrective treatment; the supply of drugs for all purposes was limited to those which could be imported from abroad, or which had been used by the Indians, none of which could be recognized as specifics, as we know the term today. Therefore, losses by death from these causes were heavy and discouraging, and there were no hospitals nor specialists to whom people could go. There were no educational facilities available, either general or professional, except such as were possible under a preceptorship system, the responsibility for carrying on which would be assumed to a large extent by those who were professionally trained. The settlements in isolated areas, including the islands off the Coast, made educational and health and treatment contacts difficult or impossible. Governmental control was located in England, and this, of necessity, made understanding of the problems difficult between the

---

1. A. B. Saye, *Georgia Government and History*, p. 117

Colony and England. A large proportion of the male population was called upon to join the army at the approach of the War with Spain, thus eliminating that relatively large group from productive activities, and consuming a large portion of the funds appropriated for the maintenance and development of the Colony.

DISEASE PROBLEMS CONFRONTING THE EARLY PRACTITIONERS

Hookworm

It is recorded that "dysentery, worms, and dirt-eating (hookworm cachexia) were common among the slaves, as was smallpox."[2] Long known as a tropical disease, and prevalent in those tropical areas where the people were primitive in character and knew no sanitary regulations or dangers, hookworm infected the people, and this was no doubt true of the slaves who came from tropical areas to the shores of America. The disease spread rapidly throughout the sandy soil section of the Colony, or whereever the use of the surface toilet prevailed. There is no evidence of the existence of hookworm disease among the American Indians prior to settlement of the Colony, and it appears to be a good guess that it was imported along with slaves. The first case of hookworm to be diagnosed and reported in Georgia was by Dr. Claude A. Smith in 1902.[3]

Smallpox

This is one of the oldest reported of the contagious diseases, having been known for many centuries. Just where it originated seems not to be determined, but when world travel or world trading began, the disease was transmitted from one section of the world to the other. However, the disease was not known on the North American Continent until after the early ships of England or of Spain began to touch the continent in various places. It has been known that the disease existed in Africa for many years, and therefore it is pretty definitely assured that the disease was brought to the Colony of Georgia by slaves who came from the tropical areas of Africa.

The disease was extensively distributed over the world, so that it was estimated that at least one out of ten people in the world had smallpox or would die of smallpox and that in the 18th

---

2. T. F. Abercrombie, *History of Public Health in Georgia*, p. 23.
3. *Ibid.*

PROBLEMS CONFRONTING THE COLONY

century every person eventually would have smallpox if he lived long enough.[4]

Smallpox had been known for hundreds of years in the Orient. Lady Wortley Montagu, wife of the Ambassador to Turkey, returning to England from China, followed the custom prevailing in the East and inoculated her children with smallpox virus, thus giving them the disease, which in turn immunized them against future attacks. She brought this process to England with her in 1718, and it became common practice throughout the known world to inoculate people with smallpox virus, this process continuing in use for the remainder of that century until Jenner's discovery in 1798. Inoculation was carried out by the use of virus or scab obtained from a person having an active case of the disease. For many years the necessity of quarantining these people who had been inoculated was not recognized, and the disease spread rapidly from those who were inoculated, as well as those who acquired the disease by infection from other exposure.

There are reports of smallpox epidemics on the North American Continent in Boston, Philadelphia, South Carolina, and possibly Virginia and Georgia early in the 18th century.[5] The process of inoculation was brought to America and carried out in almost all sections, but with no safeguard by quarantine of inoculated individuals. It is but natural that a controversy should have arisen regarding this process of inoculation. We find instances of communities prohibiting the practice of inoculation by law, and of others passing laws requiring it. A law was passed in Georgia in 1768 prohibiting the process of inoculation, with a fine of one hundred pounds for any person found guilty of inoculating others.[6]

By the time of the Revolutionary War, smallpox constituted a menace not only to the people of the Colony, but to the Army as well. And General Washington, having had the disease himself, inoculated his wife and passed regulations requiring that every recruit coming into the Army should be inoculated, but quarantined at the same time until all danger of infection was past. But for this step, the results of the Revolutionary War might have been different.

The American Indian proved to be very susceptible to infection by smallpox. The death rate among the Indians was ter-

4. *Ibid.*, p. 17.
5. W. B. Blanton, *Medicine in Virginia in the 18th Century.*
6. See also Chapter VI, page 127.

rific, and in many instances, whole tribes of Indians were erased.[7]

In 1798, Dr. Edward Jenner of England discovered the theory of vaccination by the use of cowpox virus, which gave a complete immunity to smallpox, but with none of the attendant dangers of actual smallpox. This process of vaccination was promptly carried to all sections of the world. But, as was true of the process of inoculation, some opposed it, while others favored it. And it was well into the 20th century here in Georgia before we had compulsory vaccination of people against smallpox.

Thomas Jefferson, President of the United States of America, in 1806 addressed a letter to Dr. Jenner as follows: "You have erased from the calendar of human afflictions one of the greatest. Yours is the comfortable reflection that mankind can never forget that you lived. Future nations will know by history that the dreaded disease smallpox has existed, and by you has been extirpated."[8]

Jefferson was so impressed with the efficacy of vaccination, and the need for it, and also the fact that certain of the medical profession were opposed to it or would not take the responsibility for it, that he vaccinated about 200 people, including his family and some friends and neighbors.[9]

Vaccination in the early days of the process had to be carried on by the use of virus from pustules of persons who had been vaccinated, or from the scab of a vaccination sore since vaccine as we know it today was not then available on a commercial scale, nor for many years thereafter.

Smallpox was so prevalent in Georgia well into the 20th century that almost all communities of any size had a pest-house where smallpox patients were quarantined.

"The Bloody Fluxes"

Dysentery, or "the bloody fluxes," was a problem confronting the early settlers which resulted in many deaths. But its cause was not known, and the treatment was a shot in the dark. From the symptoms described by these early practitioners, these epidemics of dysentery could have been what we now know as amoebic dysentery. And, since amoebic dysentery is typically a tropical or semi-tropical disease, the chances are that it was brought into the Colony by African slaves. The routine treat-

7. Abercrombie, *op. cit.*
8. *Journal of the American Pharmaceutical Association*, I, 693.
9. Blanton, *op. cit.*, p. 193.

ment of the disease in Colonial Georgia was "vomiting with Ipecac, or Indian Physick," and it is quite interesting to note that Emetine, the active principle of Ipecac, is one of the agents now recognized as a specific for amoebic dysentery.

Malaria

The early physician or apothecary in Georgia was to be faced with the diagnosis of, and the treatment for, a type of fever with which he was not acquainted, and which had not existed in the Colony prior to the introduction of African slaves. This disease we know now as malaria.

Dr. W. B. Blanton of Virginia writes the following report: "Malaria was a man-made disease. Its appearance in epidemic proportions awaited not only carriers from Europe, but the more numerous and more dangerous carriers from Africa."[10]

Malaria itself is one of the oldest diseases on the Continents of Europe, Asia and Africa, and by many was thought to be the cause of the Fall of the Grecian Empire and the Roman Empire, since the armies operating in malaria-infested areas had no means of protection against the disease and no knowledge of how to treat it. Now we know, of course, that malaria is transmitted through the Anopheles mosquito, which transplants the malarial plasmodium from one malaria-infected person to other persons. There is no reason to believe that the Anopheles mosquito was not already in the Colony prior to the arrival of the malaria-infected early settlers and the African slaves who constituted the medium for the transmission of the disease on a large scale. There were at that time no known means for preventing malarial infection, and no known ameliorative or curative agents other than Cinchona bark. Quinine, the active principle of Cinchona, has since come to be known as a specific in the treatment of malaria. This product, Quinine, along with sanitary measures and mosquito control measures, has, over the years, resulted in the reduction of new cases, and has made various sections of the State habitable which otherwise were not habitable in safety in the early days of the Colony.

Dr. Erwin H. Ackernecht in his treatise on "Malaria in the Upper Mississippi Valley, 1760-1900," states that "Malaria, which persecuted Louis XIV and his house, which killed James

---

10. *Bulletin History of Medicine,* XXXI, No. 5, Sept.-Oct. 1957. Article entitled, "Malaria in Virginia Brought By Slaves."

the First and Cromwell, no longer affects dramatically the great and the mighty." But he continues, "From the standpoint of prevalence, malaria appears to be the most important disease in the world today. The yearly number of cases throughout the world has been estimated at 300,000,000, and the number of deaths at 3,000,000. This would mean that one-sixth of the earth's population is suffering from malaria. Other estimates go even up to one-third of the global population."

"In the United States," he states, "in spite of thirty years of intensive anti-malarial measures, and not withstanding great successes in this field, the yearly incidence of malaria lies within one and six million cases, with 5,000 deaths per year, and economic losses of $500,000,000 and direct cost of sickness as much as $51,000,000."

With the discovery of Cinchona bark, frequently referred to simply as "the Bark," these early physicians and the public relied on it in the treatment of malaria. And when, after Quinine had been isolated from Cinchona as the active constituent, a writer has said that "next to munitions of war, few things have seemed as important as Quinine." Cinchona bark, or later, Quinine, was a "must" in the materia medica of the physicians and in the hands of the settlers themselves. No vegetable or synthetic chemical product has even yet been generally recognized as a complete substitute for Quinine, though the early settlers did resort to the use of many locally growing drugs as substitutes, particularly those substances which were bitter.

Thus malaria proved to be another of the tragedies which came as a result of slavery. The health care of these natives of Africa must have appeared to be an insurmountable problem, and the responsibility rested heavily on the government, the population, the medical and pharmaceutical practitioners.

Typhoid and Typhus Fever

Though it is not definitely proven, typhus and typhoid fevers may have been present in the early days of the Colony of Georgia, along with the other forms of fever. And some of the symptoms recorded and reported by these early physicians indicate that either or both of these forms of fever did appear in the Colony. Some of the epidemics chargeable to other types of fever may have been caused by typhoid or typhus, both being transmittable infections, and therefore contagious.

℞ PROBLEMS CONFRONTING THE COLONY

Yellow Fever

Yellow fever appeared as a problem in the early days of the Colony. It was not known by that name, but the color of the skin was a manifestation with which the physician was not familiar, and no distinction was made between this form of fever and other forms as a specific disease. There are reported epidemics of yellow fever early in the life of the Colony, extending on up the Savannah River as far as Augusta. The disease was not recognized as being contagious, and there was no known specific remedy for its prevention or its treatment.

"The offending mosquito was of African origin, and yellow fever is a disease known to have been brought to this country almost exclusively from the West Coast of Africa, where it was endemic, or from the West Indies whence it had come from the same source."[11]

Regarding yellow fever from the viewpoint of Savannah, one writer has presented the following picture:

Perhaps because of the alien nature of both the mosquito and the disease, yellow fever has occurred in spectacular epidemics in Savannah. Of the 1820 epidemic, Dr. William R. Waring said, "The scene of sickness, misery, and ruin was awful, shocking, and well-fitted to inspire melancholy sentiments of the shortness, uncertainty, and insignificance of life." He remarked further that "since the year 1807 there have been nearly 4,000 deaths, so that, calculating the average census to that number for 14 years to the close of 1820, it appears that the whole population is exterminated at the end of every revolution of 14 years, and that human life, according to that general computation, is contracted to that term. It is rare that in any part of the State that death draws so tragic a picture of its ravages in such strong colors."

Epidemics of yellow fever are reported in Savannah in the year 1801, 1807, 1808, 1817, 1819. Then came the great epidemic of 1820, with an unknown number of cases, but with 666 deaths between May and December of that year, and with only 1,500 persons of the 5,000 normal population remaining in the city on September 14th. Epidemics have occurred through the years up until 1876, which saw the last and probably the worst of Savannah's epidemics. The number of cases is, of course, unknown. LeHardy, 1894, estimates 10,000; but there were 1,066 deaths between August and December, the peak having been reached by September 20th, with 33 deaths on that day. This was recognized as the mute testimony of the tragedy of 1876.[12]

---

11. Blanton, *Medicine in Virginia in the 18th Century,* p. 459.
12. *Georgia Historical Quarterly,* Vol. XXVIII, September, 1944.

THE PROBLEMS OF DRUGS IN THE COLONY AND STATE

Attention has been called (Chapter I) to the fact that the supply of drugs in the Colony was limited to the small quantities that the settlers brought with them and the supply that came in by ship following a voyage involving three or more months. During such a voyage there was always the possibility that vegetable drugs, when stored in the hold of a ship for that length of time, would be seriously damaged.

The drugs with which the Colonists were familiar were primarily of vegetable origin, and had been in use in England or on the European Continent for generations. Many of these drugs were among those which the Trustees of the Colony hoped to find or produce in the Colony.

Unfamiliar as they were with the locally growing drugs, the settlers gradually adopted some of the drugs the Indians were using, but this required a slow process of trial by error. They remained dependent on the importation of their vegetable drugs, and 200 years later the practice continues.

Dependence on the importation of some vegetable drugs, not only in America but throughout the world, has, at times, come close to being tragic, for the stock-piling of vegetable drugs involves the probability of deterioration or of a complete loss of activity.

Most of the vegetable drug products grown for commercial purposes and export are cultivated and grown as crops in those countries where the climate, soil and labor conditions are adapted to particular drugs.

Almost every section of the world produces some drug product or products for export on which other sections of the world become dependent.

When wars or other disturbing factors arise in a country, the drug products of that country may no longer be exported, and the drug markets of the world are immediately involved. And, in the case of such drugs as quinine, opium, digitalis, ergot, belladonna, and others, the lives of people all over the world may be at stake.

In times of war, it is generally recognized that drugs along with munitions of war occupy a position of high priority and importance as imports and therefore subject to blockade and other restrictive measures at the hands of the enemy. Drugs may even take precedence over munitions of war.

PROBLEMS CONFRONTING THE COLONY

The extent to which drugs are grown or collected for export, and the wide areas of the world from which they come, is illustrated by the accompanying table. The importation of drugs in 1959 is as important and imperative as with the Colonists of 1733.

COUNTRIES WHICH EXPORT DRUG PRODUCTS ON WHICH THE WORLD DEPENDS

AMERICAN CONTINENT OUTSIDE THE UNITED STATES:

Mexico—Sabadilla, Sarsaparilla, Vanilla, Cacao (Chocolate Nut), Jalap, Cochineal
Canada—Balsam of Fir, Juniper
South America—Coffee, Soap Bark, Ipecac, Copaiba, Rhatany, Balsam of Peru, Balsam of Tolu, Coca, Guaiac, Jaborandi, Guarana, Cacao, Capsicum, Cinchona (Quinine)
West Indies—Oil of Wormseed, Oil of Orange, Oil of Lemon, Quassia, Coffee, Ginger, Copaiba

EUROPE AND THE WESTERN MEDITERRANEAN COUNTRIES:

England—Valerian, Digitalis
Ireland—Chondrus
France—Mustard, Lavender, Gentian, Rose Petals, Buckthorn, Pomegranate
Spain—Ergot, Saffron, Oil of Cade, Licorice, Oil of Orange, Oil of Lemon, Spanish Flies (Cantharides)
Germany—Gentian, Aconite, Buckthorn, Chamomile, Scopola
Switzerland—Colchicum
Italy—Saffron, Mustard, Rose Petals, Pomegranate

EASTERN MEDITERRANEAN COUNTRIES AND ASIA MINOR:

Greece—Colchicum, Nutgall, Hemlock
Bulgaria—Attar of Roses, Belladonna, Hyoscyamus
Yugoslavia—Opium
Turkey—Colchicum, Santonin, Tragacanth, Opium
Macedonia—Opium
Egypt—Senna, Malt, Acacia, Cassia Fistula, Anise, Opium
Asia Minor—Squill, Tragacanth, Storax, Opium, Prunes, Hyoscyamus, Stramonium, Almonds (Bitter and Sweet), Licorice, Manna, Scammony, Oil of Rosemary, Belladonna
Arabia—Myrrh, Acacia

AFRICA:

Aloes, Physostigma, Buchu, Strophanthus, Oil of Rosemary,

Coffee, Pyrethrum
Zanzibar—Cloves

ASIA:

Persia—Asafoetida, Nutgall, Indian Hemp, Opium
India—Senna, Aloes, Cardamom, Ginger, Black Pepper, Indian Hemp, Aconite, Opium, Kino, Nux Vomica (Strychnine), Rubber
Ceylon—Calamus, Cardamom, Spices, Tea
Burma—Calamus
Thailand—Benzoin
Russia—Ergot, Santonin

SOUTHEAST ASIA, INDONESIA, AND OTHER ISLANDS:

Indochina—Caraway, Coriander, Opium
China—Tea, Malt, Rhubarb, Opium, Camphor
Malaya—Rubber
Japan—Tea, Pyrethrum
Formosa—Camphor
Indonesia and Other Islands—Cinchona (Quinine), Cubeb, Benzoin, Oil of Santal, Black Pepper, Nux Vomica, Nutmeg, Cloves, Allspice, Cinnamon, Columbo, Cajeput, Gambir, Gamboge, Coffee

AUSTRALIA:

Eucalyptus

Beginning with the Colonial period, and following the War with Spain, the Colony and State have passed through five wars when the Coast of Georgia was blockaded for drugs, as well as for other items which might be valuable in warfare.

In the Revolutionary War, England, thinking America could not survive disease epidemics, prohibited the importation of drugs. The apothecaries and physicians, as well as the people of the Colony, had to begin a search for locally growing drugs which might be used as substitutes for those which had been supplied only by importation.

The colonists were successful in finding some substitutes for most imported drugs. And notices went out through the publications of the State, and by word of mouth, as to which local drug product might be used. One paper, for instance, published a notice to the people of the State in the case of an epidemic of fever (whether malarial, typhoid, or yellow is not known) with

℞ PROBLEMS CONFRONTING THE COLONY   49

the advice to the settlers to make and use teas or infusions out of wild cherry bark, dogwood bark, poplar bark, or any other bark, shrub, or herb, which was bitter. It was advised that a person might immunize himself against the infection by drinking these products, or he might cure himself once he contracted the disease. Reliance was placed to a large extent upon those drugs which the settlers found the Indians using,* as well as some which had been identified as being identical with, or similar to, imported products.

When the Revolutionary War was over, it was considered easier to import drugs than to find them by the slow process of experimentation. And, during the period between the Revolutionary War and the War of 1812, very little is reported of progress in the knowledge and use of locally growing drugs.

The War of 1812 came along; the Coast of Georgia was again blockaded; and the same hurry and hustle to find locally growing drugs for emergency use, similar to conditions prevailing during the Revolutionary War period, was again initiated.

In the period from 1812 to the Civil War period, the people of the State disregarded their experience with locally grown drugs and relied again upon importation for their drug needs, and for the third time in the State's history we were driven back to a consideration of our local drugs when the Civil War began. And as it progressed, with the declaration of war between the North and the South, among the first items to be embargoed by the Federal Government, so far as the South was concerned, were Morphine, Quinine and Chloroform. This embargo was to go to such extremes that no drugs were allowed to be imported for use in prisons where Federal soldiers were held — thus the great tragedy of Andersonville prison. These lines from *Ersatz in the Confederacy* just about represent the thought involved in placing an embargo on drugs coming into the South from any source for any purpose:

> No more quinine, let 'em shake,
> No more S's pills, let their heads ache.
> No morphine, let 'em lie awake,
> No mercury for Rebels to take;
> Though fever all their vitals bake,
> No nitre drops their heat to slake.[13]

---

* See Appendix for list of Indian drugs native to Georgia, page 428.

13. *Ersatz in the Confederacy*, p. 116.

Once more the wild search for drugs took place in the State. Quoting further from *Ersatz in the Confederacy*, we find the following information:

> There were three sources of drugs: One was by capture of supplies; two, by running the blockade; and three, by manufacture.
>
> Negroes being long practiced in having to find their own drugs, their remedies were frequently adopted by whites, who proceeded to manufacture them in quantity and to advertise them. Nearly every doctor and druggist had their pet remedies, most of which were as substitutes for pre-War drugs.
>
> In many places in Georgia during the Civil War drug stores had to close for lack of drugs. The woods and fields and swamps of the South then became the source of our drugs.[14]

And, from the same work, the writer states:

> The druggists of the State held a convention to discuss the problems of how to find medicines and how to secure them. The meeting was held in Augusta 1863, and a Committee of Three was appointed to accept samples of drugs and chemicals made from native substances and examine them (tests for efficacy and safety).
>
> The Confederate Government published a list of drugs, medicines, and chemicals, and laboratories were set up for their manufacture and for research in native herbs and plants.
>
> One of these laboratories was located at Augusta, Macon, Atlanta, and Milledgeville; and, heading the laboratory setup were John and Joseph LeConte [native-born Georgians and founders of the University of California].[15]

From the end of the Civil War, during the time between 1865 and the beginning of World War I, in 1914, again nothing was done toward a study of the possibilities for the use of the medicinal plants grown here in the State. Prior to the beginning of World War I, we were importing a number of drugs from various countries in Europe and from parts of Asia and Africa, most of which drugs were shut off from importation by the almost completely successful submarine activity as conducted by Germany. We were thus forced for the fourth time in our history to seek to find in our locally growing drugs those which might act as equivalents or substitutes for those we had been importing.

Following World War I, we forgot about our locally growing drugs and began our importations all over again. And when World War II loomed on the horizon, one of the first steps

14. *Ibid.*
15. *Ibid.*, p. 118.

Japan took was to capture the Island of Java, from which island comes practically 100% of the quinine of the world. American armies fighting in malaria-infested areas of the Pacific had no quinine. The stock-pile of quinine for use by the Army and Navy was so dangerously low that the Federal Government issued Conservation Order Number 131, which restricted the use of quinine to antimalarial purposes only. Wholesale, retail, and manufacturing pharmaceutical interests were requested to donate all surplus stocks of quinine to the Government. The volume of quinine to come in under this request was large enough materially to reduce the shortage and this resulted perhaps in the saving of many lives, including perhaps your son or mine. Again, we in this country were thrown into a turmoil in a search for a substitute for quinine, as well as for a number of drugs which we had been importing from Europe, Asia and Africa.

Thus, five times in our history as the result of wars we have been forced to seek for medicinal agents among the abundant plant life of the State and the Nation. But when World War II was over, we drifted back again to the importation of drugs from all parts of the world.

This story is told here in the hope that some governmental, educational, or private agency may set up some plan for a continuing program of research, running the entire gamut of our locally growing vegetable products, including drugs.

The Civil War period was a critical one in the life of the State, and, viewed from this distance, it would seem to be miraculous that the South survived the lack of those imported drugs on which we had relied for the prevention and treatment of the various diseases common to the climate.

Realizing early in the beginning of the War the importance of drugs, and that their importation would probably be prohibited by blockade, the Confederate Government recognized the necessity of finding substitutes within the South for drugs which had formerly been imported.

Dr. F. P. Porcher of South Carolina was one of the physicians trained in botany. He was a surgeon in the Confederate Army and was temporarily released (by order of the Surgeon General) from army duties to make a survey of the medicinal plants growing in the Southern States which at one time or another had been used by physicians, pharmacists, Indians, laymen and others.

Dr. Porcher's report was released in 1862 and was printed and distributed under the title, "Resources of the Southern Fields and Forests." The report was written in such language as would be interpretable by the Army surgeon in the field, the physician in his office, the apothecary in his shop, or store, the planter and the farmer and their wives. He urged that the information be distributed as widely as possible to the Army as well as to the citizenry.

Dr. Porcher's findings, along with those of Dr. Joseph Jacobs,[16] in addition to the known Indian drugs,[17] would constitute a good place to begin a systematic research program in the effort to discover or confirm the medicinal virtues of many of our herbs, shrubs, and trees.

Therefore, there is included herewith a rather detailed description of a number of the drugs that were used in the treatment of disease in the Confederate Army, as well as among the people of the South.

Some Drugs and Their Uses As Reported by Dr. F. P. Porcher

(An asterisk indicates that the drug has been reported or has been found in Georgia.)

* Aletris (Star-grass or Unicorn Root)—Remedy for colic, flatulence.

  Apocynum (Canadian Hemp or Milk Weed or Indian Physic)—Diuretic, diaphoretic, expectorant, antiperiodic, emetic. This is one of the favorite medicinal plants used by General Marion's forces of the Revolutionary era.

* Arrowroot (Maranta)—Produces a form of starch similar in character to potato starch, and therefore sometimes specified as a dietetic agent. At one time grown extensively in South Georgia for export purposes, and is yet a project which might be explored to advantage.

* Asclepias Tuberosa (Pleurisy Root or Butterfly Weed)—Diaphoretic and expectorant. Used in treatment of rheumatism, pneumonia, and consumption as a palliative.

  Barberry (Berberis)—A bitter tonic, non-astringent.

* Black Walnut—The rind of the unripe fruit is said to relieve ringworm, tetter; a fish poison. Leaves used for repelling insects: flies, fleas, mosquitoes. (A fact which explains why

---

16. Joseph Jacobs' article in *Proceedings of the A.Ph.A.*, 1898 (Vol. 49), 192, "Drug Conditions During the War Between the States."
17. See Appendix for this list of Indian drugs.

the black walnut tree is found near most of the old homes in Georgia.)
* Blackberry Root—Astringent in diarrhoea, dysentery. Also, a cordial from fruit.
* Boneset (Eupatorium)—Antiperiodic, substitute for quinine.

  Buckthorn Bark—Bark is laxative. Cherokee Indians used it as wash for cancer.

  Butternut (Juglans)—The inner bark of the root is a mild and efficient laxative. Used extensively during Revolutionary War by General Marion's army.

  Chamomile (Anthemis)—One of the old German drugs used in the treatment of hysteria, nervousness, to produce sweating and relieve pain.
* Charcoal—A form of carbon prepared from willow wood, which, being a soft wood, produces a form of charcoal in a finely divided state. Where the Pharmacopoeia specifies charcoal, reference is here to willow charcoal, it being understood that charcoal may be prepared from *any* wood. This form of charcoal is frequently given internally in the treatment of digestive troubles or may be used as a constituent of a dentifrice to purify the breath. In country districts at one time it was common practice to find pans containing lumps of charcoal in various parts of the room where a person was sick. This, for the purpose of absorbing the odors of the sickroom.
* Chenopodium (American Wormseed or Jerusalem Oak or Goosefoot)—The oil obtained by distilling the fresh plant is used primarily for the removal of round worms.
* Cedar Trees, known as Junipers, of which there are several types in Georgia (Juniper Communis or Common Juniper) —An oil is distilled from the fruit, which is diuretic, similar in action to turpentine.

  Juniper Oxycedrus—Wood is distilled producing a tar which is called Oil of Cade, used externally usually as a constituent of ointments, as a parasiticide.

  Juniper Sabina produces an oil by distillation of the tops, the leaves or needles, which is called Oil of Savin, reputed to have diuretic, emmenagogue and ecbolic properties.
* Cimicifuga (Black Snakeroot, Black Cohosh, Bugbane, or Squaw Root)—Diuretic, diaphoretic, expectorant, sedative (arterial and nervous); used in heart diseases as a substitute for digitalis; chorea, bronchitis, rheumatism, hysteria.

* Cotton Root Bark—Evidently discovered by Negro slaves. Action similar to Ergot as emmenagogue and ecbolic.
* Cypripedium (Ladies Slipper)—Used in hysteria and chorea and other nervous conditions.
* Dandelion (Taraxacum)—Cathartic, diuretic; used in sclerosis of liver, stone in bladder, jaundice.
* Dogwood Bark—Substitute for quinine; tonic, intermittent fevers.
* Elm—Inner bark yields mucilage. Used as a demulcent, emollient, poultice to boils, irritated parts. Internally, food values; demulcent in stomachic or intestinal irritation, diarrhoea, dysentery.

Euonymus (Wahoo, Arrow-wood, or Indian Arrow-wood, Burning Bush)—Laxative, diuretic, antiperiodic, antiparasitic. Leaves are poisonous to cattle; thought to be narcotic.

Euphorbia (Flowering Spurge)—Emetic, expectorant, and vesicant.
* Fig - Fruit. Unripe fruit as poultice for boils or blisters. Ripe fruit as laxative.

Gentian (Samson's Snakeroot)—An excellent bitter tonic devoid of astringency.
* Helonias (False Unicorn)—Used by Indian women to prevent abortion.
* Hop—Wild Hop of North Georgia mountains. Hypnotic, narcotic, sedative. Substitute for opium, diuretic. "Specific in asthmatic pain."
* Horehound (Marrubium)—Used in colds, asthma, hysteria, chronic rheumatism.
* Hydrastis (Golden Seal, Eye Balm, Yellow Puccoon)—Bitter tonic, antiperiodic, nerve stimulant similar to strychnine. Widely used in catarrhal conditions.
* Magnolia—The bark of the root is laxative. Used in treatment of rheumatism. (Substitute for quinine).
* Mayapple (Mandrake, Vegetable Mercury, Podophyllum)—Laxative, purge.
* Mulberry—Bark said to be purgative and vermifuge.
* Mullein (Thapsus Verbascus)—The petals of the flowers said to contain narcotic principle. The leaves of plant contain large quantity of mucilage, and hence used for poultice purposes. A syrup made of them used in the treatment of coughs.
* Mustard—Given internally as emetic; applied externally as

℞   PROBLEMS CONFRONTING THE COLONY   55

poultice to produce a blister. Also applied externally as a liniment.
* Myrica—(Bayberry or Wax Myrtle)—Astringent in diarrhoea, dysentery, uterine hemorrhage, and dropsies.
* Oak Bark—All oaks yield a form of tannin; therefore, astringent, in manufacture of leather. In manufacture of ink, boil bark with rusted iron. Black oak bark said by some to be complete substitute for quinine.
* Passiflora Incarnata (Maypop, Passion Flower, Passion Vine) —Dried flowering and fruiting top is used. Said to be narcotic anodyne in the treatment of nervous diseases and in neuralgia.
* Pennyroyal (Tickweed)—Emmenagogue, diaphoretic. The oil repels insects: fleas, flies, mosquitoes, ticks.
* Pomegranate—Bark of the root for tapeworms.
* Poplar Bark—Tonic, diuretic, diaphoretic, substitute for quinine. Used for rheumatism and gout. "Never knew it to fail in a single case of worms." Given to horses for botts. (Contains principle similar to salicylic acid and aspirin.)
* Prickly Ash (Toothache Bush, Fraxius)—Promotes saliva. Used as a blood purifier in venereal disease. Diaphoretic.
* Sage—Teas made from leaves promote sweating, and the powdered leaf is said to resist putrefaction of animal matter.
* Sanguinaria (Blood Root)—Narcotic, emetic, purge.
* Sassafras—Tea from root and leaf. Colds, measles, pneumonia, bronchitis, blood purifier. Mucilage from pith as application to irritated eye.
* Seneca Snakeroot (Rattlesnake Root, Milkwort, Mountain Flax)—Expectorant, diuretic, diaphoretic. Used in bronchitis, asthma, croup, pleurisy.
* Serpentaria (Virginia Snakeroot)—Used as a diuretic and diaphoretic in the treatment of fevers; sometimes substitute for quinine. (This plant is not to be confused with Seneca Snakeroot or Black Snakeroot or Rauwolfia Serpentina (Reserpine).)
* Spigelia (Pink Root)—Grows wild all over the South. Worm remedy of great value. In early days of the Colony, pink root was an item of export. Usually associated with senna to prevent its absorption from the intestinal tract.
* Stillingia (Queen's Root or Queen's Delight, Yaw Root)— Used as a vegetable blood purifier. Also emetic, expectorant, diuretic, and cholagogue.

- * Stramonium (Jimson Weed or Jamestown Weed)—This drug almost identical in its general action with belladonna. Powerful narcotic and poison. Reported to have value in treatment of epilepsy. All parts of the plant are poisonous in sufficient quantities.
- * Sumac (Rhus Glabra)—Bark of root is astringent. "Cures burns without leaving scar." Berries astringent, refrigerant, substitute for lemonade. Used in treatment of sore throat, dysentery.
- * Sunflower—The plants were directed to be planted around the house if the house was located in a malarial section. An edible oil may be obtained from sunflower seed, or for burning in lamps, or in the manufacture of soap.
- * Sweet Birch—Yields oil identical with wintergreen. Externally, it is antiseptic, irritant in liniments. Internally, for rheumatism, gout, as urinary antiseptic, and for fevers.
- * Turpentine—Now one of the most universally employed of all remedial agents. Almost a panacea if we accept Culbreth's materia medica, which lists its properties as follows: "Externally: rubefacient, counter-irritant, antiseptic, disinfectant."

    "Internally: stimulant, carminative, cathartic, anthelmintic, expectorant, haemostatic, diuretic, diaphoretic, antipyretic."

    "Externally for rheumatism, sciatica, lumbago, neuralgia, bronchitis, pleurisy, peritonitis, tympanites, renal colic, gangrene, sprains, wounds, scabies, ringworm, enlarged glands, burns, frostbites, colic; vapors of oil in whooping cough, diphtheria, laryngitis."

    "Internally in the treatment of bronchial catarrh, cystitis, venereal diseases, chronic urinary troubles, piles, hemorrhages, puerperal fever, inflammation of bowels, traumatic erysipelas, intestinal worms, pneumonia."

    Dr. Porcher states: "There are almost limitless uses to which turpentine may be put."
- Urtica (Stinging Nettle)—Internal or external hemorrhage, nose bleed.
- * Veratrum Viride (Itch-Weed or White Hellebore)—The root of the plant is a powerful heart depressant similar to aconite, and one of the old remedies in treatment of pneumonia.
- * Watermelon Seed, Pumpkin Seed—Administered to man and beast for worms.
- * Wild Cherry (Inner Bark)—"Fevers of scrofula and con-

sumption." Bitter tonic, dyspepsia, neuralgia, substitute for quinine. Coughs.
* Willow Tree (Salix)—Bark used as one of the best substitutes for Peruvian bark or quinine. Contains principle salicin which is similar to aspirin; hence the drug used extensively in the treatment of rheumatism.
* Witch Hazel—Indian remedy. Bark and twigs were distilled with water, giving the liquid product we know as witch hazel. The dried leaves contain tannin; therefore, astringent, haemostatic, styptic.

Dr. Porcher pleads for and advises that a continual program of study and research in plant products for medicinal or industrial uses be provided. The author enthusiastically agrees in this recommendation of Dr. Porcher, for the drug problem still confronts the people of Georgia, 1733-1959.

In recommending the possibility of an extensive research program in these old vegetable drugs, which in the minds of the practitioners proved of value, the story of MaHuang and Rauwolfia (or Snakeroot) is interesting.

MaHuang, an old Chinese drug used extensively as a panacea for perhaps thousands of years, in a comparatively recent study has yielded the active principle Ephedrine. The drug Rauwolfia, a very old drug of the East, has given us that newest and most valuable tranquillizing agent Reserpine. Our native drugs, on the basis of study with the aid of modern research, may give us some drugs comparable in value to MaHuang and Rauwolfia.

Chapter IV

SELF-DIAGNOSIS AND TREATMENT OF ORDINARY AND EPIDEMIC DISEASES BECAME A NECESSITY IN THE LIFE OF THE COLONY AND OF THE STATE, 1733-1807

THE population of the Colony was increasing, and settlers were moving into remote areas where they were out of reach of medical or pharmaceutical service, and where the need for medical treatment was ever present and frequently tragically urgent.

For drugs, the settlers were dependent on those they were able to bring in with them in the form of "medicine chests"; or on those native vegetable drugs they had been taught to identify and use; or on those they found the Indians or Negro slaves using; or on those which might be brought in by occasional contact with settlements on the rivers or the ocean.

Most of these settlers, perhaps, had received only rudimentary or no instruction in sanitation, in the recognition of disease conditions and their treatment, or in the care of wounds and injuries.

To meet the health needs of the Colonists, or at best to aid these settlers, physicians and others recognized the necessity for instruction. Some of them were prompted to publish books and pamphlets in lay language for distribution and sale, whereby the layman was enabled to recognize and treat ordinary diseases and injuries. Medicine chests, stocked with drugs of that period and with full directions for their use, were put up for sale by some of these same leading physicians, who advertised them along with their books or pamphlets, in their "medical stores" in Savannah and Augusta.

When we consider the large number of people who survived disease and hardships in the Colony of Georgia, we must recognize that these publications may have rendered a real service, or

℞ SELF-DIAGNOSIS 59

explain it in terms of the hardiness of those people who survived in spite of it all.

The instruction was so soundly done that the practice of self-diagnosis and treatment has extended through all succeeding generations, and will possibly extend into generations yet to come. It frequently happens in life that in solving one problem we create another, which may be potentially greater than the one we solve.

Those of us who were brought up in the rural areas of the State can recall the various drugs and treatments in vogue in our childhood, many of which are still in existence. Most of these originated from the remedies and treatments suggested in these and other volumes of that era.

For purposes of comparison of conditions and practices of one hundred and fifty or more years ago with present medical practices, this Chapter contains quotes from four of the many of these books which were widely distributed and used, but these are not intended for guidance or practice in this medically enlightened era of 1959.

Instruction in the Matter of Self-Diagnosis and Treatment of Ordinary Diseases.

The first of these booklets appeared in 1734 and was written by Dr. John Tennent, a prominent physician of Virginia, under the title, *The Poor Planter's Physician or Every Man His Own Doctor*. In addition to this edition of the book, it is known that at least three other editions or reprintings were published in Benjamin Franklin's printing establishment in Philadelphia. Franklin himself practiced medicine and pharmacy.

The second of these books came from the pen of John Wesley—the father of Methodism—who, in addition to his spiritual ministrations to his people, also served their physical needs in his practice of medicine and pharmacy. His book, entitled *Primitive Physic Or An Easy Way To Treat Most Ordinary Diseases*, was first published in 1747, and went through thirty-two editions and reprintings.

The third book was written by Dr. George Harral of Savannah. It is entitled, *The Medicine Chest Book*, 1807.

The fourth book was written by Dr. James Ewell. It is entitled, *Planters and Mariners Companion*, and was published also in 1807.

It is interesting to note the philosophy of Tennent and Wesley as expressed in the Preface of each volume. It is easier to agree with their philosophy than with some of the scientific counsel and advice which they give.

Quoting from the preface of Dr. Tennent's book, *The Poor Planter's Physician,* his philosophy is expressed as follows:

> The most acceptable Service we can render to God is Beneficence to Man. There are three Ways of benefitting our Fellow Creatures. We may be helpful to their Bodies, by feeding the Hungry, cloathing the Naked, and prescribing easy Remedies to the Sick; we can aid them in their Fortunes by encouraging of Industry, by relieving the Distresst, and doing all the kind Offices we are able, to our Neighbours. These are the several Ways of improving the Talents our Maker has entrusted us with; and we must every one expect, hereafter to give an Account, how we have employ'd them.
>
> I publish this short Treatise, to lead the Poorer Sort into the Pleasant Paths of Health; when they have the Misfortune to be sick, to show them the cheapest and easiest Ways of getting well again.
>
> These Considerations made me account it a Work of great Charity and Publick Spirit, to communicate to the Poor Inhabitants of this Colony (Virginia), a safe Method of curing themselves, when they shall be so unhappy as to fall into any of our common Maladies. And for their greater Encouragement, the Remedies I shall prescribe, may be procured with little Trouble and Expence, being, for the most Part, such as grow at their own Doors, or may be easily propagated.
>
> Providence has been so good, as to furnish almost every Country with Medicines proper for the Distempers incident to the Climate; and such Domestick Remedies are always sufficient for the Poor, who live upon homely Fare, and for the Temperate, who make a right Use of God's Blessings.
>
> In setting down the following Prescriptions, I have been cautious of talking like an Apothecary; that is, of using hard Words, that perhaps neither my Patient, nor my self understand.
>
> Before I mention the Cure, I shall endeavor to describe the Symptoms of each Distemper, in so plain a Manner, that any Person may be Master of his own Case, if he will but attend carefully to what he feels. At the same Time, he shall have my best Advice, to prevent every particular Ailment; which will be happier for him to know how to cure it.

PLEURISY is "the most fatal of all Distempers." [Dr. Tennent gives the symptoms. He recommends as remedies]:
1. Bleed 10 ounces; repeat 3 or 4 days.
2. Vomit with Indian Physic (American Ipecac.)
3. Give honey and Linseed Oil.

℞ SELF-DIAGNOSIS

4. Apply blister to neck and to each arm.
5. To prevent: Bleed 10 ounces if great hoarseness.

QUINSEY. If consequent to a cold, the following remedies are given: Bleed 10 ounces (prefer jugular vein and arm); or, purge with Decoction of Mallows and Syrup of Peach Blossom.

CONSUMPTION is referred to as a "Distemper slow and sure" and as "a melancholy Case." The symptoms are listed, As remedies:
"*Bleed* and blister."
"Only inward medicines" are effective.
"Chew sassafras root."
or, "Make pills of Turpentine and Deer's Dung."
As a suggested diet for the consumptive, Dr. Tennent advises: "No meat; eat plenty of turnips, roasted apples, and raisins."

THE BLOODY FLUX. The symptoms are listed. As a remedy: "*Bleed* 8 ounces; vomit with Indian Physic (American Ipecac)." Dr. Tennent speaks of the Bloody Flux as being "non-contagious."

THE WHITE FLUX. Dr. Tennent comments: "White Flux will hurry a strong man out." Remedy: Vomit and purge.

GRIPING IN THE BELLY. Remedy: "Drink a Gallon of Warm Whey."

COLIC. Remedy: "Take 2 or 3 Quarts of Warm Water, Drink a Decoction of Peach Leaves, or Sassafras Tea."

PALSEY. (Palsy) He describes the symptoms as "melancholy Tokens." As remedies: "Purge and plunge over Head and Ears into cold Water on alternate Mornings; continue for 3 Months." Or, "Cause Head, Palms of Hands and Soles of Feet to be scrubbed with Mixture of Spirit of Scurvy-Grass."*

EPILEPSY or FALLING SICKNESS. Tennent describes the symptoms: "These melancholy fits come near the full or change of the Moon." As a cure: "*Bleed*, and burn Feathers under the Nose." As a remedy to prevent the distemper: "Purge and vomit four days before and four days after the full Moon for 7 Months."

"A FEVER with violent Purging and Vomiting will hurry a Man to his long Home." To cure: "Drink 2 gallons of Thin Broth in 2 or 3 hours." "Some of it will come up and some go down."

---
* See Glossary of Terms, page 432.

FEVER and AGUE is described by Dr. Tennent: "An Epidemick Distemper in this moist and variable Climate," which unless checked, "finally ends in a Jaundice, Dropsy, Dry Gripes, or Cachexy." He urges his patients as they "tender their Health and their Looks, to disposses this Devil as soon as they can."

He calls attention to the fact that an Ague returns every day, every third day, or every fourth day; and that after the second fit, one must *bleed eight ounces*. The next day purge with Indian Physic. Then, he suggests that this treatment should be followed by "taking every morning and evening 20 grains of the Powder of Sassafras Root, mixed with 10 grains of Virginia Snake-root in 2 spoonfuls of the Decoction of Wormwood."

If the Fever Fit returns every third day "omit Bleeding," but vomit and purge and "compleat the Cure with the Powders of Sassafras and Snake-root."

"If the Fever returns every fourth day, you must vomit and purge and take a cold-water Sweat; that is, so soon as the cold Fit is off, and the Fever begins to come on." "Go into Naked Bed and drink a Pint of Cold Water; then cover yourself up, and in a little time, the Disease will be driven all out of your Pores. However, take the Powders made of Sassafras and Virginia Snake-root after this Operation for some time."

His suggestion "to prevent this Distemper" is to eat carefully, ride horseback a great deal in the hot months, to sweat out "all ill-digested Humours," and not to "chill your Bowels too much with cold Water." Avoid as much as possible "being abroad in the rain," or in the "deep dews" of the night; be cautious too of "sleeping on the ground, or with your doors or windows open."

A CONTINUAL FEVER. "Bleed immediately 10 ounces," and the day following, "vomit with Indian Physick, and purge with the same." Blisters applied to the neck and the fleshy parts of the arms are suggested. Tennent warns that "it matters not how much people eat in one of the Fevers because the Spirits requisite for Digestion are employed in struggling with the Disease."

A SLOW FEVER is described by Tennent as the "true Scorbutic Fever," and its symptoms are given. His treatment: "Take a Vomit of Indian Physick, and the next morning a Purge of the same. The mornings you do not take Physick, drink constantly a Quarter of a Pint of Sassafras Tea, fasting; and every Night, take powdered Snake-root." To prevent: one must indulge "no sloathful Inclination. But stir about your business briskly, ride as often as you can, and never take more than a pint of Water, or other Drink, in 24 hours. Breathe as much as possible in the open Air in the daytime, *but avoid it in the Night.*"

WORM FEVER is discussed. This disease is called one "principally confined to Children," and to be identified by the pain in the side or the stomach or the bowels, and sometimes accompanied by the flux and convulsions. "Like the Devil, it appears in all Manner of Shapes." His treatment: "Vomit and purge." Give the Seed of Jerusalem Oak and the juice of Wormwood for 3 mornings. Then, "Soak a cur'd Leaf of Tobacco in Vinegar, and apply it warm to the Stomach or Belly; and it will make the Worms much sicker than it doth the Patient."

Dr. Tennent philosophizes about the "Worm Fever": "It is difficult to hinder Worms from hatching, and harbouring in our bodies, for we swallow their Eggs, almost with Everything we eat; especially such as live much upon Pulse and Indian Corn, will be full of them. Three-fourths of the Children who die in these Parts die of Worms."

THE YELLOW JAUNDICE is one of those conditions which arise from "keeping the Ague too long." It evidences itself by the yellow color of the skin and the whites of the eyes, and the urine. His treatment: "A Purge of Indian Physick, and then, every morning and evening for 6 weeks a quarter of a Pint of Decoction of the Bark of Elder and the Root of Sassafras in equal quantities." His suggested diet: "To drink Beer brew'd with Sorrel Leaves, Pine Tops, Root of Ash, and a little 'old Iron.'"

DROPSY is "another one of the Consequences of Keeping an Ague too long." "This dire Calamity befalls ancient People, or to young People when they make too bold with their Constitution." Attention is called to the fact that "Loss of Blood may be one of the Causes of Dropsy." The loss of blood may come through the "Bleeding Piles," in which case he suggests purging with Indian Physick. "The Mornings you don't purge, drink the express't Liquor of Fresh Ass-Dung, sweeten'd with Syrup of Quinces."

BLEEDING AT THE NOSE. Tennent suggests that the patient "snuff up the Nose the Decoction of Comfrey Leaves," and, if it is available, add a "little 'Allom' to the Decoction of Comfrey Leaves and a Tent soak'd in the same, frequently thrust into the Nostrils."

For BLOOD IN THE SPIT OR IN THE URINE, *bleed eight Ounces,* and "the next morning, purge with Indian Physick, and drink nothing but Tea made of Comfrey Leaves and sweeten'd with Syrup of Quinces."

He indicates that VAPOURS AND HYSTERICK FITS are conditions peculiar to women. After giving the symptoms he concludes with these remarks: "In one Word, she has no Relish for any Thing, but is compleatly out of Humour, she knows not why; and out of Order, she knows not where." But his remedy for this condition is the usual one: Purge and vomit with Indian Physick.

Dr. Tennent says, "Heaven be prais'd there is little Occasion to say anything of the STONE IN THE BLADDER, for there is very little of it in this Colony." But he does say that many of us, "by sitting too long either at our Book, or our Bottle, have, now and then, some touches of the GRAVEL or STONE IN THE KIDNEYS." For this condition, he recommends: "Drink 3 or 4 Quarts of Whey, as fast as you can, in which the Root of Prickley Pear has been boil'd."

"The symptoms of the BLIND PILES are little Swellings, appearing just without the Fundament. They are occasion'd by the Flowing of corrupted Blood into the Vessels thereabouts." For this complaint he suggested as a remedy: "Every Morning, while fasting, take the Yolk of a new-laid Egg, with 12 Grains of Brimstone (Sulphur), finely powder'd, and wash it down with a small Draught of Decoction of Mallows." To prevent the Blind Piles: "Boil a Handful of Mullein Leaves in a Pint of New Milk, and sweeten with Syrup of Violets; drink this every Night for 6 Weeks, just before going to Rest."

Discussing the matter of RUPTURE, Tennent suggests that the patient "should have a Truss, and then apply fresh Cow-Dung which must be renew'd Night and Morning till the Pains are assuag'd."

Tennent describes YAWS or COUNTRY DISTEMPER as "the highest Kind of Scurvy" and the symptoms of it as "eating Ulcers in the Throat, or Palate, and filthy Sores in other Parts of the Body." He states that this disease often yields to Dr. Papa's Remedy (See Glossary of Terms and Formulas). He suggests also a remedy already referred to as "Pills made of equal Parts of Turpentine and Deer Dung."

℞   SELF-DIAGNOSIS

On the subject of the POX, Tennent states the following: "The pious Spaniards ketch'd it from their Negro Mistresses in the West Indies and had the Honor of propagating it from thence to all the Rest of the World."

He discusses CANCER, about which disease he states the following: "Some despairingly imagine it to be incurable; tho', blessed be God, there have been some Instances of Success." He indicates from his discussion of the subject that slow-healing sores of one kind or another might be "cancer." In these cases some local application might result in what he calls a "cure." He does rely heavily on a strong infusion or Decoction of Sassafras Root and Dogwood Root, and the drinking of Sassafras Tea.

The GOUT, he observes with pleasure, "grows less frequent in this country than in the time of our Fathers. His one remedy for the treatment and prevention of the Gout is "a strict and severe Temperance," both in eating and in drinking. "More in the quantity of the food and drink must be watched than in the quality of the food that is taken, as given by the example of Carnero, a noble Venetian, who tied himself down to 12 ounces of Eatables, including Bread, and 14 ounces of drink in 24 hours. He stuck close to this short allowance, using moderate Exercise, and from being a Cripple by the Gout, recovered his Health and Strength to a Wonder." Following this diet strictly, he says, Carnero "lived to the End of a long and happy Life."

Dr. Tennent calls attention to the fact that in the treatment of all these diseases no mention is made of "Mercury, Opium, or the Peruvian Bark, which have almost obtained the Reputation of Specifics." "I acknowledge the powerful Effects of these Medicines, but am persuaded they ought to be administered with the greatest Skill and Discernment. As I write only for the Poor, who are left to judge only for themselves, I was fearful of putting such dangerous Weapons into Their Hands."

He concludes his booklet with these words: "In the meantime there is no Question but *some of my Brother Quacks* will make themselves merry with some of these Prescriptions. Let them shoot their harmless Bows. I by no Means envy those Gentlemen the only Way they have of appearing Wiser than Their Neighbours. Tho' after all, it is not impossible that they may do, by some of these, just as the People of England do by the French Fashions, laugh at them first and then have the Humility to follow them."

PRIMITIVE PHYSIC
by John Wesley

John Wesley, trained as a cleric in the Church of England, during his short stay in America was much impressed with the health and hardiness of the Indians with whom he was associated, and to whom he came as a missionary. Not trained in medical science, yet he had some leaning in that direction, as witnessed by the fact that he assisted John Regnier, a Swiss nurse, in performing the first autopsy to be performed in the Colony of Georgia (1736). His contacts with the Indians and their habits of life, including the treatment of the diseases that were common to them by the use of vegetable products growing around them, made a lasting impression on him.

He returned to England, and, within a few years, established three clinics for the treatment of the poor, whereby he was prescribing for them as well as dispensing or recommending drugs. In 1747 he wrote a book entitled, *Primitive Physic Or An Easy Way To Treat Most Ordinary Diseases*. This book went through a number of editions and reprintings, totalling thirty-two. It was in common use in the Colonies of America for a number of years.

Being a cleric, it is but natural that he should introduce some theology into his book, *Primitive Physic*, as witnessed by the opening paragraph of the Preface of his book:*

> When man first came out of the hands of the Great Creator, clothed in body as well as in soul with immortality and incorruption, there was no place for physic or the art of healing. As he knew no sin, so he knew no pain, no sickness, no weakness, or bodily disorder. The habitation wherein the angelic mind, the divinae particulae aurae, abode, although originally formed out of the dust of the earth, was liable to no decay. It had no seeds of corruption or dissolution within itself. And there was nothing without to injure it: Heaven and Earth and all the Hosts of them were mild, benign, and friendly to human nature. The entire Creation was at peace

---

* Author's Note: The author is prepared to agree with a writer of Wesley's period that this book *Primitive Physic* is "a strange mixture of common sense and superstition." The reader will form his own opinion, bearing in mind that Wesley, being a minister, introduces some theology and philosophy into his discussion of these scientific matters, as witnessed by one statement he makes to the effect that if a person finds it necessary to consult a physician, he should find one "who fears God." Like Dr. John Tennent, John Wesley was, and still is, a controversial figure. We can agree with much of his philosophy and some of his scientific deductions but we can also differ with his philosophy, his theology, and his scientific deductions.

with man, so long as man was at peace with his Creator. So that, well might "The Morning Stars sing together, and all the Sons of God shout for joy."

Commenting on the Biblical quote, "By the sweat of thy face shalt thou eat bread til thou return to the ground," Wesley says that the power of exercise both to preserve and to restore health "is greater than can be conceived, especially in those who add temperance thereto." "Who, if they do not confine themselves altogether to eat bread or the herb of the field (which God doth not require them to do), yet steadily observe both that kind and measure of food which experience shows to be most friendly to health and strength."

"It is probable that physic, as well as religion, was in the first ages chiefly traditional: every father delivering down to his sons what he had himself in like manner received, concerning the manner of healing both outward hurts and the diseases incident to each climate, and the medicines which were of the greatest efficacy for the cure of each disorder. It is certain this is the method wherein the art of healing is preserved among the Americans to this day (referring to the Indians). Their diseases are indeed exceeding few; nor do they often occur, by reason of their continual exercise, and (till of late) universal temperance. But if any are sick, or bit by a serpent, or torn by wild beasts, the fathers immediately tell their children what remedy to apply. And it is rare that the patients suffer long; those medicines being quick, as well as being generally infallible."

Mr. Wesley traces the development of medicine from the beginning of time into those eras which he refers to as recommendations by the "Author of Nature" where drugs of a vegetable nature, or others, were discovered by observing animals, or perhaps people, and using them. Then comes the period of experiment in medicine. The European as well as the American said to his neighbor, "Are you sick?" "Drink the juice of this herb and your sickness will be at an end."

"Then in the process of time men of a philosophical turn were not satisfied with experimentation and accident, and they began to enquire how they might account for these things: How such medicines wrought such effects. They examined the human body and all its parts, the nature of the flesh, veins, arteries, structure of the brain, heart, lungs, stomach, bowels. What were the springs of several kinds of animal functions? They explored the various kinds of animal and mineral, as well as vegetable, substances. And hence "the whole order of physic which had obtained until that time came gradually to be inverted. Men of learning began to set experience aside; to build physic upon hypothesis; to form theories upon diseases and their cure, and to substitute these in the place of experiment."

He states: "As theories increased, simple medicines were more and more disregarded and disused until, in the course of years, the greater part of them were forgotten, at least in the politer nations. In the room of these, an abundance of new ones were introduced by reason of speculative men, and they became more and more difficult to be applied, as being more remote from common observation. Hence, rules for the application of these, and medical books, were immensely multiplied; till at length physic became an abstruse science, quite out of the reach of ordinary men."

He states further: "There have not been wanting, from time to time, some lovers of mankind who have endeavoured, even contrary to their own interest, to reduce physic to its ancient standard, and that neither the knowledge of astrology, astronomy, natural philosophy, or even anatomy itself, is absolutely necessary to the quick and effectual cure of most diseases incident to human bodies: nor yet any chemical or exotic compounded medicine, but a single plant of root, duly applied."

On the basis of such argument to himself, Wesley decides that even though many books have been written on the subject of medicine, most of them are in such language that the average person cannot interpret them. Therefore he feels that such a book as he proposes might have a place. He proposes then to write this book which is known as *Primitive Physic or How Every Man Can Treat His Own Diseases*.

He gives a long list of suggestions as to how health may be retained which he states have been transcribed from rules and recommendations made by Dr. Cheyne. Many of these rules and regulations are a part of our daily practice at the present time, so far as sanitation and health and cleanliness and even diet and exercise are concerned.

Some brief quotes from Dr. Cheyne, as reported by Wesley, may be in order.

"1. The air we breathe is of great consequence to our health.
2. The people should have those who live about them found sweet and healthy.
3. Everyone that would preserve health should be as clean

and sweet as possible, in their houses, clothes, and furniture.
4. A due degree of exercise is indispensably necessary to health and long life.
5. Costiveness cannot long conflict with health.
6. Obstructed perspiration, vulgarly called 'catching cold,' is one great source of disease. Whenever there appears the least sign of this, let it be removed by general sweats.
7. The passions have a greater influence on health than most people are aware of.
8. The love of God is the solvent remedy of all miseries, and therefore it becomes the most powerful of all means of health in our lives."

The Preface of Wesley's book, from which we have just quoted, was written in London in 1747. Following that, he states that he is surprised that the book has become so popular that a number of reprints have been called for. In 1755, from Bristol, England, the book was revised and published in larger quantities and was revised again in 1760 and in 1780.

He mentions various diseases arranged alphabetically for convenience, and gives the symptoms of those diseases, and then gives a series of remedies, these being arranged in the order of their importance, from Number 1 to Number 40, as the case may be.

Here are listed some of the diseases and the remedies:

AGUE. He defines this as an "intermitting fever, each fit of which is preceded by a cold shivering, and goes off in a sweat." Remedies are:
1. Go into a cold bath just before the cold fit.
2. Apply to the stomach a large onion, slit.
3. Apply oil of turpentine to the small of the back before the fit.

APOPLEXY, he describes as "a total loss of all sense and voluntary motion." Remedies: 1—To prevent apoplexy, use the cold bath and drink only water. 2—If the fit of apoplexy be soon after a meal, do not bleed, but vomit.

ASTHMA is described as "difficulty of breathing from a disorder of the lungs." Remedies:
1. Take a pint of cold water every morning, washing the head therein immediately thereafter, and using the cold bath.

2. Live a fortnight on boiled carrots only. It seldom fails.
3. Take an ounce of quicksilver every morning, and a spoonful of aqua sulphurate.

He says this has cured "an inveterate asthma."

BLEEDING AT THE NOSE. Drink whey largely every morning and eat much raisins. To cure it, apply to the neck, behind and on each side, a cloth dipped in cold water. Or, put the legs and arms in cold water. Or, steep a linen rag in sharp vinegar, burn the rag and blow it up the nose with a quill.

SPITTING OF BLOOD. Take a teacupful of stewed prunes at lying down for two or three nights.

BOILS. Apply a little Spanish turpentine. Or, apply a mixture of soap and brown sugar, well-mixed. Or, a plaster of honey and wheat flour.

BRUISES. Apply treacle spread on brown paper. Or, apply a plaster of chopped parsley mixed with water.

BURNS OR SCALDS. Immediately plunge the part in cold water, keeping it there for an hour or maybe four or five hours. Or, keep the part covered with a cloth, four times doubled, dipped in cold water.

He discusses the subject of CANCERS, but it is not thought wise to print here the remedies that were in use at that time.

WHOOPING COUGH.
1. Use the cold bath daily.
2. Rub the feet with hog's lard before the fire before going to bed, and keep the child warm.
3. Rub the back at lying down with old rum, which seldom fails.

CHOLERA MORBUS or FLUX AND VOMITING.
1. Drink two or three quarts of cold water, if the person is strong, or warm if he is weak.

COLDS.
1. Drink a pint of cold water lying down in bed.
2. Or, a spoonful of treacle in half a pint of water.

COLD IN THE HEAD.
Pare very thin the yellow rind of the orange. Roll it up inside out, and thrust a roll into each nostril.

COLIC (in the Fit).
1. Drink a pint of cold water.
2. Or, drink a quart of warm water.
3. Or, take Chamomile Tea.
4. Or, apply outwardly a bag of hot oats.

He discusses Bilious Cholic, an Habitual Cholic, an Hysteric Cholic, a Dry Cholic, and suggests remedies for each of these. Also, a Nervous Cholic and a Windy Cholic.

CONSUMPTION. Mr. Wesley states that "cold bathing has cured many deep consumptions." He gives a number of remedies for consumption, but we shall give his remedy number four: "Every morning cut up a little turf of fresh earth, and, lying down, breathe into the hole for a quarter of an hour." "I have known a deep consumption cured thus." (Antibiotics?)

CONVULSIONS in children. Scrape piony roots, fresh digged. Apply what you have scraped off to the soles of the feet. It helps immediately.

For the treatment of CORNS, he recommends the application of yeast from small beer spread on a rag. Or, bruised ivy leaves. Or, a chalk powdered and mixed with water. Or, apply a pitch plaster. Or, to relieve the pain of corns, steep the feet in hot water wherein oatmeal is boiled.

COSTIVENESS. Rise early every morning. Next, breakfast twice a week or oftener on water gruel. Or, take cream of tartar mixed with honey. Or, a small teacup of stewed prunes. Or, live upon bread made of wheat flour with all the bran in it.

COUGHS. Chew Peruvian Bark for as long as it remains bitter, and continue this until the cough is relieved. Or, he recommends, drink a pint of cold water lying down in bed. Or, make a hole through a lemon and fill it with honey. Roast it and catch the juice, taking a teacupful of this juice frequently.

He discusses coughs under various heads, such as the asthmatic cough, the consumptive cough, convulsive cough, the inveterate cough, the pleuritic cough, and a ticklish cough, and suggests remedies for these different types of cough.

For a convulsive cough, he recommends eating preserved walnuts.

CRAMPS IN THE MUSCLES. Take a half pint of tar water morning and evening. Or, lay a roll of brimstone under your pillow; or, hold a roll of brimstone in your hand. ("I have frequently done this with success," he says.)

CUTS. "Keep the cut closed with your thumb a quarter of an hour. Then double rag and dip it in cold water, and bind it on. Or, for deep cuts, bind on toasted cheese.

DEAFNESS. Use the cold bath. Or, put a little salt in the ear. Or, drop into it a teaspoonful of salt water. Or, two or three drops of onion juice.

He discusses the different types of DEAFNESS: Deafness with a dry ear, deafness with a headache and buzzing in the head, and lastly, a settled deafness, for all of which conditions he recommends various remedies.

SETTLED DEAFNESS. Pick out the core of a red onion, fill the place with oil of roasted almonds, let it stand a night; then bruise and strain it, and drop 3 or 4 drops into the ear morning and evening, and stop it with black wool.

DIABETES. "Drink wine boiled with ginger, as much and as your strength will bear."

THE DROPSY. "A preternatural collection of water in the head, breast, belly, or all over the body, attended with a continual thirst." He gives nine different remedies, some of which are the cold bath; rub with salad oil, or cover the belly with a large new sponge dipped in strong lime water; or apply green dock leaves to the joints, and soles of the feet; or, eat crust of bread every morning, fasting; or take as much as lies on a sixpence of powdered laurel leaves; or drink tar water; or take three spoonfuls of the juice of leeks, or elder leaves; or drink decoction of oak boughs.

EAR ACHE. "Rub the ear hard for a quarter of an hour; or, put in a roasted fig or onion as hot as may be; or, blow the smoke of tobacco strongly into the ear; or, boil rue or rosemary or garlic, and let the steam go into the ear through a funnel. Or, apply cloth four times doubled and dipped in cold water, for half an hour.

EAR ACHE FROM WORMS. His remedy is drop in warm milk and it brings the worms out.

BLEARED EYES. Drop into them the juice of crabapples.

℞ SELF-DIAGNOSIS

BLOODSHOT EYES. Apply linen rags dipped into cold water for two or three hours. Or, apply boiled hyssop as a poultice.

A BRUISED EYE. Apply a plaster made of conserve of roses.

BLINDNESS. It is often cured by cold bathing. For dull sight *the juice* (two or three drops) *of rotten apples.*

INFLAMED EYES. A poultice of roasted or rotted apples, warm; or, the white of an egg beaten up with rose water as a poultice.

SORE EYES. "Drink Eye-bright Tea," and wash the eyes with it.

WEAK EYES. "Wash the head daily with cold water."

To prevent FAINTING from letting of blood, drink broth prior to the letting of blood, and lie on the bed during the operation.

The FALLING SICKNESS, in which he describes the patient as falling to the ground, either convulsed, or quite stiff all over, with gnashing of teeth, and foaming at the mouth. Remedy: "Use the cold bath for a month daily."

FALLING OF THE FUNDAMENT. Apply a cloth covered with brickdust.

In EXTREME FAT. Use a total vegetable diet, including bread, turnips, carrots, or other roots, and milk.

FEVER. Vomit and purge, and if the pulse be hard, full, and strong, bleed. Remedy: Drink a pint of cold water, lying down in bed. "I never knew it to hurt." Or, drink tar water, or thin water gruel, sweetened with honey. Or, smear the wrists five or six inches long with warm treacle, and cover it with brown paper. Or, apply treacle plasters to the head and the soles of the feet, changing the plasters every twelve hours. In case of a high fever, he recommends plunging them into cold water. In case of a high fever with delirium, apply to the top of the head a treacle plaster.

An INTERMITTING FEVER. Remedy: Drink warm lemonade in the beginning of every fit. He also discusses a fever with pains in the limbs, a rash fever, a slow fever, and a worm fever.

To DESTROY FLEAS AND BUGS. Cover the floor of the room with leaves of black alder, gathered while the dew hangs on them. Adhering to these, the fleas are killed thereby.

FLEGM (PHLEGM). To prevent or cure flegm, take a spoonful of warm water the first thing in the morning.

A FLUX. Remedy: Receive the smoke of turpentine cast on burning coals.

BLOODY FLUX. "Take a large apple and pick out the core, fill up the space with a piece of honeycomb from which the honey has been drained out. Roast the apple and eat it, and this will stop the flux immediately."

The GOUT IN THE STOMACH. Drink dissolved Venice treacle in a glass of mountain wine. Drink it and go to bed. "You will be easier in two hours and well in ten," he says.

The GOUT IN THE FOOT OR THE HAND. Apply a raw, lean beefsteak, changing once in twelve hours.

The GOUT IN ANY LIMB. He gives a number of remedies for this condition, internal and external.

GRAVEL. Eat largely of spinach. Drink largely of warm water, sweetened with honey.

The GREEN SICKNESS. Take an ounce of quicksilver every morning. (Mr. Wesley states that quicksilver in its pure state is as harmless as water.)

To KILL ANIMALCULAE that cause the gums to waste away from the teeth. Remedy: Gargle three times a day with salt water.

The HEADACHE. "Rub the head for a quarter of an hour." Or, "be electrified." Or, "apply to each temple the thin yellow rind of a lemon." Or, "snuff up the nose camphorated spirits of lavender." Or, "snuff up the nose a little juice of horse-radish."

CHRONIC HEADACHE. Keep your feet in warm water a quarter of an hour before you go to bed, for two or three weeks. Or, wear tender hemlock leaves under the feet, changing them daily. Or, pour cold water on the head every morning.

VIOLENT HEADACHE. Remedy: Take of white wine, vinegar, and water, each three spoonfuls with half a spoonful of Hungary water. Apply this twice a day to the forehead and temples.

HEARTBURN. This is a "sharp, gnawing pain in the orifice of the stomach." Drink a pint of cold water, or drink slowly decoction of Chamomile Flowers. Or, eat four or five oysters. Or, chew five or six pepper corns a little, then swallow them. Or, chew fennel or parsley seed and swallow the spittle.

HICCUPS. Remedy: Swallow a mouthful of water, stopping the mouth and ears. Or, take anything that makes you sneeze. Or, take two or three preserved damsons. Or, three drops of oil of cinnamon on a lump of sugar. Or, 10 drops of chemical oil of amber dropped on sugar.

HOARSENESS. Rub the soles of the feet before the fire with garlic and lard, well beaten together, every night. "The hoarseness will be gone the next morning," he says. Or, "take a pint of cold water, lying down." Or, "swallow slowly the juice, of radishes." Or, "take half a pint of mustard whey, lying down."

For hypochondriac and hysteric disorders. Use cold bathing. Or, take an ounce of quicksilver in the morning, or ten drops of elixir of vitriol in the afternoon in a glass of cold water.

JAUNDICE. Wear leaves of celandine upon and under the feet. Or, take a small pill of castile soap every morning for 8 or 10 days.

ILIAC PASSION. "In this violent kind of cholic, the excrements are supposed to be thrown up by the mouth in vomiting." Apply warm flannel, soaked in spirit of wine, or hold a live puppy constantly on the belly. Or immerse, up to the breast, in a warm bath. Or, take ounce by ounce a pound or a pound and a half of quicksilver.

THE ITCH. "Wash the part with strong rum." Then, "anoint them with black soap or a poultice of powdered brimstone."

THE KING'S EVIL is discussed at length, and remedies suggested, none of which would be recognized or permitted to be advertised at the present time.

THE LEGS SORE AND RUNNING. Remedy: Wash in brandy and apply elder leaves, changing them twice a day.

LUNACY. Give decoction of agrimony, four times daily. Or, "rub the head several times a day with vinegar, in which ivy leaves, ground, have been infused." Or, "take daily an ounce of distilled vinegar."

A RAGING MADNESS. Keep the head close-shaved, and frequently wash it with vinegar. Or, apply to the head cloves dipped in cold water.

THE BITE OF A MAD DOG. "This disease can be cured even after the hydrophobia has begun by plunging into cold water daily for 20 days, and keeping there as long as possible."

On the subject of MEASLES, he says that this disease is "appreciated" by a violent cough fourteen days before the red spots come out. Remedy: Drink only thin water gruel or milk and water, the more the better. Or, toast and water.

NERVOUS DISORDERS. The one medicinal remedy he recommends is Valerian, which, if it is the wild Valerian, he says "has no bad smell." But if it does have a smell, cats have urined upon it, which they will do, he says, if they come upon it. (Author's note: This must have happened to all the Valerian with which he is familiar.)

NETTLE RASH. (Called in Georgia the PRICKLY HEAT.) Remedy is to rub the parts strongly with parsley.

OLD AGE. Remedy: Take tar water morning and evening. Or, decoction of nettles. Either of these will probably renew their strength for some years. Or, "chew cinnamon bark daily and swallow the spittle."

Wesley describes and names remedies for a number of other diseases including: Stubborn Pain in the Back, A Palsy of the Hands or Mouth, Piles, Pleurisy, Polypus in the Nose, Ptyalism (or Continual Spitting), A Purge, A Strong Purge, Quinsey, A Quinsey of the Breast, The Rheumatism, The Rickets, Ringworms, Running at the Nose, A Rupture in Children, A Windy Rupture, A Scald Head, The Sciatica, A Scorbutic Atrophy, Scorbutic Gums, Scurvy, Shingles, Morning Sickness, A Long-running Sore Leg, Sore Mouth, Sore Throat, Inflamed Sore Throat, A Sprain, A Venomous Sting, Bee Sting, Nettle Sting, Wasp Sting, Stomach Pain with Coldness and Wind, Kidney Stone, The Strangury, Sunburn, Passage of the Stone with Raging Fit, To Ease the Stone, Profuse Sweating, Night Sweats, Swelled Glands in Neck, To Fasten Teeth, To Clean the Teeth, To Cure the Toothache, Teeth Set on Edge, Thorns, Swelled Tonsils, Twisted Guts, Tympany, or Windy Dropsy, Vertigo, An Ulcer, Bleeding Varicose Ulcer in Leg, An Easy and Safe Vomit, Warts, Worms, Flat Worms, Wounds of All Kinds,

℞ SELF-DIAGNOSIS

Torpor, Vein or Sinew Cut, Inability to Sleep, Bite of Viper or of the Rattlesnake, Urine by Drops, Involuntary Urine, A Soft Wen.

THE MEDICINE CHEST BOOK
by Dr. George Harral

Dr. George Harral practiced at various times in Savannah and in Augusta, Georgia. In 1803 he advertised the 53rd edition of his book entitled, *The Guide to Health,* price $1.00. A few years later, he published another book entitled, *The Medicine Chest Book*, which was advertised in the newspapers and by other means for sale to planters, to ship owners, or to other persons who found themselves out of contact with medical help.

Quoting from the Preface of Dr. Harral's *Medicine Chest Book:*

When the study of a science is rendered easy and intelligible, every person of sense and education can form an opinion on the subject of it. As health and the comforts of it are the greatest and best blessings of mankind, so, in sickness, medicine is a most necessary and essential requisite.

I hope, therefore, by committing to the care of such intelligent persons a few choice and efficacious medicines, with some instruments and necessaries comprised in a small compass, that such advantage and assistance will accrue; especially to those who have families, many domestics, or to captains of vessels who may not have any other assistance.

By such an assortment, I flatter myself that the frequent use of frivolous and ineffectual, as well as dangerous, medicines will be prevented, and expense avoided. This assortment will, I hope, be further satisfactory because no preparations are admitted but such as have long been approved. No nostrums nor family secrets, but such only as have stood the test, the inquiry, and have the approbation of learned and eminent men in the profession. The number in this collection is forty-three, exclusive of instruments and necessaries, which are eleven, and this book of directions.

Dr. Harral's address is given as follows: "George Harral, M. D. Sign of the Man and Mortar, Market Square, Savannah, Georgia." The book was printed in Savannah by Thomas G. Collier, in 1807.

In addition to this book, Dr. Harral was advertising his medicine chests, about which he stated the following: "The medicine chests are put up at various prices and on improved plans, from ten dollars, to one, two, and three hundred dollars and upwards. Each chest ought to contain the medicines here enumerated, but the price and size of the small ones will not admit of the whole being put up; therefore, a few of the instruments, and some of the medicines, will be unavoidably omitted." His list of medicines is given in the following pages, each carrying a number, so that in discussing the diseases for which they are to be used, Dr. Harral is able to suggest remedies by number.

The list of medicines includes:

1. Best Bark
2. Flake Manna
3. Glauber Salts
4. Magnesia
5. Sulphur
6. Laudanum
7. Spirit of Lavender
8. Spirit of Hartshorn
9. Goulard's Extract
10. Friar's Balsam
11. Paregoric
12. Antimonial Wine
13. Elixir of Vitriol
14. Salt of Wormwood
15. Dover's Powder
16. Cream of Tartar
17. Rhubarb
18. Ipecac
19. Jalap
20. White Vitriol
21. Nitre
22. Camphor
23. Oil of Peppermint
24. Tartar Emetic
25. Tincture of Rhubarb
26. Blue Vitriol
27. Turner's Cerate
28. Yellow Basilicon
29. Calomel
30. Court Plaister
31. Corrosive Sublimate
32. Drawing Plaister
33. Adhesive Plaister
34. Mercurial Ointment
35. Purging Pills
36. Powder for Injection
37. Senna
38. Sweet Spirit of Nitre
39. Castor Oil
40. Blistering Plaister
41. Balsamic Drops
42. Linseed
43. Opodeldoc

Note at bottom of this list: "By the above table, the eye will be immediately directed to any medicine wanted. As each medicine is numbered to correspond with the book of directions, as well as marked by name, the facility of getting at the history and use of the article is more readily come at."

The instruments and necessaries included in the medicine chest:

1. Lancet, to bleed or open a tumour, etc.
2. Bolus knife, a round pointed knife to mix or lift powders with, to spread plaisters, or make boluses, etc.
3. Syringe, with which we inject or throw fluids up the urethra, the vagina, or the ears.

℞ SELF-DIAGNOSIS 79

4. Glyster-bags and pipes, for giving glysters.
5. Glass pestle and mortar.
6. Scales and weights from one grain to 2 drachms.
7. Graduate measure, a glass graduated from ½ drachm to 2 ounces.
8. A skin for spreading plaisters, as blistering plaisters, etc. Any soft leather, such as an old glove, will answer in lieu of it.
9. Lint, to clean and dress sores, and to apply to wounds. It is the most soft, easy, and eligible for the purpose.
10. Tow may be used as lint, but is chiefly to make compresses of, to suck up superfluous matter, for cleaning the skin around sores; but a good sponge, soaked up in warm water, is preferable for this latter purpose.

He describes the medicines according to the number which appears on each of them in the chest:

1. Contains BARK (CINCHONA), a medicine much and deservedly approved of; particularly in all intermittent fevers and periodical pains. It may be taken in any fluid, or in any form, as pill, bolus, or electuary. In Agues, which are the chief as to distinctness, of all the intermittents, it is an unerring medicine. The doses in Ague should be large and often repeated; the stomach being the sole index as to quantity. You may begin to give it the moment the feverish fit is off, although sometime we are forced to give it in nervous or low fevers, attended with great weakness particularly, even while the fever exists. But it is not given to any certain or satisfactory advantage until the stomach and bowels are first well cleansed by emetics and purges.
2. FLAKE MANNA, which is an agreeable, mild purgative used mostly by delicate or pregnant women and children—dose from one to two ounces, and that repeated until it operates; however it is most generally quickened by salts or senna tea, etc.
3. GLAUBER SALTS, though a common, is yet a good and easy purgative. It is generally given with equal parts of Manna. And when so joined, they will make an effectual and speedy purge.
4. MAGNESIA is a mild and gently aperient medicine. It is very serviceable in heartburn, which always proceeds

from acidity or a weak state of the stomach. It is the best of all purgatives for infants and delicate frames.

5. SULPHUR also proves gently opening. It much promotes insensible perspiration, and is highly valued by some in the piles. However, its great use is in the cure of the Itch, in which it seldom or never fails. It is for this purpose made into an ointment of hog's lard or butter, and rubbed on the parts affected. The rubbing may be frequently repeated, and clean changes of linen or bedclothes should be indulged in while using it. Unless the case is a very bad one, a very few days will give a cure; however the friction with it is to be persisted in until it has the desired effect.

6. LAUDANUM is a solution of Opium, with aromatics, in spirits. In irritations, spasm, or pain, it will be found an excellent medicine. It cheers the spirits, procures sleep, and promotes perspiration and sweat. Opium enters into numberless medicinal preparations. But the best and most common liquid opiate is Laudanum. The dose of Laudanum is from 10 drops to 50 drops in any fluid. Although small doses is the mode of administering it; yet when great pain urges, it may be given in large quantities. It is given to greatest advantage in violent pains of the gout, gravel, rheumatism, sciatica, and in all pains or painful sores; after all violent accidents; after operations in surgery, and in cases of violent retchings, or pain in the stomach or bowels; in short, wherever pain, restlessness or anxiety exists, it is an excellent remedy. In hysterics it is given with great advantage. The only caution requisite it is to begin with small doses, and increase them as pain or restlessness urges. (Author's note—The abandon with which Opium was given is terrible to contemplate.)

7. SPIRITS OF LAVENDER. This is a grateful, reviving cordial, much and deservedly used in all kinds of languor, weakness of the nerves, and lowness of the spirits.

8. SPIRITS OF HARTSHORN (AMMONIA). This is a volatile alkali. It is serviceable in languors or faintings. It is very useful in lethargic, hysteric and hypochondriac complaints, and in "sizeness" of the blood, as it is a good attenuant.

℞ SELF-DIAGNOSIS

9. GOULARD'S EXTRACT. A solution of litharge (lead oxide) in vinegar, used only externally.
10. FRIAR'S BALSAM (TURLINGTON'S BALSAM) stands highly and deservedly recommended for cleansing and healing fresh wounds.
11. PAREGORIC ELIXIR, which he says is a strained solution of opium and camphor in rectified spirit. It is not so nauseous to some as laudanum.
12. ANTIMONIAL WINE possesses the virtues of antimony, and may be so given as to perform all that can be effected by any antimonial preparation.
13. ELIXIR OF VITRIOL (SULPHURIC ACID). A valuable medicine in weakness and relaxation of the stomach.
14. SALT OF WORMWOOD (POTASSIUM CARBONATE). An alkaline salt which, when saturated with fresh lime juice or vinegar, makes an excellent cooling medicine in fevers.
15. DOVER'S POWDER (a mixture of IPECAC AND OPIUM). He calls it a most powerful and efficacious sudorific.
16. CREAM OF TARTAR (POTASSIUM BITARTRATE) is cooling and antiseptic. It quenches the thirst and corrects the tendency to putrefaction.
17. RHUBARB. A gentle purgative, and in small doses an excellent astringent, and strengthens the tone of the stomach and bowels.
18. IPECAC. One of the mildest and safest emetics we are acquainted with.
19. JALAP. A strong and excellent purgative.
20. WHITE VITRIOL (ZINC SULPHATE). When dissolved in water in the proportion of a grain and a half to an ounce, it is an excellent wash in inflamed eyes or any inflamed membrane.
21. NITRE (POTASSIUM NITRATE). It is an excellent diuretic, and much used in gargles and in inflammation of the throat.
22. CAMPHOR is esteemed as a most efficacious diaphoretic and antispasmodic. It sometimes produces sleep when Opium fails.
23. OIL OF PEPPERMINT. Good in colics attended with coldness and wind.
24. TARTAR EMETIC. A preparation of Antimony, given to produce vomiting.

25. TINCTURE OF RHUBARB is an excellent aperient for children.
26. BLUE VITRIOL (COPPER SULPHATE) is used externally as an escharotic, or destroyer of proud flesh.
27. TURNER'S CERATE is an ointment for application to sores.
28. YELLOW BASILICON is an ointment for application to boils.
29. CALOMEL (MERCUROUS CHLORIDE). The virtues of calomel in a number of instances are extolled.
30. COURT PLAISTER (ICHTHYOCOLLA). A neat application for trifling cuts, or scratches about the face and hands.
31. CORROSIVE SUBLIMATE (BICHLORIDE OF MERCURY) is another mercurial preparation more powerful and more violent than Calomel, one grain of which, when dissolved in half an ounce of spirits, and with two ounces of water added, made an excellent wash in venereal sores.
32. DRAWING PLAISTER. To cover and keep warm, sores and hurts, as they stick firmer than ointments.
33. ADHESIVE PLAISTER. This is frequently used as it fits easy to the skin, and is most commonly used to hold on other dressings.
34. MERCURIAL OINTMENT (BLUE OINTMENT). To be used as a dressing for venereal sores after they are well washed with number 31.
35. PURGING PILLS. An excellent purgative. One or two at bed-time will be found in general to answer very well.
36. POWDERS FOR INJECTION. Used in the treatment of gonorrhea.
37. SENNA. A mild and effectual cathartic.
38. SWEET SPIRIT OF NITRE (ETHYL NITRITE). Quenches thirst, promotes urine, and expels flatulency.
39. CASTOR OIL. A very excellent medicine for obstructions in the bowel and for violent pains across the belly.
40. BLISTERING PLAISTER (CANTHARIDAL) is used for blistering in paralytic and rheumatic cases.
41. BALSAMIC DROPS. Used in seminal weakness or gleets.
42. LINSEED. A useful medicine in obstructions.
43. OPODELDOC. Of great use, for rheumatism.

Dr. Harral lists the disease and remedies, including the following:

BLOOD. *To Stop:* Apply pressure with fingers or compress dipped in number 10, or a solution of number 26.

BLOOD. *To Let:* "Tie a bandage a little above the elbow of the right arm. Press the vein you mean to open with the thumb of your left hand, and cut it obliquely with a lancet, betwixt the thumb and the bandage. Blood-letting is the first and most essential remedy in all accidents from external violence. Blood ought to be taken away in the beginning of fevers when there is a strong, quick, pulse, the eyes red and inflamed with great heat and thirst, but never when the fevers are in the decline; as they are often at this period degenerated into the nervous kind. Bleeding is proper after all falls, blows, bruises, or any violent hurt, received either externally or internally. Secondly, in asthmatic complaints. Thirdly, in coughs, if the pulse is quick, full, with an oppression in the breast, or difficulty in breathing. Fourthly, in colics, if the pain is violent, the bowels inflamed, and no stools easily procured. See number 39. Fifthly, in fits, if the spirits are hurried and overpowered, and the patient full of blood. Sixthly, in swimming, dizziness, and pains of the head. Seventhly, in stitches, and pleuritic disorders of the side and breast, particularly if it gives pain to respire freely. Eighthly, in sore throats, when there is a strong, quick, pulse, and the throat greatly swelled and inflamed."

"The quantity of blood to be drawn must always be regulated by the strength, age, constitution, manner of living, and any other circumstance relating to the patient. The common quantity is from one-half pint to a pint."

(Author's Note: What a pity there were no blood banks then! Could all of the blood that was let for therapeutic purposes have been preserved through the years, it is intriguing to speculate that the blood of some forebear of generations back might now serve as a transfusion and be circulating in our system. The blood of some of the notables of that era would probably be in demand *and at premium prices.*)

BLOOD. To thin; take number 8.
BLOOD. Spitting of it. Use number 13.
BOIL. To poultice, number 28 or 27.
BROKEN BONES. He gives directions for setting a leg or arm or thigh.

BRAIN. Brain injuries, he says, are too hard to handle except for professionally-skilled men.

BRUISES. Use number 9 and number 43.

CARBUNCLE. Use number 36.

AGUE. Number 1 and 14.

ANODYNE. As an allayer of pain, use number 6, 11, or 22.

ANTISPASMODIC. That is, against cramps, stitches, or sudden and violent pains, use number 6, 8, 11, and 22.

APOPLEXY. To bleed largely, evacuate, and blister. Number 12, 20, and 40.

APPETITE. To create it, see number 1 and 13. If occasioned by foul stomach, take an emetic.

ASTHMA. During the fit, bleed and open the body with gentle physic, and see number 11.

BARK. See number 1.

BILE. Puke when it is redundant, and purge with jalap.

CHILBLAINS. Poultice if in much pain, and dress with number 27.

CHOLIC. Empty the bowels and stomach, and see number 18 and 24, for emetics. And see number 3, 17, 19, and 39 for cathartics. When the bowels are cleansed, see number 6 for relieving the pain.

COLDS. Procure perspiration, clothe well, keep quiet, live low, and empty the bowels, and bleed, if uneasiness or pressure is violent. See number 11.

COMPRESS. A bit of rag, lint, tow, or flannel, folded up in the form of a square pad. It is used with a cut vein, for stopping the blood after bleeding.

CONSUMPTION. Live on milk and vegetable diet. Bleed often, but in small quantities. Get into a warm climate, and use generous exercise. Get rest by number 6 or number 11.

CONVULSIONS IN CHILDREN. Generally arise from bad matter in the bowels. Let them be emptied with number 40 or number 17. Even give an emetic if requisite.

COUGH OR COLD. See the remedies for a cold. If caused from consumption, see that. If from asthma, see it. If nervous cough, see number 6 and number 11.

CUTS. Apply lint, drenched in number 10, and use compress, if needed.

DEBILITY. Use bracing medicines, such as Bark, Elixir of Vitriol, etc.

DIGESTION. To make it good, use Bark, Bitters, etc. Live on

℞ SELF-DIAGNOSIS 85

light foods, drink mineral or chalybeate waters, and take air and exercise.

DIURETIC. See number 21, 38, and 42.
DIZZINESS. See nervous drops. Number 7 and 8.
DROPSY. See number 16 and 19.
EMBROCATION. See number 43 and 22.
EMETIC. See number 12, 13, 20, and 24.
FAINTING. See number 7 and 8.
FEVER. See number 1, 14, and 29.
FITS. See 7 and 8.
FOMENTATION. See number 9.
FLUX. See number 17, 18, and 25.
GLYSTERS. See number 35.
GRAVEL. See number 6, 38, and 42.
GRIPING. Empty the bowels with number 17 or 39. Then use number 6, 11 or 25.
HEADACHE. If from the stomach, empty it. If from a nervous cause, see 7 and 8 and apply blisters.
HEARTBURN. To cure or alleviate, use 4 and 14.
HOARSENESS. See number 11.
HYSTERICS. Use 6, 7 or 8.
JAUNDICE. Use repeated emetics, with physic, and exercise on horseback.
INFLAMMATION OR SORE THROAT. See 15 and 38.
ITCH. See number 35.
MORTIFICATION. See number 1.
NERVOUS COMPLAINT. See 6, 7, and 8.
PAIN. To relieve, see 6, 22, and 11.
PILES. See 5 and 9.
PURGING. To stop, see number 6.
RHEUMATISM. See 15 and 43.
SCALDS AND BURNS. See number 9 and 27.
SORES. See number 1, 27, and 28.
STOMACH SICKNESS. If from bile, an emetic should be taken. See 21, 18, and 24.
STOMACH STRENGTHENERS. See number 1 and 13.
STRAINS OR SPRAINS. See number 43.
SWEAT. To procure, use warm drinks with 12, 15, and 38.
VOMITING. See number 14 and 6.
WATER. Suppression of, see 42.
WIND. To expel, see 23.
WORMS. To expel, see 29.

WOUNDS. For fresh wounds, cleanse them with warm water and sponge.

PLANTERS AND MARINERS MEDICAL COMPANION

Treating according to the most successful medical practice: first, the diseases common to warm climates and on shipboard; second, common practices in surgery, as fractures, dislocations, and so forth; and third, the complaints peculiar to women and children; to which are subjoined a dispensatory, showing how to prepare and administer family medicines, and a glossary giving an explanation of technical terms.

by Dr. James Ewell

After having read the preface in Tennent's, Wesley's, and Harral's books as quoted in this Chapter, it is not difficult to recognize in James Ewell's work a writer of more and better medical education, and also some progress in the knowledge of disease and of medicinal agents which has come about during the period from 1734 to 1807.

All four of these books—Tennent, Wesley, Harral, and Ewell —and a number of similar works which followed, however, were conceived and written in the hope that those who were out of contact with professionally-trained people might be instructed how to recognize disease conditions and apply the then-known-and-thought-to-be-best remedial agents.

That the life span of many was increased, and the lives of many saved, as a result of the instruction thus put into the hands of the layman cannot be questioned. The danger, however, lay in the fact that self-diagnosis and self-treatment, once established, would prove definitely fixed in the minds of many of our people, and can be eradicated only by the long, slow, tortuous process of education.

We cannot deny—and we must not forget—that instruction in the matter of diagnosis and of the use of drugs served a useful purpose during those years when medical and pharmaceutical services were not available to the people of the Colony and of the State in its early days.

To His Excellency, Thomas Jefferson, President of the United States.

I beg leave to present this book to Mr. Jefferson, not because he is the President, in 1807, but because he was the patriot of 1776; and, still more, because through the whole of a long and glorious life, he has been philosopher and friend of his country; with all the ingenuity of the former, exposing the misrepresentations of liberal foreigners; and with all the ardor of the latter, fanning the fire of American science, and watering the roots of that sacred olive, which sheds her peaceful blessings over our land.

To whom then, with equal propriety, could I dedicate a book, designed at least to promote health and longevity? And to whom am I so bound by the tenderest ties of affection and gratitude, as to Mr. Jefferson? The early classmate and constant friend of my deceased father, and instrumentally the author of my first acquaintance with the first characters of the State of Georgia, among whom, with peculiar pleasure, I would mention the honored names of Milledge, Troup, Bulloch, and Flournoy.

That you may long direct the counsels of an united and wise people, steadily pursuing health, peace and competence, the main pillars of individual and national happiness, is the fervent prayer of your Excellency's most obliged, and very grateful servant.

James Ewell

Preface

On the important subject of domestic medicine, many books have been written, which, though excellent in other respects, have greatly failed of usefulness to Americans, because they treat of diseases which, existing in very foreign climates and constitutions, must widely differ from ours.

The book now offered to the public has, therefore, the great advantage of having been written by a native American, with a long successful practice in these Southern states, and who for years past has turned much of his attention to the composition of it.

The professed object of his book is to treat in the most clear and concise manner of most every disease to which the human body is subject—to give their common names and surest symptoms—to point out the causes whence they originate with the most approved method of treatment—and lastly to prescribe a suitable means of prevention.

A publication like this cannot but be of exceeding use to all, and especially to those who live in the country, or who go to the sea, where regular and timely assistance cannot be always obtained.

Among the many and great services which may be rendered by such a book, we may fairly state is its tendency to prevent that dangerous officiousness of ignorant persons, as also that equally pernicious neglect of the patient at the onset of the disease, whereby so many lives are lost. These, with many other evils resulting from the want of such a work, constituted the motives which first led the author to the publication of this work to his countrymen. It is not for him to determine whether it be happily executed or not. But whatever may be the general opinion as to its merit, he has the high satisfaction to know that it not only flows from the purest motives, but also contains a faithful relation of facts, founded principally from his own experience, and what is not his own has been selected from authors of the greatest celebrity.

As to language, he has not, he confesses, been over-studious of ornament. Having made it his prime object to convey instruction, he has employed the style which, for him has made it the most intelligible; so that in all cases of disease, the patient might be directed in the plainest manner possible to the appropriate remedies.

The reader will find in the latter part of the work a table of such medicines as are almost constantly called for in families, with an adaptation of the doses according to the age of the patient; together with directions how to prepare and administer them.

To have those articles always in readiness, would not only save a great deal of time and expense of sending on every trivial occasion to a distant physician, but must also afford to attend the parent, or master, an infinite satisfaction, because of the very great advantage it gives him over a disease which he can meet with a suitable remedy at the first moment of its first attack. For there can be no doubt that thousands have perished, not because there were no remedies, but because these remedies were at such a distance, that the patient was lost before they could be brought to him.

On the whole, the author flatters himself that the "Planters and Mariners Medical Companion" will prove highly useful to his fellow citizens, and under this pleasing impression, he submits it to their perusal and patronage.

Preliminary Observations. Contemplating the numberless diseases to which man is liable, and which may cause him to drag out a protracted life of distress, or to suddenly cut him off in the bloom of his existence, and amidst his usefulness, we must adore that divine excellence which has, in medicine, given us the means of counteracting those dreadful evils, which otherwise would have severely molested our temporal condition.

Some observations which Dr. Ewell makes at this point are the following:
1. The value and necessity of medicine.
2. He reports continued progress in medical science.
3. He sets up Hippocrates, Sydenham, Jones (of Savannah), Rush, Craik of Alexandria; Weems of Georgetown; Stevenson of Baltimore, and Chapman of Philadelphia, as approaching the ideal in medicine.
4. He encourages laymen to seek a greater knowledge of health.
5. Of all the sciences, medicine is the most inviting and that which opens the largest treasures.
6. He criticizes empiricism and the empiric practitioners, and the use of nostrums by physicians as well as by the laity.
7. Medicine should be adapted to the nature of the disease, the age and condition of the patient.

℞ SELF-DIAGNOSIS 89

8. He lauds the lancet, but says: "It is mischievous when wrongly applied."
9. He glorifies opium, but cautions against its imprudent use.
10. He urges the use of the bath in its different forms for treatment of headaches and other conditions.
11. He urges cleanliness of person and surroundings, particularly applying to children and slaves.
12. He gives a dissertation on diet.

Dr. Ewell states: "Medicine is the digest of human knowledge. It is the greatest reservoir into which every stream of science pours a tribute, which in return spreads its fertilizing water over every field that brings forth its ripe and abundant harvest."

In discussing FEVERS, Dr. Ewell divides them into several groups: Ague or Intermittent, the Remittent or Bilious Fever, the Summer and Autumnal Fever, and Nervous Fevers.

Remedies: INTERMITTENT or AGUE, whether quotidian or tertian or quartan: Give an emetic, or a dose of calomel and jalap, followed later by the Bark (Peruvian Bark). "It must afford much pleasure to the benevolent to learn that the black oak bark of America possesses the same virtues as the Peruvian Bark, as has been verified by repeated experiments, not only in the cure of intermittents, but other diseases hitherto treated by the Peruvian Bark. When the black oak bark is not available the red oak bark could be substituted. And, when that is not available, dogwood bark is recommended by Professor Barton. Also, the columbo root."

Remedies for the remittent or bilious fevers: *Bleeding*, cathartics, emetics, and diluents.

The "Nervous" Fever, he says, has been described by various authors under different names; such as the "slow fever," the "gaol" fever, the hospital fever, the "petechial" fever, the putrid fever, and the malignant fever. Remedy: On the first appearance of the symptoms, give 5 or 6 grains of the tartar emetic. Use glysters or laxatives such as rhubarb or cream of tartar.

PHRENSY OR INFLAMMATION OF THE BRAIN. Treatment: *Blood-letting* is "the anchor of hope in this disease." This should be repeated as the symptoms and the strength of the patient will permit. The bowels must be kept open by cooling cathartics or glysters.

THE COLD. At times epidemic, when it is known by the name Influenza. Remedy: Antiphlogistic or cooling remedies are recommended; bathe the feet and legs before going to bed, in lukewarm water, and drink freely of diluted liquors, as flax-seed, balm, or ground-ivy teas. In violent cases, blood-letting in a larger or smaller quantity should be employed. The steam of hot water, or vinegar and water, should be inhaled.

QUINSY OR INFLAMMATORY SORE THROAT. Remedies: *Bleeding,* purging and other cooling means.

PUTRID SORE THROAT. He says: "This is a contagious disease, and appears more generally in autumn after a hot summer. It often attacks children and persons of relaxed habits than those of vigorous health." (This disease might have been diphtheria). The treatment: Give the bark; gargles should be employed if the disease is mild (common or astringent gargles), but if more severe, the detergent gargle.

MUMPS. A contagious disease affecting the glands and muscles of the neck, externally. Treatment: Keep the head and neck warm with spare diet, and a laxative state of the bowels. In case of a high fever, *bleeding* and blistering behind the neck may be necessary.

SORE EYES. Remedy: When the disease is moderate, cure is perfectly easy, requiring little more than external applications such as washing the eyes frequently with warm milk and water, mixed with a little brandy. Or, use a lotion like simple rose water, or about 8 grains of white vitriol (zinc sulphate) dissolved in a gill of spring water. In severe cases, *bleeding,* blistering behind the ears or the nape of the neck, with purgatives, and the cooling regimen.

PLEURISY. Bleeding, blistering, keeping the bowel open, are the suggested remedies.

PERIPNEUMONY, or the Inflammation of the Lungs. Antiphlogistic means are used, and the *taking of considerable blood from the arm.*

INFLAMMATION OF THE LIVER. Treatment: The same means to take off inflammation as advised in the Pleurisy should be carefully observed. In the chronic the stimulant purgative pills, which contain mercury, must be applied.

INFLAMMATION OF THE STOMACH. Treatment: *Copious bleeding* is almost the only remedy to be depended on.

INFLAMMATION OF THE INTESTINES. Treatment: Fresh olive oil in the dose of a tablespoonful is perhaps the only medicine that can be admitted with certainty.

INFLAMMATION OF THE KIDNEYS. Treatment: Bleed copiously. Keep the bowels open with castor oil, and emollient glysters. Use the warm bath, or foment the part with a hot decoction of chamomile, or bitter herbs, or hot water alone; give mucilaginous and diluting liquors, as flax-seed tea, etc. with the camphorated powders, or small portions of nitre.

INFLAMMATION OF THE BLADDER. Treatment: As in the treatment of Inflammation of the Kidneys. The patient should drink no more than is absolutely necessary.

HEADACHE. Treatment: Give an emetic, after which take Columbo three times a day. Or, in certain conditions, *bleeding may be necessary,* and purgatives.

EARACHE. Frequently produced from living insects getting into the ear. To get rid of them, blow in the smoke of tobacco, or pour in warm sweet oil. Or, inject warm milk and water into the ear. Or, drop in a little laudanum or volatile liniment.

TOOTHACHE. Is best removed by extracting the tooth. To prevent, or to preserve the teeth perfectly sound and the breath sweet, dip the toothbrush in warm water, and then in charcoal powder; should be used constantly every morning. The charcoal powder, an invention of the celebrated Darwin, is good at whitening the teeth and at correcting bad breath. The toothpick and tumbler of pure water should never be forgotten after every meal. Dr. Ewell states that "young people who wish to carry fine teeth with them through life must take care never to sip their tea scalding hot, nor to drink water freezing cold."

INFLAMMATORY RHEUMATISM. In the inflammatory rheumatism, *large and repeated bleedings are necessary,* as indicated by the fullness of the pulse, to be followed by a free use of diluent drinks, such as flax-seed or balm tea, or rice-water, with a little nitre dissolved in each draught. Or, the antimonial mixture in small doses. He states that "in some cases of the most obstinate Rheumatism, I have witnessed the happiest effects of taking for some time a teaspoonful of flowers of sulphur, night and morning." "In others again, I have found nothing equal to the pokeberry bounce (wine), in doses of a wine-glass full morning, noon, and night." He believes cold bathing and the use of flannel next to the skin are the most effectual means of preventing the recurrence of both acute and chronic Rheumatism.

THE VACCINE DISEASE, OR COWPOX. He extols the virtues of vaccination for the prevention of smallpox. But he includes a statement on the subject of smallpox and its treatment, and prevention.

MEASLES. "This disease attacks persons only once in life." Treatment: Keep the bowels open with a cathartic mixture or castor oil. Or, in case of high fever with measles, *bleed,* blister the breast, and inhale through the spout of a teapot the steam of hot water.

ST. ANTHONY'S FIRE. Remedy: Keep the bowel open with small doses of cream of tartar and sulphur. Or, in case of a violent attack, *bleed,* bathe the feet in warm water. Apply sinapisms (mustard plasters) to the extremities.

BLEEDING-AT-THE-NOSE. Remedy: Give cold, acidulated drinks, and apply cloths dipped in vinegar and water, to the face and the back of the neck. A piece of metal, as a key, for example, applied cold to the naked back, is a familiar remedy, and often succeeds.

CONSUMPTION. Various suggestions are made, none of which would be accepted at the present time as being of any value. Though Dr. Rush suggests (given here by Dr. Ewell) that he has often succeeded by giving small doses of calomel until a slight salivation is excited.

INCONTINENCE. A blister applied to the os sacrum, or lowermost part of the backbone, will be found highly beneficial, and often effects a cure.

SUPPRESSION AND DIFFICULTY OF URINE. Treatment: *Bleed* and administer emollient glysters and cooling laxatives, such as castor oil.

PILES. Remedy: Bleed, and live abstemiously. Keep the body gently open with molasses and water, or equal parts of flowers of sulphur and cream of tartar.

DYSENTERY OR BLOODY FLUX. Evacuate the bowl by calomel, castor oil, or a cathartic mixture; *blood letting* will also be required.

APOPLECTIC FITS. "He is to be *bled most copiously* to the amount of a quart or more, and this is to be repeated after a short time until relieved."

EPILEPTIC FITS. "The patient should be placed on a bed; the clothing should be everywhere loosened, and the head moderately elevated. A slip of wood should be placed between the jaws to prevent their closing on the tongue."

FAINTING FITS. "The patient should be placed in a reclining posture, and every part of the clothing which, by its tightness, is likely to interrupt the free circulation of blood must be immediately loosened." Plenty of fresh air is given the patient. "Sprinkle the face with cold water often, or vinegar, and apply volatiles, or burnt linen, or burnt feathers to the nostrils."

THE PALSY. Treatment: A tablespoonful of horseradish, scraped, or the same quantity of mustard seed swallowed three or four times a day will have a good effect. The volatile alkali is also of infinite service in large doses (volatile alkali being ammonia).

A CRAMP. "A painful spasm of the calf of the leg or muscles of the toes, and sometimes of the stomach." Treatment: Stand up and throw the weight of the body on the toes. If it is a cramp of the stomach, treat it by a large dose of ether or laudanum, accompanied with friction on the part, he says.

LOCKED JAW. Remedy: Give on the first appearance of this disease two or three teaspoons of laudanum, or three or four grains of opium. If these should fail to relieve the spasm, give from 20 to 30 drops of the tincture of Cantharides every hour until it produces strangury, or difficulty of urine. "Cold water poured copiously on the shoulders has sometimes done admirable service."

PALPITATION OF THE HEART. "If the heart action is violent, *bleeding* is indispensable, which should be followed by a cooling cathartic."

HICCUP. Remedy: If the hiccup is due to acidity, give 20 drops of hartshorn, with a teaspoonful of magnesia in a cup of mint tea. Or, a spoonful or two of milk and lime water. To prevent, take 10 grains of the rust of steel twice or thrice a day. If occasioned by poisons or improper foods, an emetic will be proper.

NIGHTMARE. If the patient be of a plethoric habit, bleed, purge, and use a spare diet.

ASTHMA, he says, is often hereditary, and when attended with an expectoration of phlegm, it is termed "moist" or "humoural," and when with little or none, it is called "dry" or "nervous" asthma. Treatment: On the first attack of asthma, *bleeding* is serviceable. Or, an emetic will be found serviceable if the asthma comes from a loaded stomach. Or, a cup of strong coffee has oftentimes afforded great relief. Or, when the disease proceeds from the irritation of mucous, a spoonful or two of vinegar in a glass of cold water is a good remedy.

HEARTBURN. Treatment: May be relieved by taking a teaspoonful of salt of tartar; or a tablespoonful of magnesia; or a wine-glass full of lime water and new milk; or a tumbler of mucilage of gum arabic; or flax-seed tea taken cold. But to cure the disease effectually, after an emetic give 10 grains of the rust of steel twice a day for some time, and keep the bowels moderately open with magnesia or the root of rhubarb chewed occasionally, or the tincture of it taken in small doses.

INDIGESTION OR WEAKNESS OF THE STOMACH. Treatment: If the patient complains of oppressed stomach with nausea, give a vomit with ipecac, and afterwards the Columbo.

THE COLIC. A violent pain in the bowels originating from constriction, attended by costiveness, and sometimes by vomiting. Treatment: If the symptoms are due to wind or gas on the bowels, give hot drinks of ginger. But if the pain is acute, bleeding is advisable. Then, give purgatives, such as castor oil, calomel, and jalap; or salts, senna, and manna, aided by stimulating glysters. (In the present era, all of these items would be barred from use due to the possibility of appendicitis existing).

CHOLERA MORBUS, OR VOMITING AND PURGING. Treatment: Endeavour as early as possible to expel the acrimonious matter which affects the alimentary canal by large and repeated draughts of chicken water, beef tea, barley or rice water, or thin gruel. After cleansing the stomach and intestines, give a teaspoonful of ether or 30 or 40 drops of laudanum in mint water or tea. Repeat this dose every hour or oftener, as the frequency of the evacuations or the urgency of the pain may require.

DIARRHOEA, or looseness. A purging, without sickness or pain, caused by acid or putrid aliment, obstructed perspiration, acrid bile, drinking bad water, worms, violent passions, or a translation of morbid matter of other diseases to the bowels. *Remedy:* Give an emetic and an opiate at bedtime, and again on the succeeding day.

DROPSY. Treatment: Like other diseases, the treatment must vary according to circumstances. If the pulse is hard, full and quick, blood-letting constitutes one of the principal remedies, and must be repeated once or twice a week until the action of the arterial system is considerably diminished. Brisk purges, as calomel and jalap in four doses; cream of tartar, half an ounce to an ounce, dissolved in a pint or more of water; and any other similar laxative.

GOUT. Treatment: "No matter what part of the body that disease first seizes, the lancet (that is, *blood letting*) will be required in every case where there is an increased action of the pulse."

Remedy: Nitre with diluting liquors, given in such quantities as to excite a gentle perspiration. Any person who is subject to gout should keep always a vial of ether or laudanum, or a case of good old French brandy, he says, the latter of which "is admirable for chasing the gout from the stomach." He says that General Wayne was cut off long before his eye was dim or his natural heat abated because of the lack of good French brandy at the proper time.

Dr. Ewell gives a long series of treatments for Veneral Diseases, none of which would be useful in the present era. Therefore no mention will be made here in this brief study of his treatments.

Dr. Ewell does make one statement in regard to "The Pox." He says: "Happily for mankind the Governor of the world is 'a father who pitieth his children,' and afflicts them not to kill but to cure. In mercy He has appointed *a medicine* for this dreadful malady." This medicine to which he refers is mercury.

SCURVY. Causes: Cold, moist air; vitiated or scanty diet, an indolent life with luxurious indulgences. Treatment: Raw and fresh vegetables of every description, particularly those of the acid kind, such as fruits like limes, lemons, apples, etc., this being the most effectual remedy.

ITCH. Remedy: Sulphur used internally and externally is considered as the certain specific.

TETTER OR RINGWORM. A saturated solution of borax with lemon juice is an excellent remedy without producing the least pain on its application. Local. One dram to two ounces.

JAUNDICE. Treatment: Remove the obstructions of the bowels, as it originates from different causes. Remedy: *Bleed,* then give an emetic; then a day after, a dose of calomel and jalap. Or, if it be a chronic condition of jaundice, give night and morning a pill of mercury.

INTOXICATION. Remedy (but not to prevent): Emetics and cold applications.

TO RECOVER PERSONS APPARENTLY DROWNED OR KILLED BY LIGHTNING OR NOXIOUS VAPORS. Also, he gives a treatment for persons poisoned, bitten by mosquitoes, or by "venomous animals," or by mad dogs.

He discusses the Guinea worm. He says: "This disease is frequent among the Negroe, and is pretty uniform in appearance. It is a condition that affects the skin, apparently." He gives remedies for chilblains, scalds and burns, hernia, prolapsus ani, warts and corns, whitlow, tumors or boils, scirrhus or cancer, common ulcers, wounds, sprains and bruises, dislocations, injuries to the head, fractures of the limbs.

He gives an intimate, detailed discussion of blood-letting, so that the layman could perform this operation without too much danger.

Dr. Ewell also discusses pregnancy and gives practical advice and warnings on this subject. And, in the same style and language he discusses "progress of labor" and "management of childbed" and management of infants, diseases of infants, including worms, convulsive fits, teething, watery head, croup, hives, whooping cough, rickets, and fevers.

CHAPTER V

WITH THE APPEARANCE OF NEWSPAPERS IN GEORGIA IN 1763, THE VALUE OF ADVERTISING IS DISCOVERED AND IS PROMPTLY ADOPTED BY THOSE HAVING MEDICINAL PRODUCTS OR MEDICAL SERVICES TO OFFER THE PUBLIC, (1763-1820)

FOLLOWING the period when self-diagnosis and self-treatment were aided, abetted, encouraged and taught by apothecaries, physicians and surgeons, the newspapers, books on the subject, or word of mouth, these same agencies, or most of them, were to go still further away from what we now (1959) recognize as ethical principles and practices. They proceeded to advertise to deliver professional services and products, both of which, judged by modern standards, would be considered as lacking in quality, be it service or product.

Prior to, during, and in the post-Revolutionary War period, the population of Georgia ranged between 53,000 in 1773 and 162,000 in 1800. It was during this period that there were estimated to have been less than 200 physicians, apothecaries, or drug dealers in the State, even at its highest peak of population.

Since there was no legal standard of measurement to determine who was to be entitled to be called "physician", or "apothecary", many came into the practice of one or both of these professions by adoption, by necessity of conditions in the community, or through the preceptorship-apprentice system.

Various writers have estimated that fully 90% of those who were practicing medicine in Georgia prior to 1825 were nongraduates of a medical college, and that the 10% who may have been graduated from some medical college were probably no better trained, and conceivably not so well trained, as many of those who came through the preceptorship system. The medical college curriculum extended over two terms of four months each, whereas apprenticeship may have extended over a much longer period of time, with instruction under apprenticeship on a more intensive and thorough basis when under a competent and conscientious preceptor.

Considering these conditions in addition to those created by the encouragement of self-diagnosis and treatment, it is not difficult to understand how the practices outlined in the advertisements and contributions from newspapers (1763-1820) as cited here could exist.

The reader of these advertisements and published notices will question perhaps the integrity or knowledge on the part of the advertisers in the freedom with which claims are made as to "cures" for various diseases. It appears that unless a medicinal product were advertised as a "cure" it would not justify the investment in advertising.

The reader will have noted from the books by Tennent, Wesley, Harral, Ewell, et al, and lists of "medicine chest" items, the reckless abandon with which Opium or the preparations which contained it was made available to the public along with encouragement in its indiscriminate use. Some of the more popular and better known of these ready-for-use products included the following: Opium itself in the form of Gum Opium; Laudanum; Paregoric; Bateman's Drops; Godfrey's Cordial; Black Drop (Vinegar of Opium); Sydenham's Laudanum (Wine of Opium); Daffy's Elixir; Dalby's Carminative; Squire's Elixir; Venice Treacle; and in some of the older formulas for the following: British Oil; Harlem Oil; Elixir of Vitriol; Turlington's Balsam, or Friar's Balsam.

This reckless and indiscriminate use of opium and its derivative products was to continue not only in Georgia but in the United States until the passage of the Harrison Anti-Narcotic Law in 1914. Here in Georgia, however, the pharmacists of the State, recognizing the dangers inherent in the situation, passed a State Law in 1907 confining the distribution of opium and its products to prescriptions written by licensed physicians. (The reference to opium here is intentionally a repetition to impress the fact that, but for timely legislation, America might have become a nation of narcotic addicts.) It is well known that up to the time of this restrictive legislation, many of the advertised medicinal products contained opium or one of its derivative pro-

℞ ADVERTISEMENTS

ducts as the chief, *and sometimes the only,* medicinal agent of value.

Mysticism has, from the beginning of time, been associated with drugs and the practice of medicine and pharmacy. Gullibility as to the claims made for medicinal agents is not confined to lay people, but may also apply to some practitioners of medicine and pharmacy. The advertisers of a medicinal product prepared under a secret formula constituted, and constitutes, a fertile field in which to appeal to the mind which is receptive and responsive to mysticism.

Since there was no educational deterrent, no ethics to be infringed, nor legal restrictions to be observed, the sky was the limit when claims for efficacy were to be made. The newspapers of the period 1763-1820, responsive then as now to the practices of the times, made their contribution to the current popular practice of self-medication and passed on to the public information which may or may not have come from any professional source.

The advertisements and newspaper items which appear here are arranged in three groupings, each of these also appearing generally in chronological order. One group depicts typical newspaper "cures" offered to the readers; a second shows several of the early dental advertisements by the dentists themselves; and a third grouping represents many of the physicians' and druggists' own advertisements placed as insertions in early Georgia newspaper columns.

These advertisements and newspaper items represent a period in the life of drugs, medicine, and pharmacy in Georgia, and thus are judged to be of sufficient interest to warrant a place in the present volume.

THE NEWSPAPERS OF THE PERIOD MAKE A CONTRIBUTION TO THE CONFUSION REGARDING THE EFFICACY OF DRUGS WHEN THEY RECOMMEND CERTAIN PRODUCTS OR PRACTICES AS "CURES."

Witness No. 1: *The Georgia Gazette,* Savannah, Georgia, June, 1768.

CURE FOR THE CRAMPS

To these afflicted with the cramps, the following will be found a very easy

Author's Note: Other newspaper "cures" named for Cancer, Asthma, Hydrophobia, Colds, Ague, Sore Throat, Epilepsy, are not thought wise to be published.

and immediate remedy. Extend or rather turn back, as much as possible, the fingers or the toes, of the limb affected. This may be easily done, when it may not be in one's power to move the whole limb. I have ever found it to give immediate relief; and it is much more effectual than friction, which may not at any time be easily performed.

Witness No. 2: *Augusta Herald,* Augusta, Georgia, November 11, 1801.

A Certain Cure for Corns

Take two ivy leaves, put them into vinegar for 24 hours, apply one of them to the corn, and when you find its virtue extracted apply the other, and it will effectually and speedily remove the corn without the least pain.

Witness No. 3: *The Augusta Chronicle and Gazette of the State,* September 14, 1805.

Cure for Consumptions

By a temperate mode of living (avoiding spirituous liquors wholly) by wearing a flannel next the skin; and taking every morning half a pint of new milk, mixed with a wine-glass full of the expressed juice of green hoar-hound, the complaint will not only be relieved, but the individual shall procure to himself a length of days beyond what its mildest form could give room to hope for, I am myself, a living witness of the beneficial effects of this agreeable, and, though innocent, yet powerful application. Four weeks use of the hoar-hound and milk relieved the pains of my breast; gave me power to breath deep, long and free; strengthened and harmonized my voice; and restored me to a state of better health than I had enjoyed for many years.

Witness No. 4: *Augusta Herald,* Augusta, Georgia, April 3, 1806.

Infallible Cure for the "Hooping" Cough

Dissolve a scruple of Salt of Tartar in a gill of water: add ten grains of Cochineal finely powdered: sweeten this with fine sugar. Give to an infant the fourth part of a tablespoon four times a day; and from 4, upward, a spoonful may be taken. The relief is immediate, and the cure in general effected within 5 or 6 days.

Witness No. 5: *Augusta Herald,* Augusta, Georgia, July 24, 1806.

Cure for the Dropsy

To the Editor of the London Sun.
Sir, in your paper a few weeks since, I observed that Bohea Tea, and the

℞ ADVERTISEMENTS 101

leaves to be eaten, were recommended as a cure for the above fatal disorder; and as I had a pauper in the house at that time, who was given over by the visiting surgeon, I ventured the experiment, and to my astonishment found an almost instant relief. I repeated the dose but once, and the woman in the course of a week, was able to go out to hay making and will begin reaping for me Monday next, if the weather continues fine. The woman's name is Elizabeth Austin, her age forty-two.
I am, sir, yours, etc.
T. H. Shrimton, Gov.
House of Industry

Witness No. 6: *Columbian Sentinel,* Augusta, Ga., Sept. 6, 1806, Vol. 4, No. 163. From the London Magazine.

A Cure for the Rheumatic Pain and Deafness

Mr. Urban, So simple a thing as brown paper has, from my knowledge, been so beneficial in several instances, that I am induced to request your inserting this in your useful Magazine.
The Countess of S. for a long time has recommended it with success. A Mrs. R. of Oxford-street was cured of rheumatic pains in a few days by wearing a waistcoat of brown paper.

Witness No. 7: *Farmers Gazette,* Sparta, Ga., May 30, 1807.

The Gout

A new cure has been proposed for that disease in France; by an author of some celebrity, M. Cadet de Vaux. The remedy is to drink 48 glasses of warm water in 12 hours, a glass at the end of every quarter of an hour, taking nothing else during the time. This remedy is in pretty general use in France, and has had great success. It is supposed that the profuse perspiration which this process in general occasions is the cause of the cure.

Witness No. 8: *Georgia Express,* Athens, Ga., February 25, 1809.

Cure for the Croup

A disorder among children, commonly called the Croup, has of late been very prevalent among them:
We beg to name, for the information of the parents an effectual remedy. The daughter of J. Walker Esq. of Mile End, was severely attacked, and pronounced irrecoverable by the medical aid called in; her father thereupon immerged her up to her chin in water as hot as she could bear it, and kept her in that state for a quarter of an hour, till she nearly fainted, after which a small portion of rum and oil was given her; she was then wrapped in a blanket and put to bed—by which means she was perfectly restored. On the dissection of children dying of this disorder, a thick

glutinous matter has been found covering the lungs, which prevented due respiration. Liverpool paper.

Witness No. 9. *Columbian Sentinel,* Augusta, Ga., Nov. 25, 1809, Vol. 7, No. 331, P. 3.

WHOOPING COUGH

Dissolve a scruple, or twenty grains of Salt of Tartar in a quarter of a pint of water, add 10 grains of Cochineal, and sweeten this with loaf sugar. Give a child within a year, a teaspoonful 4 times a day; with a tablespoonful of barley water, or any other mucilaginous water.
A child two years old, two teaspoonful.
A child 4 years old, a tablespoonful.
Boiled apples put in warm milk may be the chief food. This has been applied in various instances with uninterrupted success.
Copy this in the front leaf of your day-book.

. . . Mentor.

Witness No. 10: *Georgia Journal,* Milledgeville, Ga., April 24, 1810.

A CURE FOR ULCERS

Mr. Richard Walker has published, in the Medical Journal, some observations which demonstrate the extraordinary effects of carrots, in the cure of sores and ulcers of every species, by correcting their morbid disposition. The method of preparing the roots is as follows: The carrots having been previously cleaned, by scraping and washing, are cut into thin, transverse slices, and boiled until they are quite tender; after which they are taken out of the water, beaten in a mortar, to the consistance of a soft pulp. This may either be applied in portions with the hand, and kept on with a cloth or roller, or it may be spread upon a cloth, and laid on like a common poultice. It is best when fresh prepared, and should be changed twice a day. This simple application corrects the fetor of ill conditioned sores, and reduces them to a perfectly healthy, or good conditioned state and thickness; and diminishes the discharge.

Witness No. 11: *The Augusta Chronicle,* Aug. 30, 1811.

RHEUMATISM

It is the "indispensible" duty of every mortal traveler to make the world happier, better, and wiser by every possible exertion. The subscriber has prevented several fits of Rheumatism by using violent exercise on the part affected, the instant pain was felt; he begins with easy blows with the end of the finger or knuckle and increases the forces to the number of 100, and in half an hour repeats the exercise; and if the pain returns he observes the same rules, and has never had occasion to repeat a third experiment. The body must be kept open, and the parts additionally clothed, thick shoes should be worn, and plenty of pepper used as preventatives. The Flesh brush does not go sufficiently deep. Provided you have neglected the above cautions, and the pain increases, put a handful of fat lightwood splinters into a quart of rum, and take a table spoonful in water three times a day until cured.—Shake the bottle.

. . . Mentor.

Witness No. 12: *Augusta Herald,* July 9, 1812.

RHEUMATISM

It is said to be a specific for the Rheumatism, to apply a Cabbage leaf to the part affected. Choose a perfect leaf cut off the protuberant stalk at the bark, and place it on the part with a bandage of flannel at going to bed. It will produce a local perspiration, and on two or three repetitions effect a cure.

(Note: Cato's favorite remedy as a panacea.)

Witness No. 13: *Augusta Herald,* Oct. 1, 1812, Vol. 14, No. 14.

A COMPLETE AND SIMPLE CURE FOR THE RHUMATISM

Take a pint of good Rum, and infuse in the same, a small quantity of the bark of the Prickly Ash,—and the person afflicted by taking a wine glass full of the same, every morning will soon get relief.

A person in whose possession the above Receipt had been for some time, having occasion lately to make trial of it found it effectually answered the end proposed. This simple preparation for the Rhumatism, was for several years sold at a high price, by the person from whom the Receipt was obtained, and who increased both his wealth and reputation by administering this alone in all Rhumatic cases, while he carefully concealed the composition from his patients.

Witness No. 14: *Augusta Herald,* March 21, 1816.

CURE FOR A FELON

(Taken from the Orange County Republican of November, 1806). The following was taken from the paper of Deacon I. C. Lumberland, and published at his expressed request. Take a piece of rock salt about the size of a butternut, wrap it in a cabbage leaf, if to be had, if not, in a piece of wet brown paper; cover it with coals, as you would to roast an onion; after it has been roasting about twenty minutes, take it from the fire, and powder it very fine; mix it with as much common soap as will make a salve; if the soap be not pretty strong of turpentine, (which may be known by the smell) then add a little more of it. Apply the salve to the part affected, in the course of a few hours, and sometimes in a few minutes the pain will be relieved. After this, if a suppuration has taken place, it must be healed like a common sore.

Witness No. 15: *Augusta Herald,* May 30, 1816.

Cure for Hydrophobia
Scullcap—Scutellaria Galerieulata

Description. This is a perennial Plant, and rises about two feet in height. Leaves are on a square stem, opposite each other, the same as Boneset, and spear-shaped toward the end; flowers blue, or rather of a violet color.

History. It grows about the borders of ponds, and on the banks of rivers, and flowers in August.

Medical virtues. It is a good astringent, and has been found an infallible cure for the bite of a mad dog, either in man or beast.

The following secret preparation I procured from a physician in New Jersey, who brought me the herb; and which I now communicate for the general good of my fellow creatures, that, in case of their meeting with such a misfortune they may know how to apply a remedy that has never failed, on one instance, when applied according to the following.

Preparation. Gather the leaves of the plant about the last of July; dry them carefully in the shade; and, after being pulverized, sift the powder through a hair sieve, and put it in bottles, well corked, for use. As soon as a person has been bit by a mad dog, he must take a gill, four times a day, every other day, of the tea, made by pouring a pint of boiling water on a tablespoonful of the dry herb or powder; and the day it is committed, he must take a tea spoonful of the flour of sulphur in the morning fasting and at bed-time, in new milk, and apply the pounded green herb to the wound every two hours, continuing the prescription for three weeks.

To cattle or horses, give four times the quantity prescribed for a man.

Dentists Begin to Advertise

No. 1: *Augusta Herald,* April 9, 1812, Augusta, Georgia, Vol. XIII, No. 41.

B. T. LONGBOTHAM, *Surgeon Dentist*

Informs the inhabitants of Augusta, and its vicinity, he is now in this city, and may be consulted in the line of his profession, at the House of Messrs. Calffrey & Bustin's in Reynolds Street; those desirous of his attendance at their own residence, will please to intimate the same to him personally or by message in writing, as his stay will be very limited. Persons purposing to employ him are requested to be immediate in their application. His Dentifrice can at all times be had by application at the Augusta Book Store.

Advertisement.

℞ ADVERTISEMENTS 105

No. 2: *Augusta Herald,* Dec. 15, 1818, Augusta, Georgia, Vol. XX, No. 48.

JAMES BATES, *Physician, Surgeon, Surgeon Dentist.*
Having extensively practiced in the several branches of his profession for six years (two of which were spent in the Military Hospitals of the United States), offers his services to the citizens of Augusta; and confidently hopes by constant and careful attention to business, so far to merit the patronage of a liberal public, as to induce him to make this the future residence of himself and family. Being informed there is no settled Scientific Dentist in this place, he assures the public that he will perform every operation on the Teeth, in a style equaling any thing of the kind in the United States; and unless perfect satisfaction is given, no pay will be received. Numerous references can be given to Gentlemen of the highest respectability in town and elsewhere. He will reside for the present at the Globe-Tavern.
— *December 11. Advertisement*

No. 3: *The Augusta Chronicle,* March 26, 1821, Augusta, Georgia, Vol. XXXV, No. 1987.

A. J. SHYMANSKI—*Dentist*
Respectfully informs the ladies and gentlemen of Augusta, and its vicinity, that he will remain in this place for a few weeks, during which time he will attend to the different branches of his profession.
He will INSERT TEETH, real or artificial, from one to the entire set. Also, he will EXTRACT, CLEAN, SEPARATE, PLUG, and REGULATE TEETH.
He will either attend at his Room, at the Globe Tavern, or wait on them at their respective Dwellings.
— *March 15. Advertisement*

No. 4: *The Augusta Chronicle,* May 9, 1822, Augusta, Georgia, Vol. 36, No. 60.

Three Weeks Longer,
   DR. C. S. BREWSTER, *Surgeon Dentist*
Will continue in Augusta this season, to assist those who require the assistance of a Dentist, to furnish new Teeth, or to assist in the preservation of the natural Teeth.
All advice given gratis, and Teeth not too far decayed, so loaded that they shall never decay or give pain.
Office in M'Intosh-Street. North of the Post-Office.
— *May 6. Advertisement*

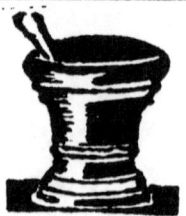

New Medicine Store.

THE Subscriber respectfully informs his Friends and the Public, that he has just received an additional supply of warranted Fresh and Genuine

Drugs, Medicines, &c.

Which with his former Stock on hand, renders his Assortment complete as any in the City. Planters and Families, that will favour him with their custom, may rest assured of being always supplied with MEDICINES of the very first quality, and at the most reduced prices.

Some few are the ARTICLES:

Crude Antimony,
White & Yellow Arsenic,
Double Aqua-Fortis,
Arnatto,
Quick-silver,
Alium,
Bole Armeniac,
Borax,
Camphor,
Calomel,
Cochineal,
Best red Bark, in quill,
Do. & common Manna,
Corrosive Sublimate,
Red and white Precipitate,
Best powder'd Jalap,
Do. Hippo,
Do. & Root Rhubarb,
Castor Oil,
Columbo Root,
Volatile & Crude Sal Ammoniac,
Best Glauber & R.
and powder,
Do. pale do.
Cream of Tartar,
Roll & root Liquorice,
Camomile Flowers,
Sulpher in roll & powder,
Best Sena,
Gum Ammoniac,
Arabic,
Alloes,
Benzoin,
Assafœtida,
Guaicum,
Myrrh,
Opium,
Scammony,
Tragacanth,
Best Magnesia in lumps and powder,
Salts,
Hartshorn,
Sweet spt. Nitre,
Tartar Emetic,
White Vitriol,
Blue & green do.
Glass of Antimony,
Green & white Vials, assorted,
Nipple Pipes & shells,
Smelling Bottles,
Essence Bergamot, Lavender and Lemon,
Prussian Blue, from No. 1 to 3,
Vermillion,
Rose Pink,
White Lead,
Gamboge and Indian Ink,

PATENT MEDICINES.

Anderson's Pills,
Bateman's Drops,
British Oil,
Daffy's Elixir,
Essence of Peppermint,
Godfrey's Cordial,
Hoopers Pills,
James Fever Powders,
Squire's Elixir,
Turlington's Balsam,
Harlem Oil,
Balsam of Honey,
Dalby's Carminative,
Stoughton's Bitters.

——— ALSO, ———

Neat MEDICINE CHESTS, with suitable directions for Shipping and Plantation uses.

N. B. Wanted an attentive Youth, as an Apprentice, whose morals will be strictly attended to, and every exertion made towards his speedy progress.

Sign of the Mortar & Pestle, next door to Messrs. J. & M. Clelan, Duke-street, Market-Square.

G. HARRAL.

September 22.   n.50.

Columbian Museum & Savannah Advertiser
Savannah, Georgia, September 22, 1797

JAMES CUTHBERT

Has imported in the Polly, Capt. Quince,
A FRESH ASSORTMENT of MEDICINES; also lancets, surgeons instruments, &c. &c. which he will sell reasonably. He will fit up boxes of medicines for plantation use, with directions.

The Georgia Gazette
Savannah, Georgia, December 29, 1763

ANDREW JOHNSTON

Has imported, in the Polly, Capt. Quince, from London,
A FRESH ASSORTMENT of MEDICINES.—He has also to sell, hyssop tea in lb. and qr. lb. canisters, prunes, currants, raisins, preserved citron, ginger, sweetmeats, white and brown sugar candy, Anderson's pills, small steel trusses, surgeons pocket instruments, middle sized and small brass and marble mortars, lawn sieves, &c. &c.

The Georgia Gazette
Savannah, Georgia, December 29, 1763

℞ ADVERTISEMENTS

ADVERTISEMENTS OF PROFESSIONAL MEDICAL SERVICES AND PRODUCTS

The Georgia Gazette, Savannah, Georgia, June 16, 1763.

The subscriber gives notice, that he hath opened shop in Mrs. Campbell's house near the church in Savannah, where he will practice physick and surgery; he will particularly cure the 'burstedness or rupture of the guts' and others. He hath to sell . . . Godfrey's cordial, Turlington's balsam, Bateman's drops, Squire's elixir, Daffy's elixir, Stoughton's bitters, plain & golden spirit of scurvy-grass, single & refin'd British oil.

HENRY LEWIS BURQUOIN

Georgia State Gazette or Independent Register, Augusta, Georgia, Saturday, September 8, 1787.

DR. BURKE

Takes this opportunity of informing the public, that he intends practicing in Augusta, and that he has lately brought in with him from Europe, a select assortment of fresh Medicines expects the efficacy of them will answer his wishes. His charges of assiduity shall not be complained of, as he wishes to render universal satisfaction. He may be seen at Mr. Fox's, where he has his medicine store.

N. B. Paper medium or produce will be taken in payment.
Advertisement.

Columbian Museum & Savannah Advertiser, Savannah, Georgia, Friday, Feb. 2, 1798.

THE SUBSCRIBER

Respectfully informs the Public, that he has commenced the practice of PHYSIC in Liberty County at Newport bridge and flatters himself with the pleasing expectation that he shall meet with the confidence of the people. Should he be so fortunate, he hopes from several years devoted to that science (through divine assistance) to have in his power to give relief to his fellow creatures, as nothing can afford more tranquillity to a sympathizing and benevolent mind. I am with esteem, the public's most obedient servant.

JESSE BOUCHELL

Advertisement

Just imported,

To be sold on the most reasonable terms, by

BUTTON GWINNETT,

At the store lately occupied by Messrs. Johnson and Wylly,

THE FOLLOWING GOODS, viz.

RHUBARB,—Turlington's balsam of life,—Dr. James's powders for fevers,—flake manna,—glauber salts,—Florence oil,—mustard,—tin ware,—ironmongery,—plain, silver, and gold laced hats,—breeches pieces,—silk and thread hose,—jewelery,—pickles,—cutlery,—saddlery,—earthen and delft ware,—mould candles,—fine beer,—glass,—shoes,—sheeting,—canvas,—oznaburgs,—Irish linens,—cheques,—paint,—cheese,—butter,—nails,—cyder,—Scots barley,—English manufactured tobacco,—vinegar,—bed furniture,—and many other articles too tedious to insert.

The Georgia Gazette
Savannah, Georgia, September 12, 1765

ANDREW JOHNSTON HAS TO SELL,

Orange-flower water, rose water, Rhenish wine, tamarinds, saltpetre, oil of turpentine, Fryar's balsam, smelling bottles, bougies, gold and silver leaf, a few surgeon's instruments and shop utensils, viz. cases of needles, small pewter syringes, steel-spring trusses for ruptures, splints for fractures, a large brass mortar and iron pestle, large and small scales and weights, &c. Likewise a small assortment of fresh garden seeds, and a few pots of sweetmeats and bottles of pickles. All which, with most kinds of medicines, and family medicines, he will dispose of on reasonable terms.

The Georgia Gazette
Savannah, Georgia, November 3, 1763

Doctor DYSART,

Respectfully informs the public, that he has just received from Philadelphia and Charleston,

A SUPPLY OF Fresh DRUGS,

Which will be sold on a very small advance, for cash, tobacco or ginned cotton.—Handsome horses will be taken in payment.

February 2, 1796.

The Augusta Chronicle and Gazette of the State
Augusta, Georgia, February 4, 1797

DOCTOR HULL,

Informs his friends and the Public,

THAT HE HAS RECEIVED

A FRESH SUPPLY OF DRUGS,

PATENT MEDICINES, &c.

DIRECT FROM LONDON,

Which he will sell on the most reasonable terms.

January 22.   (tf. 28.)

Augusta Herald
Augusta, Georgia, February 5, 1800

CUTHBERT and BRYDIE,

HAVE JUST IMPORTED,

A PARCEL of FAMILY MEDICINES, which they will sell very cheap. Cash will be given for pink root and Virginia or small snake root.

The Georgia Gazette
Savannah, Georgia, January 10, 1765

To be Sold,

On reasonable terms, for Cash, Tobacco, Negroes or Horses,

A very large & general Assortment of

MEDICINES,

Just imported from Europe, which are as follow, viz.

PERUVIAN Bark
Cascarella bark
al. Polychrist.
Spanish flies
Flowers of Sulphur
Gentian root
White lead
Anth. flowers
Aloes
Jalap in powder
Glauber salts
Epsom salts
Magnesia
Camphire
Litharg. Aur.
Manna
Myrrhæ
Hellabor
Gum. Thus.
Chamomile flowers
Aloes
Red lead
Gum. Arabac
Galbanum
Rheubarb
Gum. Fragacanth.
Guiacum
Burgundy pitch
Laps. Calamin.
Sennæ
Zedoary
Ginger
Long pepper
Crude sulpher

Tart. emetic
Alum. Rupm.
Calomel
Corrosive sublimate
Cinnabec ppt.
Sal. absynth.
Copperas
Borax
Ipecacuanha
Turmerick
Radx. Columbe.
Cummin seeds
Mace
Cloves
Best Cinnamon
Chrystal. tartar
Cinnella Alb.
Sal. ammon. crud.
Radx. galangal.
contrayerva.
Terra Japon.
Creta. ppt.
Foenugreek seeds
Resina flav.
Laudanum
Opium
Oil of amber
Spirits of lavender
Sapo. liquid
Huxham's tincture bark
Volatile spirits
Balsam capivi
Oil of spike
Valerian root
Cassiæ fistulæ
Liquerice root

Oil of vitriol
Aqua fortis
Ratbane
Nitri

Many other Articles too tedious mention.

C. Dysart.

Augusta Herald, Augusta, Georgia, December 18, 1799, No. 23, Vol. I

YELLOW FEVER
LEE'S Genuine New-London Patent
BILIOUS PILLS,

Which were greatly successful in preventing and curing Epidemical, Bilious, Inflammatory, Yellow and Malignant Fevers in New-York, Philadelphia, Norfolk, Baltimore, Charleston, etc. etc. and the West-Indies. Prepared by SAMUEL H. P. LEE, M.D.

New-London, (Connecticut). Patent rights secured according to law of the United States. For sale, Wholesale & Retail, by ISAAC HERBERT, —Augusta. They are approved by eminent Physicians, and others for their virtues as an easy, safe, mild and efficacious remedy for all those complaints which arise from a redundancy of Bile in the Stomach and first passages of Men, Women and Children: Such as Jaundice, Remittent, Intermittent, and Ague Fevers; Yellow Fevers, Cholera Morbus, Dysentery, Diarrhea; sick Head Aches, Foul Stomachs, Indigestion, etc. etc.

They are also found very useful in Worms, Dropsy, Gravel, suppression of Urine, Obstructions, obstinate Costiveness, and all those complaints where purging is indicated—also for restoring the loss of appetite after eating or drinking to excess over night; for recruiting the habit in the spring season, and may be safely used in all constitutions, ages, and sexes.

(Signed) SAMUEL H. P. LEE, *July 21, 1799.*

Advertisement.

The Augusta Chronicle and Gazette of the State, September 5, 1801, Augusta, Georgia, Vol. XV, No. 778.

DOCTOR JAMES EWELL

Having fixed on Augusta, as his future place of abode, RESPECTFULLY offers to the inhabitants and those of its vicinity, his MEDICAL SERVICES, assuring those who may call upon him that every attention may be rendered, to merit his full approbation. The poor will find him ready to attend them gratis.

N. B. He may be found at his Shop (Broad-street) near the City-Hotel, where he intends keeping a general Assortment of Medicines, which he will sell on moderate terms, and warrant them to be genuine.

September 2.

Advertisement.

The Augusta Chronicle and Gazette of the State, September 25, 1801, Augusta, Georgia, Vol. XVI, No. 781.

DOCTOR BIBB

Having returned from Philadelphia, offers his Medical Services to the Citizens of Petersburg and its vicinity, and hopes by his attention to gain

IMPORTED, in the FRIENDSHIP, Capt. HORTON,
A Compleat Assortment of MEDICINES, &c.
TO BE SOLD BY
Lewis Johnson,
At his Shop in Broughton-Street, next Door to the Printing-Office.

Amongst which are the following:

- ALUM
- Antimony
- Distilled vinegar
- Verdigrease
- Balf. capivi
- Balsam of sulphur
- Borax
- Juniper berries
- Peruvian bark
- Ditto powdered, in pound bottles
- White wax
- Best saffron
- Cream of tartar
- Spanish flies
- Camphor
- Sweet mercury
- Burned hartshorn
- Shavings of ditto
- Elixir vitriol
- Liquorice juice
- Chamomile flowers
- Gum guaiac
- Isinglass
- Manna
- Nux vomica
- Oil of amber
- Oil of turpentine
- Oil of mace
- Oil of sweet almonds
- Oil of anise
- Oil of lemons
- Oil of lavender
- Oil of rhodium
- Oil of cinnamon
- Cold drawn linseed oil
- Pil. cochiæ
- Pil. ex duobus
- Ipecacuan
- Jalap
- Rhubarb
- Spermaceti
- Saltpetre
- Glauber & Epsom salts
- Crude sal armoniac
- Volatile ditto
- Salt of hartshorn
- Spirit of ditto
- Senna
- Spirit of lavender
- Spirit of sal volatile
- Rectified spirit of wine
- Sweet spirit of nitre
- Venice treacle
- Tartar emetic
- White and Roman vi-

- Sago
- Barley sugar
- White sugar candy
- Brown ditto
- Candied citrons
- Vermicelli
- Jordan almonds
- Currants
- Turkey figs
- Prunes
- Cinnamon
- Mace
- Cloves
- Nutmegs
- Ginger
- Black pepper
- Poland starch
- Plain and perfumed hair powder
- Pomatum
- White wine vinegar
- Flour of brimstone
- Copperas
- Prussian blue
- Best cut tobacco
- Ditto pigtail
- Ditto Scots snuff
- Strasburgh rappee
- Lancets
- Instruments for drawing teeth
- Vials and gallipots
- Pill boxes
- Iron, bell metal, and marble mortars
- Copper scales
- Boxes of scales & weights
- Flint bottles, different sizes, with ground stoppers
- White and red leather
- Steel spring trusses for ruptures
- Glyster syringes
- Small ivory and pewter ditto
- Gold leaf
- Flesh brushes
- Family medicines, viz.
- Duffy's elixir
- Squire's ditto
- British oil
- Stoughton's bitters
- Jackson's cordial ditto
- Godfrey's cordial
- Turlington's balsam

- James's powders
- Jesuits drops
- Essence of pepper-mint
- Eau de luce
- Magnesia
- Rose water
- Orange flower ditto
- Lavender ditto
- Honey ditto
- Hungary ditto
- Spirit of scurvy grass
- Beaume de vie. This medicine is in great repute all over Europe for disorders of the stomach and bowels, gout, gravel, and rheumatism, but particularly for diseases incident to the female sex.
- A compleat assortment of Dr. Hill's medicines, viz.
- Balsam of honey, for coughs, consumptions, asthmas, &c.
- Tincture of centaury, a stomachick bitter for loss of appetite and bad digestion;
- Tincture of valerian, a cordial nervous medicine, for fits, convulsions, lowness of spirits, and all paralytick disorders;
- Elixir of bardana, for the gout and rheumatism;
- Tincture of sage, a rich cordial and stomachick, well adapted to relieve the infirmities of age;
- Essence of water-dock, for the scurvy, leprosy, and all obstinate diseases of the skin;
- Tincture of spleenwort, for the cure of hypochondriacal disorders and obstructions in the bowels.
- ——&c. &c. &c.——
- Boxes of medicines

The Georgia Gazette

Savannah, Georgia

October 4, 1769

a part of the public confidence. He expects soon to receive a general supply of

FRESH DRUGS AND MEDICINES

Which he will dispose of on as low terms as they can be sold by any other person in the upper part of this state.

September 21, 1801.

Advertisement.

Augusta Herald, Augusta, Georgia, November 11, 1801, Vol. III, No. 122.

The evidence of the efficacy of Perkin's Tractors, of late the subject of so much controversy and speculation, is at length considered as decisive and medical characters of high reputation are now recommending their use. The idea entertained by some that their good effects were ascribable to imagination is proved to be erroneous, since they are found to cure infants and horses as readily as any other subjects. Indeed, the utility of the Tractors, as a remedy for inflamed eyes, sprains, contusions, and consequently lameness of horses, is now so well established that they are rapidly adopting in Gentlemen's Stables, etc. . . .

Advertisement.

The Augusta Chronicle and Gazette of the State, Feb. 18, 1804, Augusta, Georgia, Vol. XVIII, No. 907.

CORDIAL BALM OF GILEAD

The Subscribers have received a supply of this Valuable Medicine, which is prepared (only) by the sole proprietor and inventor, S. Solomon, M.D. author of "The Guide to Health," and other valuable works, at his house, Soloman's Place, Brownlow-Street, Liverpool.

The train of melancholy disorders which affect the human frame, under the denomination of nervous diseases, are the principal source of human misery in the privation of health. Those disorders proceed from such an infinite variety and complication of causes, as to render it impossible, if even it were always necessary, to trace them to their true source. The effects however are but too well known and too severely felt amongst too great a portion of mankind; and to these effects it may without exageration be asserted, that any remedy superior or more celebrated for efficacy than Dr. Solomon's Cordial Balm of Gilead, never has been discovered. In all delicate, weakly and relaxed constitutions; lowness of spirits, hypochondria, horrors, tremblings, loss of memory, impaired vigor, tabes dorsalis, nervous consumptions, and the numberless symptoms of impaired and tottering constitutions, whether arising from a life of inactivity, intemperance or inattention to health. By the strict perseverance in its use it cheers, braces, and invigorates the whole nervous system, and gives a new tone to all the vital functions, of which numberless instances can be avouched. Thousands at this day live to bless the day they first applied to this ad-

mirable remedy, and enjoy the blessings of health, who might otherwise have dropped into an untimely grave, the victim of an early imprudence. Also: DR SOLOMON'S GUIDE TO HEALTH, Wray & Childers, *Feb. 11.*
Advertisement.

The Augusta Chronicle and Gazette of the State, March 24, 1804, Augusta, Georgia, Vol. XVIII, No. 912.

DOCTOR HARRIS

Takes this opportunity to inform the public, that he is at length returned, to Augusta, the place of his nativity, after an absence of nearly seven years, which time he has spent in the most celebrated schools in Europe, viz. the Universities of Edinburgh, Paris and Mont Pellier, at which last place he took his degrees as Doctor of Physic, and has proper vouches of his attendance at each of the other places.

Dr. H. flatters himself, from having been born and raised in this climate, and from his having performed his first studies in this place, under one of the first Physicians of the day, as well as from his entire acquaintances with the diseases incident to the climate, as his well known steadiness and temperance that he will meet that favorable reception, a continuance of which, will be his greatest ambition to merit.

Dr. H. during his stay in London, made it his business to establish a correspondence with the best Druggists, Book Sellers and Surgical Instrument Makers there, that he might have it in his power to answer the demands of his friends in each of these branches, on the shortest notice and cheapest terms. He has now on hand, at his shop, in the Brick House, next, Door below Captain Kennedy's, a general Assortment of the best
MEDICINES,
Just from London, which he will dispose of on the most reasonable terms.
March 17.

Advertisement.

Augusta Herald, Augusta, Georgia, Vol. VII, No. 43, May 1, 1806.

> *Facts are stubborn things!*
> *Riches, without health, no pleasure brings.*

It is a fact that most of the complaints of the spring and summer seasons, arise from accumulated billious juices, distending the involuntary organs, and thereby predisposing the system for the induction of such species of diseases as accidental circumstances may occasion. It is also a fact that by clearing the stomach and bowels occasionally, predisposition may be removed and good health restored. It is, furthermore, a fact, that nine tenths of diseases, in their various forms and stages, are cured, if cured at all, by the agency of purgative medicines, blood-letting excepted. Does not the

METALLIC TRACTORS.

DR. PERKINS's METALLIC TRACTORS, which have gained such immense repute in England, Germany, Copenhagen, (Denmark) and almost every part of Europe, for their unparalelled efficacy in the cure of rheumatic and gouty affections, inflammations, and various topical diseases—and for the invention of which a public vote of thanks was passed by the Royal Society of Medicine, FOR SALE, at this OFFICE.

The Augusta Chronicle
and Gazette of the State
Augusta, Georgia, July 12, 1800

DOCTOR MURRAY

Respectfully begs leave to inform the public that he has just received from London,

AN EXTENSIVE SUPPLY OF

Fresh Drugs & Genuine Medicines,

ALSO,

Patent Medicines, Shop Furniture, And Surgical Instruments.

The quality and price of which he flatters himself will on trial be found equal to any ever offered for sale here; and which he hopes will entitle him to that share of the public favor he has heretofore received.

Medical practitioners, and country store keepers, who take a general assortment, will be supplied on liberal terms.

The Augusta Chronicle
Augusta, Georgia, September 14, 1799

Augusta, June 1, 1798.

DOCTOR HULL,

Has removed to the store lately occupied by Messrs Birch and Owey, next door to Messrs. Urquhart and Tait; he has received a complete assortment of

DRUGS & MEDICINES,

Which he will sell on the most reasonable terms. Gentlemen of the profession or store keepers can be supplied very nearly as cheap as in Charleston: he will put up small medicine chests for planters, with directions.

He has a small quantity of each of the following PATENT MEDICINES:

DAFFY's elixer
Godfrey's cordial
Norris's drops
James' powders
Bateman's pectoral drops
Stoughton's bitters
Pectoral balsom of honey
Dolby's carminative
Nuxham's tincture of bark
Turlington's balsam
Gowland's lotion
La Blache's military drops
British oil
Squires's elixir
Anderson's pills
Opodeldoc
Essence of peppermint.

June 1, 1798.

The Augusta Chronicle
and Gazette of the State
Augusta, Georgia, June 2. 1798

C. W. & H. R. J. LONG,

Wholesale and Retail Druggists,

ATHENS, GA.

Keep constantly on hand, a large and well selected stock of

Paints, Oils, Varnishes, Dye Stuffs, Brushes, Window Glass, Putty.

—ALSO—

Dealers in

American, French and English Chemicals,

DRUGS, MEDICINES, PERFUMERY, AND FANCY ARTICLES.

☞ Physicians, Dealers and all others, can depend upon their orders meeting prompt attention, upon the most accommodating terms. Their goods are selected with great care, and will be warranted as represented.

Jan 26—46—ly.

Southern Banner
Athens, Georgia, February 2, 1854

Wanted,

A Quantity of Pink Root,

For which a good price will be given by
MONTGOMERY & BIRD.

Augusta, May 11, 1792.

The Augusta Chronicle
and Gazette of the State
Augusta, Georgia, May 11, 1792

HENRY LEWIS BOURQUIN,
HAS TO SELL,
A fresh and large Assortment of MEDICINES,
Just imported in the last vessels from London.

Amongst which are,

SOME very good for plantation use, such as, Best Rhubarb; Ipecacuana; Epsom Salts; Camphire; Manna; Spermaceti; Julap; Flour of Sulphur; Jesuits Bark; Camomile Flowers; White Vitriol; Turner's Cerate; Seneca Rattle-snake-root; Anderson's Pills; Lockyer's Pills; Pill Coché; Turlington's Balsam; Pectoral Balsam of Honey; Bettu's British Oil single and refined; Jackson's Bitters; Hunter's Drops; Plain and Golden Spirit of Scurvy-Grass; Amber & Castor Oil; Squire's Grand Elixir; Daffey's Elixir; Bateman's Drops; Stoughton's Bitters; Hungary and Lavender Water; Rose Water; Orange Flower Water; Honey Water; Nuc. Vomic. vulgarly called Hog's Vomit; Isinglass; Gold Leaf; Tamarinds; Preserved Ginger; Dried Ginger; Best Mustard in bottles; Raisins; Currants; Barley Sugar; Pearl Barley; Sagee; Jordan Almonds; &c.——He likewise prepares Medicine Boxes for plantation use with directions.

The Georgia Gazette
Savannah, Georgia, November 12, 1766

Apothecary's Hall.

FOR SALE,

5 Hhds. 1 Tierce and 4 Cases Vials, consisting of White, Green, Specie, Essence and Patent VIALS, assorted.

—*ALSO*—

20 Barrels Salts,
300 lbs. Pale Peruvian Bark
100 lbs. Yellow ditto do.
20 lbs. Red ditto do.
50 lbs. English Calomel,
100 lbs. Powdered Jalap,
200 lbs. Camphor,
100 Bottles Castor Oil, W. I.
6 Dozen cold strained American, for family use,
6 Do. Henry's Cal'd Magnesia, (London)

With an extensive and general
ASSORTMENT OF
DRUGS, SPICES, DIES, PAINTS AND PATENT MEDICINES, SHOP FURNITURE.
BY
Cunningham & Dunn.
—*Constantly on hand*—
White WINE VINEGAR.

January 20   58

Augusta Herald
Augusta, Georgia, February 27, 1818

Notice.

THE Public are respectively informed that the subscriber has engaged himself in the stand lately occupied by Doctors CUNNINGHAM & MEIGS, in the capacity of an APOTHECARY, where a constant attendance to all prescriptions will be given day and night.

MEDICINES will be Retailed on the lowest terms, and every attention will be paid to give public satisfaction.—The Institution will select the Choicest MEDICINES, and preparations made with care and exactness.

One or two more Physician's exclusive business can be received, and their commands attended to with punctuality and promptness, at the charge of their patients.

Families can be supplied on the lowest terms, but written orders will always be required, to prevent errors of servants, accidental or intentional.

MEDICINE CHESTS made and repaired agreeable to orders for Planters at APOTHECARIES HALL, immediately opposite the *Augusta Book Store*.

Charles C. Dunn.
May 7.   tf

The Augusta Chronicle
Augusta, Georgia, May 7, 1817

physician depend more on this indication than all his pharmacopeal preparations besides? Does he not consider all others as the mere medendi of fanciful and, sometimes, visionary theories; which may or may not answer the desired objects? Does he not know, that unless he is really a master of the science, and keeps this object in view, he may (innocently, no doubt) kill more than he may chance to cure? He certainly does; and every honest one will confess it. As to the opinions of dishonest and ignorant empirics, they may be believed by those who are fond of long fits of sickness, long bills, ruined constitutions, or premature death.

Purging is found to be the most effectual method of relieving over distended vessels or intestinal congestions, of any in use. The choice of these is often misjudged, from traditional prejudices, habitual customs, or a fear of doing wrong. But certain and effectual purgation can never do harm; the use of them often prevents the necessity of calling in the attending physician, and if called upon, his work is more than half done. There is no preparation now extant, to answer as a purgative for all ages and sexes, and for safety, convenience and ease, as the "Patent New London Billious Pills." Seven years general and increasing use of them, by physicians of respectability and integrity, by families who have found great expenses saved thereby, by their introduction into the Navy of the United States as well as among seamen generally; in short, as the only medicine which will admit of universal success in all hands; are the best evidences of their real virtues, and promise to secure to mankind a remedy valuable in the extreme.

Samuel H. P. Lee, *Physician and Member of the Connecticut Medical Society*

Advertisement.

The Augusta Chronicle and Gazette of the State, August 30, 1806, Augusta, Georgia, Vol. XX, No. 1039.

Just received a Fresh assortment of Medicines & Medicinal Drugs

THOS. I. WRAY

Having just arrived with a general assortment, laid in under his own inspection, at the best American Markets; which he will dispose of on really moderate terms.

He has added to his former articles a fine assortment of nice Confectionaries, Henry's patent Magnesia, essence of Spruce, indelible Ink for marking clothes, two Electrical Machines, and lately appointed agent for Doctor Solomon, having brought with him a large supply of genuine Balm of Gilead and Anti-Impetigines. A judicious writer remarks, that, "to live with satisfaction to one's self and others, to procure as many comforts of life as are consistent with our mental and bodily constitution, and to avert impending danger, or, in other words, to preserve our selves from the injurious attacks of what relates to the practical part of human life." If then to live with satisfaction to ourselves and others is so desirable how can we accomplish it when deprived of that which is more to be esteemed than gold and treasure? That which enlarges the soul—that which, when possessed, leaves little more to be wished for—that which when wanted is the greatest of wants—even that which is the greatest of all blessings, namely Health! The principal source of misery, then, being the loss of this great jewel, it behooves us to find a remedy for those diseases which have hitherto baffled the skill of the Faculty, namely nervous, consumptive, and hypochondriac. If any one man has ever been more successful than another, it is Doctor Solomon, who has brought his Cordial Balm of Gilead to such perfection that it never fails removing the worst and most crabbed disorders of this nature. It always exhilarates and cheers the spirits, braces and invigorates the whole frame. Such a medicine, for its healing, balsamic, friendly and sanative qualities upon the debilitated constitution deserves the wondrous encouragement it meets with from all ranks, who have been fortunate enough to have recourse to it. Pamphlets on its efficacy delivered gratis by the agent, And sold in bottles, price Three Dollars each.

Augusta, Aug. 30.

Advertisement.

Georgia Express, Athens, Georgia, August 13, 1808.

DOCTOR GERDINE

Has now on hand a good assortment of DRUGS and PATENT MEDICINES, which he will sell on as good terms as can be procured in the country: He resides at his plantation six miles below Athens and on the main road leading from Watkinsville to the Cherokee Corner, where those having need of his professional services may find him.

Advertisement.

Augusta Herald, Augusta, Georgia, Vol. X, Whole No. 497, January 19, 1809.

JUST RECEIVED
And for Sale at the Augusta Book Store,
The Following Valuables,

PATENT MEDICINES

Thompson's Celebrated Eye-Water, So salutary and effectual in all complaints of the eyes, and the virtue of which, is now extensively known and well established.—Price 50 cents a bottle.

CHURCH'S COUGH DROPS
For colds, asthmas and consumptions. Price 75 cents.

THOMPSON'S FEBRIFUGE ELECTUARY
Or a safe and effectual remedy for ague and fever, and every kind of intermitting fever. Price 1.00. a box.

DR. ULMO,

Next door above Mr. Murren's Store,
BROAD-STREET,

LATELY arrived in this city, where he intends to make his residence, has the honor to offer his services to the public, in his capacity of PHYSICIAN and SURGEON.

HE HAS FOR SALE,
A LARGE AND GENERAL ASSORTMENT
OF

MEDICINES,

—Among which are—

Flake & Calabrian Manna	Gum Arabic
Glauber salts	Hemlock extract
Epsom do.	Isinglass
Rochel do.	Juniper berries
Sulphur in rolls	Ipecacuanha in powder and root
Ditto flower	Magnesia alba
Senna	Opium
Cream of tartar	Quick silver
Camphor	Turkey Rhubarb
Castor oil	White sugar candey
Chamomile flowers	Spirits of nitre
Borax	do. do. dulcified
Agaric	Muriatic acide
Aloes socotrine	Salt of tartar
Alum	Tartar emetic
Antimony	Tartar vitrioletic
Coperas	Vitriol white and blue.
Gentian root	

PATENT MEDICINES,

British oil	Turlington
Opodeldoc	Dalby's carminative
Squiers's elixir	Daffy's elixir salutus
Essence of peppermint	Hooper's pills
Stoughton	Anderson's do.
Godfrey's cordial	

And a number of other articles too numerous to mention, warranted genuine, and of the best quality, which he will sell wholesale or retail, at the lowest prices.

Nov. 13.

The Augusta Chronicle and Gazette of the State
Augusta, Georgia, November 15, 1800

Apothecary's Shop

NEWLY ESTABLISHED IN MILLEDGEVILLE

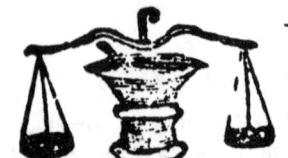

JUST received in addition to former supplies, the following articles, to wit:

Alum,	Nitre Refined,
Borax,	Oil of Vitriol,
Calomel,	Opium,
Camphor,	Peruvian Bark,
Cinnamon,	—— Yellow,
Cloves,	Quicksilver,
Copperas,	Salts Glauber,
Cremor Tartar,	—— Rochelle,
Flowers of Benzoin,	Sapo Caudia,
—— Sulphur,	—— Castile,
Flake Manna,	—— Windsor,
Indigo, Carolina,	Senna,
Ipecac,	Sugar Candy,
Jalap,	Spirits Turpentine,
Magnesia,	Verdigris,

PATENT MEDICINES.

Anderson's Pills,	Dalton's Caminrative,
Coit's do.	Opodeldoc,
Hooper's do.	Turlington's Balsam,
Lee's do.	
Bateman's Drops,	Wheaton's Jaundice Bitters,
British Oil,	
Cheltenham Salts,	—— Itch Ointment,

MISCELLANEOUS:

Black Lead Pencils	Snuff, Scotch,
Beast Pipes,	—— Macauba,
Camel Hair Pencils,	Teeth Brushes,
	—— Common,
Court Plaister,	—— Silver Wired,
Nipple Sheth's	Wafers,
Patent Lint,	Walkdens Ink Powder.
Paint Brushes,	
Pomatum,	

Also, on consignment, several hundred weight of good Copperas, 1500 lbs. of extra Heat Salt, all of which are offered low for cash.

William Sturges, & Co
December 22   9—tf.

Georgia Journal
Milledgeville, Georgia, January 5, 1814

TO BE SOLD,
By Lewis Johnston,

BOXES of MEDICINES for the use of plantations and families, containing such as are the most useful, and best adapted to the diseases of this country, with printed directions.

May 9, 1782.

The Georgia Royal Gazette
Savannah, Georgia, May 30, 1782

℞ ADVERTISEMENTS

STEER'S CHEMICAL OPODELDOC
So universally esteemed for its superior efficacy in all rheumatic complaints, gout, sprains, bruises, wounded or contracted tendons, etc. Price 50 cents bottle.

BRITISH OIL
So much esteemed as a valuable remedy for scorbutic and rheumatic disorders, contusions, contraction of the nerves, strains, withered limbs, ulcers, old sores, wandering or fixed pains, wounds, cuts, scalds, burns. Price 37½ cents a bottle.

ESSENCE OF PEPPER-MINT
A preparation well known for its virtues in cases of cholic, flatulencies, retching, sickness of the stomach, loss of appetite, etc.—Price 25 cents a bottle.

RAWSON'S CELEBRATED ANTI-BILIOUS AND STOMACHIC BITTERS
Which have been so long esteemed and highly approved of in all parts of the United States, as a remedy against bilious complaints, pains in the head and stomach, debility, lowness of spirits, indigestion, fainting, numbeness, coldness of the limbs, etc. etc. Price 50 cents a bottle.

HINKLAY'S INFALLIBLE REMEDY FOR THE PILES
A preparation now of established reputation and an easy and effectual cure for a complaint which often proves extremely tedious and troublesome.—Price 50 cents a box.

RAWSON'S WORM POWDERS
A medicine perfectly safe for persons of all ages, and a salutary remedy for many complaints of the bowels to which children are often particularly subject.—Price 50 cents packet.

DUNHAM'S CELEBRATED JAUNDICE BITTERS
So valuable in affording relief, in cases of sickness of the stomach, vomitings, want of appetite, costiveness, flatulency, jaundice, melancholy and hypochondriac affections, as well as in restoring the tone of the stomach, and giving the usual vigor and sprightliness to the system, after an indiscreet intemperance or drinking too freely, over night. It is an elixir of nature, being prepared from roots, plants, and flowers, and will be found a useful remedy for all disorders of the stomach.—50 cents a box.

THOMPSON'S WELL KNOWN, AND MUCH ESTEEMED AROMATIC TOOTH PASTE
For whitening the teeth, and curing the scurvy in the gums, correcting that badness of the breath which proceeds from decayed teeth, and removing all foulness from the teeth and gums.—Price 50 cents a box.

LEE'S WINDHAM BILIOUS PILLS

The first pills ever patented in the United States, and the superior efficacy of which have been proved by experience. They are recommended as the most valuable and safe anti-bilious medicine ever yet discovered.—Price 50 cents a box.

COOLEY'S VEGETABLE ELIXIR

For coughs, asthmas, consumptions, spitting of blood, shortness of breath and other diseases to which the lungs are exposed. The proprietor states that the efficacy of this Elixir is established by "many well authenticated testimonies."—Price 75 cents a bottle.

COOLEY'S ANTI-PESTILENTIAL, ATTENTUATING AND RESTORATIVE PILLS

Esteemed in rheumatic complaints and bilious diseases.—Price 50 cents a box.

RAWSON'S GENUINE AND CELEBRATED ITCH OINTMENT

Curing eruptions, pimples, and cutaneous distemper, as well as being a safe, easy and certain cure for Itch.—50 cents a box.

THOMPSON'S SPECIFIC DROPS

For Tooth Ache.—37½ cents a bottle.

RAWSON'S ANTI-BILIOUS PILLS OR FAMILY PHYSIC

For relieving headache, swoonings, dizziness, pains in the stomach and bowels, etc.—Price 25 cents a box.

SIGNUM SALUTIS

A sure preventative against a loathsome disease.—Price 100 cents a bottle.

January 19.

Advertisements.

The Augusta Chronicle, May 5, 1810, Augusta, Georgia

DOCTOR HOWARD

Late of Camden, (South Carolina)
Most respectfully informs the public in general, that he is now settling in this town at the house lately occupied by Mr. Zachariah Bell, in Reynolds street, where he intends holding himself in readiness to attend on those who may favor him with their calls. The subscriber flatters himself, that for nine years past, he has had unparalleled success in the treatment of most chronic or lingering diseases, of which numerous respectable references may be had; and he hopes, by a careful and regular attendance on all slaves put under his care, to have a continuation of his former success, and thereby to merit and have such a share of public patronage as to enable him

Drugs, Medicines
AND
PATENT MEDICINES,
Wholesale & Retail,
On the lowest terms for Cash, at
APOTHECARY'S HALL,
Opposite the Herald Office, Broad-Street, Augusta.

LOTION, which removes blemishes from the face, making the skin delicately soft and clear, improving the complexion, and restoring the bloom of youth,
Essence of Mustard, for the gout, rheumatism, sprains, &c.
Elixir, for colds and coughs,
Doctor Hahn's German Eye Water,
Lee's Antibillious Pills,
Coit's Family Pills,
Hooper and Anderson's Pills
Sovereign Itch Ointment,
Opodeldoc, Bateman's Drops,
British Oil, Haarlem Oil,
Turlington's Balsam, Balsam Honey,
Henry's Calcined Magnesia,
Cheltenham Salts,
Ink Powder, Tooth Powder in Boxes,
Godfrey's Cordial,
Dalby's Carminative,
Teeth Brushes,
Race and Powdered Ginger,
Cinnamon, Cloves, Mace, Nutmegs,
Allspice, Pearl Barley, Arrow Root,
Anniseed, Fennel Seed,
Windsor Soap, Wash Balls, Fancy Soap, Castile Soap,
Camel's Hair Pencils,
Copal Varnish, Red Lead,
Vermillion, Prussian Blues,
Purple Brown, Patent Yellow,
Rose Pink, Gamboge,
Alum, Brimstone, Coperas,
Arnatto, Spanish and common,
English Camomile Flowers,
Flour Sulphur, Aloes, Camphor,
Salts, Jalap, Rhubarb, Æther,
Cream Tartar, Calomel,
..... quares, ... cal.

ANTICIPATED SHORTLY.
Shop Furniture, Vials, white and green,
Assorted Mortars
Teeth Instruments,
Lancets, thumb and spring, assorted, with all the variety suited for practitioners' use and this market.

Cunningham & Dunn.
June 21.

The Augusta Chronicle
Augusta, Georgia, June 25, 1817

DOCTOR COCKE,
Has Just Received from PHILADELPHIA,
A FRESH SUPPLY OF GENUINE
Drugs & Medicines,
WHICH HE IS NOW OPENING
At his SHOP Front of the HERALD PRINTING-OFFICE, WASHINGTON-STREET.
Among which are the Following, VIZ.

GUM ALOES,   Flake Manna
—— Ammoniac,   Common do.
—— Myrrh,   Oil of Cloves
—— Opium,   —— Cinnamon
—— Tragacanth   —— Olives
—— Kino   —— Amber
—— Scammony   —— Lavender
—— Gamboge   —— Mint
—— Guaiacum   —— Vitriol
—— Assafoetida   —— Aniseed
Flowers Benzoine   Yellow Resin,
Sal Ammoniac,   Tamarinds
—— Tartar,   Nitric Acid
Glauber Salts,   Aqua Fortis
Best powd. red Bark   Marine Acid
—— Pale do.   Spirit Lavender
—— Rhubarb   —— Turpentine
—— Ipecac.   —— Hartshorn
—— Jalap.   —— Nitre
—— Gum Arabic   —— Wine
Orange Peel   Alum
Roots.—Gentian   Tartar Emetic
—— Marshmellows   Sugar Lead
—— Pink   Sponge
—— Seneka   Senna
—— Colombo   Squills
—— Sarsaparilla   Essence PepperMint
Borax   —— Lemon
Camphor   —— Bergamot
Chamomile Flowers   Verdegris
Sulphur   Balsam Copaiva
Cantharides   Nitre
Liquorice Ball   Vitriolic Æther
White Vitriol   Galls
Roman do.   Digitalis
Spermaceti   Prepared Chalk
Magnesia,   Aniseed
Lunar Costic   Grained Sago
Castor Oil   Litharge
Quicksilver   Glass of Antimony
Calomel, ppt.   Uva Ursi
Corrosive Sublimate   Red Saunders
Red Præcipitate   Vials assorted, &c.

Also a General Assortment of
PATENT MEDICINES,
Which ... ers for sale on the most moderate ... ms.
January 29.   (tf. 29)

Augusta Herald
Augusta, Georgia, February 5, 1800

ere long to realize his views in the establishment of a private infirmary, Botanic Garden, Distillation, etc. etc.

Chronic white persons will be attended to, as may be previously agreed on. Five dollars will be required with each slave sent from the country for their support while in the hospital. Cures will be warranted permanent. Bleeding and extracting teeth and stumps will be attended to at any hour, and done in the most ample manner.

JESSE HOWARD

Augusta, Georgia.
Advertisement.

The Augusta Chronicle, August 23, 1816, Augusta, Georgia, Vol. XXX, No. 1459.

DOCTOR SAVIGNE

Respectfully informs the public in general, that he wishes to commence the practice of physic in this place. He hopes by his attention to business to merit a liberal support from his fellow citizens. He has practiced in the following places, Viz.—Charleston, Richmond, Virginia, Baltimore, Philadelphia and New York, and binds himself to make a sound cure of the following diseases, if patient will follow his directions, viz.—

The Consumption, Bloody Flux and vomiting blood, Fits, Gravel, Asthma, the Venereal Diseases (without using mercury), Gout, Rheumatism, the Sciatic Pains, all kinds of ditto, all kinds of old sores, wounds and Cancers, all detention of Urine, all kinds of sore eyes, all kinds of putrified fevers, the Influenza, etc.

Dr. S. may be found at Mr. Jermans, on the cross street back of Mr. Silvero's brick building.

August 16.

Advertisement.

The Augusta Chronicle and Ga. Gazette, Dec. 2, 1818, Augusta, Georgia, Vol. XXXIII, No. 1676.

DOCTOR W. S. PARROTT

Will resume his former practice in Augusta and its vicinity, for three ensuing months, and the probability is he will make this his permanent residence. He cures Cancer, Wens, Ring or Tetter Worms, Scurvy, White-swelling, or any Scorbutick or Chronical humours on the surface of the human body, are infallibly cured by my cancer powder.

No. 2—He also officiates in the capacity of Dentist in all its branches, makes and inserts artificial teeth, which are durable, equal in beauty to the natural ones, transplants teeth, cleans teeth, plugs the hollow ones with gold or lead, which method not only puts an end to the pain but preserves the teeth a great while, he prepares a powder much to the purpose for cleaning the teeth which preserves the gums and restores a sweet breath, he has had a late supply of implements and the best Hippopotamus for the purpose of making artificial teeth. He has taken a room at the Eagle Tavern where he will be every day found unless absent on his professional duties.

N. B. Ladies will be waited on at their private Rooms if requested.

December 2.

Advertisement.

Chapter VI

PUBLIC HEALTH, ORGANIZATION, MEDICAL AND PHARMACEUTICAL EDUCATION, AND LEGISLATION BEGIN A SLOW BUT DEFINITE PROCESS OF EVOLUTION (1760-1828-1959)

REGARDLESS of all the self-diagnosis, self-treatment, and indiscriminate advertising that went on in the Colonial as well as in the post-Colonial period, there were some bright spots along the way which indicated proper thinking on the part of practitioners of medicine and pharmacy and governmental officials who were struggling through an era when contagious and infectious diseases were rampant, and the causes and treatment of them were unknown.

Public Health

It was in the minds of the Colonists as early as 1760 that disease might prove to be a community rather than an individual problem, and therefore measures had to be provided which it was hoped would bring some degree of protection for the public against infectious or contagious diseases. These thoughts were then—and are even today—expressed in what we know as public health measures. It was recognized even then that if all health agencies were to discharge their full responsibility to the public in matters concerning their health and welfare, all scientific knowledge must be coordinated toward this end.

No doubt encouraged and urged by the physicians and surgeons and apothecaries of the period, the Government of the Colony, in the hope of preventing the introduction of contagious diseases, sponsored the adoption of health legislation which had to do primarily with quarantine of ships coming into the harbor of Savannah.

PUBLIC HEALTH, ORGANIZATION, EDUCATION

It is interesting to note that even at that early date the welfare of the public was given preference over that of the individual, and that all succeeding health legislation has accepted this principle as a precedent. It is further significant that steps to protect the health of the public should have taken priority over the matters of organization, education, and legislation as witnessed by the series of laws governing public health matters as recorded in *Digest of Georgia Laws—1800*.

From this "Digest" of Georgia laws come the following items:

1760—An Act to require incoming ships to observe quarantine. (Savannah)
1763—An Act to strengthen quarantine regulations and "to prevent the harboring of sick sailors and others." (Savannah)
1764—(May)—An Act "to prevent the further spreading of smallpox" in Savannah and other ports.
1764—(December)—An Act "to prevent as much as may be the spreading of smallpox in this Province."
1765—The above law (1764) was re-enacted.
1767—An Act "to purchase 104 acres of land on Tybee Island for a Lazaretto." (Pest-House)
1767—An Act "to prevent the introduction of malignant distempers into the Colony."
1768—Inoculation against smallpox was made illegal, with £ 100 fine for those who administered inoculation, and a like fine for those who submitted to inoculation.
1770—Additional smallpox legislation was enacted.
1786—An Act creating a Health Officer for the port of Savannah.
1793—More quarantine regulations.
1803—Recording of deaths and burials in Savannah was provided for.
1804—A City Board of Health for Savannah was created.

It is well to note that during this period in which inoculation with smallpox virus was practiced, there were occasions when communities prohibited by law the practice of inoculation while other communities—and even the Revolutionary Army—were enforcing inoculation, as the only step which had shown some promise of bringing the disease smallpox under control. (Distinction must be kept in mind between the term "inoculation" as used in 1700 and "vaccination" of the present era.)

In addition to the public health regulations establishing quarantine and other measures for the prevention of the spreading of infection, other health regulations were adopted to inspect premises, to establish (in Savannah at least) a system of registration of births and deaths, and to provide for the inspection of meats.

Following are some public health notices which appeared in the newspapers of the era, some of which were classified as "Acts" but most of which were local in character.

The Georgia Gazette

Savannah   Public Notice
Thursday, April 14, 1763
Savannah, Council Chambers, April 7, 1763
Acts Passed Last Session of Assembly

An Act entitled, An Act to prevent the bringing into and spreading of contagious Distempers in this Province; and to oblige vessels going out of any Port within the same, first to produce, for that Purpose, a Passport from the Governor or Commander-in-Chief for the Time being, and to prevent the harbouring of sick sailors and others.

The Georgia Gazette

Savannah, May 12, 1763   Advertisement

Whereas it has become a custom for travellers to pass and repass through my plantations, and to leave down my fences and bars; and whereas the small-pox is now in Carolina, which I am greatly afraid may be brought into my plantation by travelling people, no reasonable person will be offended by my desiring them to make use of the publick road.

(Signed) Joseph Gibbons

The Georgia Gazette

Savannah, Ga.   News Item
Thursday, July 7, 1763

Monday died at Tybee of the small-pox, Capt. Benjamin Ware, of the sloop Savannah Packet, from Charleston. He was taken with them just as his quarantine was out; the vessel is not permitted to come up to the harbour. Same day a passenger on board said sloop got up to town, but was immediately taken and committed to prison.

The Georgia Gazette

Savannah   News Item
July 21, 1763

We hear from Charlestown, that by the resolution entered into by the physicians there not to inoculate, a stop is almost put to the small-pox in that place.

PUBLIC HEALTH, ORGANIZATION, EDUCATION

The Georgia Gazette

Savannah *Public Notice*
December 20, 1764

An Act to prevent spreading of small-pox in the Province. Put sign on house signifying same. Make no hospitals.

The Georgia Gazette

Savannah *Public Notice*
April 19, 1764

To be sold at the Printing Office. A few copies of the following Acts of the General Assembly of this Province, Viz. - An Act to prevent the bringing into and spreading of contagious distempers in this Province and to oblige vessels going out of any port within the same, first to produce, for that purpose, a passport from the Governor or Commander-in-chief for the time being; and also to prevent the harbouring of sick sailors and others.

The Georgia Gazette

Savannah *Public Notice*
May 3, 1764

To be sold at the Printing-Office. A few copies of the following Act of General Assembly of this Province, - Viz. An Act to oblige ships and other vessels coming from places infected with epidemical distempers to perform "quarantain."

The Georgia Gazette

Savannah, Georgia No. 61
May 31, 1764

A severe epidemic of small pox prevailed in Savannah and throughout the Colony. Due to the practice of inoculation then prevailing (without the precaution of isolation) the disease was being spread very rapidly.

The General Assembly of the Colony, in an effort to arrest the spread of the disease, passed some very restrictive legislation covering the subject of inoculation and general precautions to be observed, as follows:

1. A fine of £ 100 was to be assessed any individual who inoculated another person.
2. A fine of £ 100 was assessed against any person who willfully submitted to inoculation.
3. A similar fine was assessed against any person who opened a hospital or other place where persons affected with small-pox might be harbored.
4. Any house wherein small-pox prevailed was required to have displayed on the outside a white flag, whereby the public could be notified of the existence of the disease in that house, and a guard was to be placed outside the house to confine the person or persons who had become infected with small-pox.

5. A public notice was to be placed in all public buildings, including churches, stating the warning that small-pox existed on this plantation or in that home.
6. Provision was made for this law to be repealed, or exceptions made thereto, by the Governor of the Colony.

The Georgia Gazette
Savannah, May 24, 1764   *Advertisement*

As I have been informed of a report being spread that I would not inoculate for the smallpox, which, with other reports of equal veracity and tendency must certainly have been propagated industriously by some of my good friends, (tho' I doubt, not with an intention of serving me) for I am positive I never gave any grounds for them:

This is to acquaint such as are really my friends, that I will inoculate as soon as permission is given; with regard to others, I equally despise and deny what they can be capable of.

(Dr.) Andrew Johnston.

The Georgia Gazette
Savannah
Thursday, May 30, 1765

It is with pleasure we can acquaint our readers, that upon enquiry we find the small-pox is now only in one house in town.

The Georgia Gazette
Savannah   *Public Notice*
Wednesday, July 30, 1766

Whereas the butchers in and near Savannah have for some time in the past sold beef, veal, mutton, lamb etc. at their houses contrary to law, this is therefore to desire all whom it may concern to refrain from that practice for the future, and that all beef, pork, mutton, veal, etc. killed within one mile of Savannah, and all beef, pork, mutton, etc. brought from other parts to Savannah for sale, be brought to the publick market, and there exposed to sale, strictly observing the market act which has been publickly read in the market for that purpose, as I am determined to take notice of all transgressions without distinction in order that they may be dealt with according to law.

David Zubly, Clk.

Augusta Herald
Augusta, Georgia   *Public Notice*
June 18, 1800

CITY COUNCIL, Augusta, 9th June, 1800.

Whereas the City Council has received information that the Small Pox is now prevalent in Savannah, and having determined to prevent if possible its contagion from spreading in the city:

℞ PUBLIC HEALTH, ORGANIZATION, EDUCATION

It is therefore Resolved, That it shall be the duty of the Marshall and Constables to examine all persons coming from the City of Savannah, either by land or water, as well as all Places where they may have reason to suspect any person or persons having the Small Pox may be; And upon any infested person being so discovered, to give information of the same to the Intendant, or some member of the board, who shall direct such person to be removed immediately to some proper place without the limits of the Corporation: And upon such person or persons refusing to comply with such directions, the Marshall and Constables are hereby ordered, to remove such person or persons immediately to such place as may be pointed out by the City Council.

Joseph Hutchinson, Clk.

Columbian Museum and Savannah Advertiser
Savannah *Public Notice*
August 13, 1802
IN COUNCIL, Savannah, August 2, 1802

Information being laid before Council that the Yellow Fever has made its appearance in the City of Philadelphia; It is ordered, that the Health Officer be directed to order all vessels coming from the Port of Philadelphia to be brought to at Cockspur, and there to perform a quarantine of fifteen days . . . and remain until they shall receive a certificate of health from the health officer.

Extract from the Minutes.
Health Office Port of Savannah
Wm. Cocke, M.D. Health Officer

The Augusta Chronicle and Gazette of the State
Vol. XVI, No. 801 *Public Notice*
Feb. 13, 1802

The Physicians of Augusta feel it a duty incumbent on them, to notify the citizens at large, that they have commenced the Inoculation for Cow- or Kine-Pox. So much has been published on the importance of this discovery, and the many advantages resulting to mankind from its introduction, that little remains for them to comment on. It may be proper here to remark, that those who are not disposed to receive this mild disease by Inoculation cannot contract it in any other way; and when a patient has once gone through Kine-Pox, he is forever exempt from that horrid scourge Small Pox. N.B.—The poor will be inoculated and attended gratis.

The Augusta Chronicle and Gazette of the State
Vol. XVIII No. 914 *Advertisement*
April 7, 1804

KINE-POCK

Doctor Childers takes this method of informing the citizens of Augusta and its vicinity, that he has received a supply of the genuine Kine Pock infection, with which he is ready to inoculate.

The efficacy of Vaccination, as a preventative of the Small-Pox, is now so generally known, that it would be superfluous to offer any observation on that head. To those who have not seen the disease, it may be necessary to observe, that it is attended with little or no sickness at all; that it does not hinder attention to business, as before; that it may be taken with the most perfect safety by all ages; in short, that the most loathsome of diseases may be certainly prevented by the mildest of all remedies. To say nothing of the late accounts of its efficacy in preventing the Plague.

Possessing these advantages, Dr. C. rests assured, that it will meet a general reception in this place.

Georgia Republican and State Intelligencer (Savannah)
Savannah, Georgia, Tuesday, Oct. 2, 1804. *Public Notice*
BOARD OF HEALTH, Savannah, Oct. 1, 1804

RESOLVED that the members of this Board will on Tuesday, the first day of November next, proceed through the city to examine all yards, enclosures, and privies, and that public notice will be given in the newspaper.

Extract from the minutes, John H. Harris, Clerk.
September 18.

Georgia Republican and State Intelligencer
Savannah, Tuesday, August 13, 1805 *Public Notice*
A COMMITTEE OF THE GEORGIA MEDICAL SOCIETY appointed to keep correct registers of the births and deaths in Savannah, take this method of notifying the inhabitants that they will go round from time to time, in the wards to which they have been respectfully appointed, for the purpose of collecting the information necessary to carry into effect the intention of the Society; and considering the utility of the measure, it is hoped every person will willingly aid them in the undertaking, and be prepared when called upon, to furnish an account of the births and deaths since the 8th June last (the period it is intended the registers shall take date from) which have come immediately within their knowledge. The Wards have been assigned to the members of the committee for the above purpose, as follows, viz.

Elbert, Liberty to Dr. Henry Bourquin
Oglethorpe, Franklin to Dr. Moses Sheftall
Heathcote & Percival to Dr. Peter Ward
Decker & Darby to Dr. James Ewell
Reynolds & Anson to Dr. William Cocke
Columbia & Greene to Dr. George V. Proctor
Warren & Washington to Dr. William Parker
August 9.

℞ PUBLIC HEALTH, ORGANIZATION, EDUCATION

Augusta Herald

June 4, 1812 — *Advertisement*
Augusta, Georgia

DOCTOR L'HOMME

Informs the citizens of Augusta, that he has received FRESH VACCINE now operating in some healthy children. Those who wish to take advantage of this opportunity for Inoculation (VACCINATION), may apply to him, at Messrs. Bignon & Son. June 4.

Georgia Express

Athens, Georgia — *Public Notice*
August 13, 1812 (Vol. V, No. 2)

VACCINE MATTER

The undersigned having been appointed by the President of the United States, as Agent for Vaccination, hereby gives notice, that genuine VACCINE MATTER will be furnished to any physician or other citizen of the United States who may apply to him for it.

The application must be made by post, and the requisite fee, five dollars, (in the current bank paper of any of the Middle States) forwarded with it. When required such direction how to use it will be furnished with the matter, as will enable any discreet person, who can read and write, to secure his own family from the Small Pox with certainty, without any trouble, danger, or expense. All letters on this subject, to and from the undersigned and not exceeding half an ounce in weight, are carried by the United States mail, free of any charge for postage, in conformity to a late Act of Congress, entitled "An Act To Encourage Vaccination."

(Signed) James Smith, U. S. Agent for Vaccination, Baltimore,
May 27th, 1813.

Augusta Herald

Augusta, Georgia — *News Item from Savannah*
March 14, 1816
Item from Savannah, March 5.

We regret to state, that cases of the small pox have appeared in Savannah, notwithstanding the vigilance of the constituted authorities.

The Council have removed them—but, citizens! be on your guard! To 'make assurance doubly sure', adopt proper measures to oppose the spreading and the ravages of this destructive disease! Vaccination furnishes an infallible means of prevention. There is plenty of the vaccine virus in town. We entreat you to recur promptly to the advise given below.

'Dr. Proctor, the Health Officer for the Port of Savannah, recommends and urges to have families and negroes vaccinated. He calls upon his medical brethren throughout the State to urge every person .... That a person once undergoing it can never have the small-pox is now placed beyond a doubt.'

The Augusta Chronicle

September 19, 1820   Augusta, Georgia
City of Savannah   Post Office, September 14, 1820.

I feel it my duty to announce to my fellow citizens, and to all whom it may concern, that a mortality prevails in this city, never before experienced; and that the character and type of the fever, is of a malignancy which renders it prudent for any person, who can make it convenient, to remove beyond the city's atmosphere.

I feel myself also authorized to say, that the fever which is carrying off our people, is not contagious, and that no apprehension ought to be entertained of its being communicated by persons leaving the city.

                                                             (Signed) T. V. P. Charlton, Mayor.

Augusta Herald

November 23, 1815   Vol. XVII No. 22   Augusta, Georgia

The following periods have been noticed when the Influenza prevailed in North America: 1647, 1655, 1697-98, 1732, 1737, 1747, 1756-57, 1761, 1772, 1781, 1789, and 1790, 1802, 1815. From which it appears that the longest interval has been 43 years, and the shortest interval 4 years, while the average interval is 14 years.

These first steps toward the establishment of health regulations led gradually, over the years, to the creation of sentiment for a state-supported program of public health, as represented by the present Public Health activities under the direction of Dr. T. F. Sellers, who followed Dr. Abercrombie, Dr. Harris, and others as Director.

Dr. T. F. Abercrombie, Director Emeritus of the Georgia Department of Public Health, has given us an excellent record of the development of public health in Georgia from 1733 to 1950 in his *History of Public Health in Georgia.*

It was deemed desirable, however, in addition to Dr. Abercrombie's work, to include in this volume something about public health in the Colony and in the State since it was associated with medicine and pharmacy in that period as well as now.

For a fuller discussion of public health in its early days, as well as its development into an important and integral part of the State Government, the reader is referred to Dr. Abercrombie's volume.

Organization

From the beginning of time, it has been the custom of those whose interests were held in common to band themselves together as an organization for mutual protection and benefit. But where professional groups organize, the matter of self-protection and benefit becomes secondary to their responsibilities to the public, since professional groups are set apart from other groups under a franchise granted to them by the public because of their qualifications in the specialized field in which each functions. In accepting the franchise, these professional groups commit themselves to high ethical standards in their practices, and to function at all times and under all circumstances and conditions in the interest of the public health and welfare.

It is interesting to note that the first step following the setting up of a professional organization is to specify standards of character and professional abilities of those who are to be admitted to the profession and organization, and who would participate in disseminating professional knowledge and practices in the interest not only of the profession but of the public whom they serve.

No doubt these motives prompted those who had come through the Colonial period and the early years of Georgia as a State.

Among the earliest records of any trend toward organization of those who were practicing pharmacy and medicine in the Colony and State, there appears a published notice in the *Augusta Chronicle and Gazette* of December 16, 1797, which is signed by a group of "subscribers and practitioners of physic and surgery," whereby a fee bill is agreed upon and the public is so notified.

Bearing in mind the fact that there were no educational or legal restrictions applying to those who were professional practitioners, some individuals were entering the professions who were prompted by ulterior motives, and were charging a fee for their services which in some instances was either absurdly low or excessively high. This group of "subscribers and practitioners" felt it their responsibility to acquaint the public with what they considered reasonable fees for professional services rendered, there being no anti-trust law to be violated by such an agreement.

This first fee bill of 1797 was to be followed by another in 1818, and still another in 1829. The newspapers of Augusta carried notices of the itemized statement of the fee bills as they were promoted or promulgated by the profession of medicine.

A FEE BILL

Published in *The Augusta Chronicle and Gazette of the State* on January 6, 1798, and dated Augusta, Georgia, December 16, 1797. Published by the subscribers and practitioners of physic and surgery in the Town of Augusta.

(From *Georgia Historical Quarterly,* Vol. XXI, 1937).

Visits per day in town	$ 1.00
Visits per day from bed	3.00
Visits per day in country per mi.	1.00
A call from bed and visit not necessary	1.00
Advice per letter without medicine	5.00
Attendance for 24 hours	10.00
Attendance for 12 hours	5.00
Consultation	5.00
Bolusses (common, per doz)	1.50
Bolusses (anodyne, each)	.50
Bolusses (with musk, each)	1.00
Cathartic	.50
Draught	.50
Emetic	.50
Liniment (per oz.)	.50
Linctus (per pot)	1.00
Lotion (per lb.)	1.00
Mixture (per ½ lb.)	1.00
Mixture (per lb.)	1.50
Ointment (per oz.)	.50
Pills, per dozen	1.00
Powders, per dozen	1.50
Powders, vermifuge, each	.25
Plasters, each	1.00
Tinctures, per ounce	.50
Ingredients for common decoction	.50
Ingredients, bitter (qt.)	1.00
Ingredients, with bark	1.50
Amputating thigh, leg or arm	40.00
Amputation of finger, or toe	10.00
Blood Letting	1.00
Cupping, etc.	2.00
Dressing wound, each time	.25
Extracting a tooth	1.00
Extirpating polypus	10.00
Introducing catheter, first	5.00
Introducing catheter, each	2.00
Inserting issue	1.00
Opening abscess and dressing	1.00
Reducing fracture of thigh, leg or palm	20.00
Jaw	5.00
Operation for aneurism	40.00
Operation for cataract	40.00
Operation for fistula	20.00
Operation for hernia	40.00
Operation for hydroceli	20.00
Operation for trepan	40.00
Cases in midwifery	30.00

All other charges in same proportion

(Signed by Cornelius Dysart, John H. Montgomery, Dennis Smelt, George Graves, John Murray, William Brazier.)

☞ The rapid diminution in the comparitive value of money, has rendered it necessary that the Physicians of Augusta, should, in justice to themselves, again revise their Charges for Medical Services. At a meeting held for this purpose, they have adopted the following Prices, to take effect from the first day of July next:—

	D. C. to D. C.	
Visiting each day		2
Ditto from bed		5
A call from bed without visit		2
Mileage in the country, by day		1
Do. do. after dark		2
Advice by letter	5	10
Do. oral	1	5
Consultation		10
Attendance by desire of patient, per hour		2
Bleeding		1
Cupping		2
Extracting tooth	1	2
Lancing gum		1
Cutting frænum linguæ		1
Scarifying eye		2
Do. tonsil		5
Opening abscess	1	5
Dressing wound or ulcer	1	5
Introducing seton or issue		2
Do. bougie or catheter	2	10
Cases of gonorrhœa	10	50
Do. syphilis	50	100
Paracentisis of abdomen		10
Do. of thorax		20
Reducing luxation of thigh	20	50
Do. other luxations	10	30
Do. fractures	20	50
Do. hernia by taxis	5	20
Operation for hernia	50	100
Do. hydrocele		20
Do. polypus	10	20
Do. hair lip	10	30
Do. cataract		80
Do. trichiasis		30
Do. pterygium	10	30
Do. fistula lachrymalis		20
Do. do. in ano	20	50
Do. trepan	40	50
Do. aneurism	20	80
Do. Lithotomy		100
Amputation thigh, leg or arm		50
Do. finger or toe		15
Extirpating female mamma	30	50
Obstetric cases	30	50
Cathartic, emetic & draught each		50
Boluses com. each		25
Do. Anodyne each		50
Do. musk each		1
Pills per dozen		1
Powders per dozen		1 50
Do. vermifuge and alterative each		25
Tinctures per oz.	50	1
Linctus per oz.		50
Liniment per oz.		25
Mixture per ½lb.		1
Ditto per lb.		1 50
Lotion per lb.		1
Ingredients for decoction	50	2
Ointment per oz.	25	1
Plasters each	1	3

Vaccination to be without charge.

D. Smelt,
A. Watkins,
J. G. M'Whorter,
T. H. M. Fendall,
J. B. Cumming, M. D.
Carter, M. D.
A. Cunningham, M. D.
M. Galphin, M. D.
W. T. Young, M. D.
E. Brux,
J. Dent.

June 5   r3t   97

AUGUSTA FEE BILL
Augusta Herald, Augusta, Georgia, June 26, 1818

FEE BILL IN BY-LAWS OF MEDICAL SOCIETY OF AUGUSTA, 1829

For each visit during day .. $ 1.00	Extirpating a polypus 5.00 to 25.00
For each visit from dark until 9 P.M. 2.00	Extirpating tumours . 5.00 to 50.00
For each visit during the day in inclement weather 4.00	Extirpating female mamma ...... 50.00 to 100.00
For each visit from dark until 9 P.M. in inclement weather 4.00	Extirpating other parts .... 5.00 to 50.00
	Reducing fracture of the nose .... 5.00 to 10.00
For each visit after 9 P.M. in inclement weather ... 6.00	Reducing fracture of lower jaw ...... 10.00 to 20.00
For oral advice ..... 1.00 to 4.00	A clavicle .... 10.00 to 20.00
For written advice.. 5.00 to 10.00	Scapula .... 10.00 to 20.00
Each prescription 1.00	Ribs .... 5.00 to 10.00
Each consultation 5.00	Arms .... 10.00 to 20.00
Remaining in town per day by desire 10.00	Hands .... 5.00 to 10.00
	Thigh .... 25.00 to 50.00
Attendance per hour by desire 2.00	Patella .... 10.00 to 30.00
	Reducing a fracture of leg .... 20.00 to 40.00
Each mile under 11 during day 1.00	Reducing a fracture of foot .... 5.00 to 10.00
Any distance over 5 miles, charges to be discussionary	Reducing other fractures .... 5.00 to 20.00
For each mile under 11 at night 2.00	For reducing a dislocation of lower jaw 10.00
For each mile during day in inclement weather 2.00	For clavicle .... 10.00 to 20.00
	For shoulder ...... 10.00 to 30.00
For each mile at night in inclement weather 4.00	For elbow joint .... 10.00 to 20.00
	For wrist or fingers . 5.00 to 10.00
Extracting a tooth 1.00	For hip joint ...... 20.00 to 50.00
Venesection 1.00	For patella 10.00
Introducing catheter or Bougie 5.00	For ankle or foot .. 10.00 to 30.00
	Other dislocations .. 5.00 to 30.00
Opening an abscess ... 1.00 to 2.00	Amputation at hip joint ... 100.00
For Cupping .... 3.00 to 5.00	Amputating thigh or leg .... 25.00 to 50.00
For introducing a seton or issue .... 1.00 to 2.00	Amputating shoulder joint .... 50.00 to 100.00
A pessary .... 2.00 to 5.00	
For scarifying ...... 1.00 to 5.00	Amputating arm or forearm .... 20.00 to 40.00
Removing foreign bodies from esophagus ... 2.00 to 10.00	Other amputations .. 5.00 to 25.00
Dressing wound, each time .... 1.00 to 10.00	Reducing a hernia (taxis) .... 5.00 to 20.00
Dressing ulcers ...... 1.00 to 5.00	

℞ PUBLIC HEALTH, ORGANIZATION, EDUCATION 137

Reducing hernia (operation) .... 25.00 to 50.00
Trepanning skull .. 20.00 to 50.00
Trepanning other bones .... 10.00 to 20.00
Operating for entrossium .... 5.00 to 10.00
Operating for ptygerium .... 5.00 to 10.00
Operating for fistula lachrymalis 25.00
Operating for cataract .... 20.00 to 50.00
Operating for harelip 10.00 to 20.00
Operating for aneurism ...... 10.00 to 100.00
Operating for hydrocele .... 5.00 to 20.00
Operating for fistula in perineo .... 10.00 to 20.00
Operating for fistula in ano .... 10.00 to 20.00
Performing lithotomy .... 100.00 to 200.00
Puncturing bladder . 10.00 to 30.00
Paracentisis thoracis .... 10.00 to 25.00
Paracentisis abdomenis ...... 10.00 to 20.00
Attending case nat. labor .... 10.00 to 20.00
Attending case preternat. labor .... 30.00 to 100.00
Removing the placenta alone .... 5.00 to 15.00
Charges for services not specified in the foregoing to be discussionary.

There are some interesting points concerning these fee bills. First, in the item of 1797, the fees themselves were low in comparison to the fees of the present era. Advice by letter, but without medicine, cost a fee of $5.00. Noteworthy is the fact that frequently a physician was called upon to spend 12 hours, or at times an entire 24 hours, with a patient, due to the fact that there were no hospitals and there were no nurses available. Thus the physician had to take the place of the nurse.

Second, if the physician was called into consultation; that is, with other physicians, the fee was $5.00.

Third, the item "boluses." A "bolus" is a large pill. In 1797 there were no manufactured pills available for use, but pills were made up extemporaneously. As the items here indicate, a common "bolus" was usually a laxative; but if the "bolus" contained morphine or opium, it was supposed to be a stimulant and somewhat of an aphrodisiac.

Fourth, the item "linctus." The term is applied to very thick viscous liquids, too near the consistency of jelly to be poured, and intended to be licked from the spoon rather than swallowed as a body.

Fifth, the item "plaisters" or "plasters." Plasters were extensively used, not only at this time but for many years thereafter, to get the external effect of certain drugs, as well as to provide for the absorption of certain drugs by way of the skin. These plasters were made extemporaneously in the drug store or doctor's office of that time.

Sixth, "amputation of thigh or leg" or other "amputation." The fee was very low, and it must be borne in mind that this operation was done without anaesthesia, since there was no such thing known at that time.

Seventh, the item "extracting a tooth." The charge was $1.00. There was no general practice of dentistry during this period, and the physician frequently was called upon to extract a tooth when the layman was not equipped for this operation.

Next, looking at the fee bill of June 26, 1818, in the *Augusta Herald,* shown in illustrations p. 135: The explanation for the advancing fees is interesting, particularly at this time when, 140 years later, the same argument is used for advances in professional fees and for medicinal agents as was given in these fee bills. The item of 1818 refers to "the rapid diminution in the comparative value of money," which is something about which we hear quite a bit nowadays.*

These fees which came about in 1818 were almost double the fees that applied in 1797, a period of 21 years having elapsed between the publication of the two bills. Here again, the physician was doing dental work and also nursing work, as well as selling pharmaceuticals in the form of cathartics, emetics, boluses, pills, powders, vermifuges, tinctures, linctus, liniments, mixtures, lotions, et cetera, and ointments and plasters.

The fee bill of 1829 is published after an interval of 11 years. It is interesting to note that the fees were reduced approximately to what the fees had been in 1797. A startling and very interesting observation is the fact that in this fee bill of 1829 there are no charges listed for medicines of any kind. This might indicate that a separation between medicine and pharmacy existed at that time, or was contemplated.

But even so, a complete separation into their specialized fields of pharmacy and medicine, though contemplated at that time, has never been consummated, for there are still some physicians who dispense their own drugs, and some pharmacists who recommend drugs to patients. Neither practice is in the interest of the health and welfare of the public. If the public is to be best served, a complete and permanent and distinct separation of the two professions into their specialized fields must be consummated and enforced. Especially is this desirable since specialization in the

*Another example of devaluation is shown in a Fee Bill published in 1865. See Appendix 6, page 438.

present era is an absolute necessity, not only in medicine in its varied branches, but in pharmacy and dentistry and other health professions as well. With expanding knowledge of scientific matters, it is inconceivable that any one individual or any one group of individuals, whether physicians, pharmacists, dentists, or others, could know all that is to be known about the identification, the manufacture, the uses of medicines, or the treatment of diseases or of surgical practices, even though it was of necessity attempted in the early years of the Colony and State.

A step which gradually led to the establishment of a statewide medical association occurred in Savannah in 1804, when the medical practitioners of that city organized and incorporated themselves under a local law. The organization was known as a "medical board of examiners," who were to concern themselves with the qualifications of those who were to enter the practice of medicine and/or pharmacy.

This local law specified the qualifications and the necessity for licensure of those who were to practice medicine or to dispense medicines. A severe penalty was applied to those who practiced any phase of medicine without due license given by the medical examining board.

In 1822 a similar organization to the Savannah body was created in Augusta, Georgia. It was known as the Medical Society of Augusta. As was true of the Savannah group, this local law placed in the hands of the Medical Society responsibility for granting licenses to practice medicine, and for enforcing regulations having to do with the control of epidemic diseases. The names and officers and members of this Augusta Medical Society were as follows: Dr. Anderson Watkins, President; Dr. Alexander Cunningham, Vice-President; Dr. Milton Antony, Dr. T. J. Wray, Dr. W. T. Young, Dr. William Savage, Dr. John Dent, Dr. P. B. Thompson, and Dr. Thomas N. Fendall.

In 1825 the Legislature adopted a law which set up ways and means for creating a Medical Board of Examiners on a statewide basis, whose responsibility it was to examine applicants for license to practice pharmacy or medicine, and to require examination before said Board.

About 1835 a statewide medical society was organized under the name, "Central Medical Society of Georgia," which was chartered in 1836 under the name, the "Georgia Medical Society." This was the organization which no doubt constituted the nucleus for the creation of the Medical Association of Georgia, which came in 1849.

A summary of the professional health organizations of Georgia, especially as to the date of organization, is given below:

    1849   The Medical Association of Georgia organized
    1859   The Georgia State Dental Society created
    1875   The Georgia Pharmaceutical Association organized
    1907   The Georgia State Nurses Association organized
    1929   The Georgia Hospital Association organized

The professional health organization, acting under its ethical responsibilities, must concern itself not only with the immediate problems which confront the profession but also with plans for expanding, perfecting and extending the activities of the organization in its future operations and functions. These responsibilities include plans for education and legislation.

Education, general as well as technical, was and is accepted by professional health organizations as a primary objective in establishing professional status and standards, as witnessed by the establishment of the first medical college in Georgia in 1828, which followed the formation of the Medical Society of Augusta which had come about in 1822. It was the hope and plan of the Medical Society that training in this medical college would supersede or replace the preceptorship-apprenticeship system which had been the only training medium for physicians up to that time. This system of training had operated through the years without any formal or basic educational requirement, because little or none was available.

Over the years other medical schools were organized in Georgia. Two of these (rather short-lived) were in Savannah, one in Atlanta (which eventually became divided into two schools, both of which were later to be merged and absorbed by Emory University), and one "Botanic" or "Thomsonian" school organized in Forsyth and later moved to Macon.

The standards for medical education have been gradually raised, with the result that today the two medical colleges in Georgia are comparable in quality to any in the United States.

The Georgia State Dental Society was first organized in 1859; but, due to the interruption caused by the Civil War, ten years elapsed before a permanent organization was effected. In 1869 the Georgia State Dental Society came into existence.

Though dentists, like other professional health groups, were aware of the need for educational advantages, both general and technical, for their practitioners, it was not until 1891 that the Southern Dental College was established in the State—a college which for many years operated as a proprietary and independent school, but which later was absorbed by Emory University.

For further details concerning professional education, the reader may see Supplement A of the present volume.

The Georgia Pharmaceutical Association was organized in 1875. It must be borne in mind, however, that pharmacy as a profession was practiced in some form from the beginning of the Colony in 1733 and from the day when Dr. Samuel Nunez opened and operated what came to be the first apothecary shop in Georgia, located in Savannah. But in those early days pharmacy came under domination of medical practitioners who were also practicing pharmacy, and this domination by the medical practitioners was to continue until 1875 when the Georgia Pharmaceutical Association came into existence.

The preceptorship-apprenticeship method of training pharmacists was for at least 100 years to be the accepted practice. But when pharmacists began to recognize the value of education in its broadest sense, this preceptor-apprentice method seemed to be unbreakable as a system, for it was not until 1933 that a college diploma became the legal requirement for license to practice pharmacy in Georgia.

For several years prior to the college requirement for licensure, there were four schools of pharmacy and one or more "Quiz" schools in operation in the State. All of these schools, with the exception of the Southern College of Pharmacy in Atlanta and the College of Pharmacy of the University of Georgia at Athens, have ceased to exist. But, like medical education in the State, pharmaceutical education is now on a high level of quality, comparable in character to pharmaceutical education in any other state.

For a fuller discussion of pharmaceutical education the reader is referred to Supplement B of this volume.

The Georgia State Nurses Association was organized in 1907, but prior to that time there were several hospitals in the State which offered training for nurses on a preceptorship basis. The educational requirements for license to practice nursing have risen from time to time and are comparable in character to those of the other health professions.

LEGISLATION AFFECTING PROFESSIONAL HEALTH ORGANIZATIONS

In addition to the responsibility of setting up proper educational requirements, professional health organizations have the added responsibility of establishing proper laws to govern professional activities, and to provide for the enforcement of these laws. Such laws are in the interest of and for the safeguarding of the public health and welfare, and not for purposes of creating a monopoly.

The professional groups of pharmacy, medicine, dentistry, and nursing in Georgia have every reason to be proud of the laws which they have been instrumental in placing on the statute books of the State.

In many instances our Georgia laws represent pioneering, particularly in the matter of narcotics and other dangerous drugs; and in all instances they compare favorably with the laws of the other states governing the practices of professional health organizations.

Supplement C of this volume gives a chronological synopsis of all the Georgia laws from 1820 to 1958 which have to do with the organization and practices of our professional health organizations.

THE GEORGIA PHARMACEUTICAL ASSOCIATION

The reader must visualize the vast changes which had come into the State from the early days of 1733, with the expanding knowledge of medicine and pharmacy, and with the introduction of many diseases which were not previously known in the Colony, which, with the ever-increasing population, multiplied rapidly the health problems of the State.

In the interest of the public's welfare it was recognized by all groups of professional people that a higher and still higher degree of specialization was necessary. There was a growing tendency on the part of those who had been practicing medicine and pharmacy, or practicing pharmacy and medicine, to separate their activities into the respective fields.

In 1852 the American Pharmaceutical Association had been formed in Philadelphia, and a number of outstanding Georgia pharmacists (some of whom were physicians as well) became members of the Association. Prominent among these people was Dr. Robert Battey, of Rome, who was a pharmacist as well as

PUBLIC HEALTH, ORGANIZATION, EDUCATION

a physician of international fame. Among those who joined Dr. Battey in membership in the American Pharmaceutical Association in the early days of its life were Dr. John S. Pemberton, of Columbus and Atlanta, (later to become famous as the originator of Coca-Cola), and John M. Clarke, of Milledgeville, (who was to become the first President of the Georgia Pharmaceutical Association). This group of Georgia pharmacists who were active in the national organization were responsible for developing a sentiment in Georgia for a state pharmaceutical association.

Dr. Battey served as Third Vice-President of the American Pharmaceutical Association in 1856, and was likewise the first Georgia pharmacist to serve as an official of that Association. He reported at this third annual meeting of the Association, "Pharmacy in Georgia is in a sad state; in Rome and Floyd County there are 21 places selling drugs, only two of which are served by licensed pharmacists; 'quackery' in Western Georgia is on the increase; in the cities and the State physicians are gradually discontinuing the practice of dispensing drugs; and there are 127 drug stores in the State." How this figure was determined Dr. Battey does not state, and this seems to be the only instance up to that time where the number of drug stores is referred to during a long period.

During the late '50s and during the early '60s Dr. Battey, Mr. Clarke, and Mr. Pemberton were joined in membership in the A.Ph.A. by various other Georgians whose names are familiar: A. A. Solomons; W. W. Solomons; W. H. Warner of Rome; J.D.W. Nowlin, Rome; Fleming Grieve, Milledgeville; J. A. Taylor; W. A. Langsdale; Robt. A. Massey; D. M. Smith—all of Atlanta; J. Henry Zeilin, Macon; R. H. Land, Augusta. In the year 1860 Mr. Theodore Schuman, of Atlanta, was added, and his name proved to be that of the last Georgian to join the American Pharmaceutical Association prior to the Civil War. During the Civil War period there were no additional members from the State.

However, following the War, in 1869 and during the early '70s, William A. Cotting of Milledgeville, and J. B. Huddart of Macon, and John B. Daniel of Atlanta, were added. Frederick F. Peacock, of Atlanta; and Leonard W. Hunt, of Macon; and Frederick S. Mason, of Rome, joined in the late '70s; and somewhat later Foster S. Chapman joined the others, as well as Homer S. Tarrant, both of Augusta. W. A. Taylor, of Atlanta, and John Ingalls, of Macon, followed.

Well into the 70's physicians were still controlling the issuance of license to pharmacists, and most of the physicians themselves were practicing pharmacy. At this time a discussion arose in the State over some incidents having to do with poisons. The physicians and the Board of Health were considering introducing in the Legislature a Bill to be known as a Poison Law. This seemed to be the focal point around which the druggists of Georgia might rally to form an association, for it was their contention that since the law affected the sale of poisons in the drug stores of the State, the druggists themselves should have some voice in the choice of the items named to go into the Poison Law, and the framing of the Law.

Promptly thereafter, a group of pharmacists got together, in the summer of 1875, and sent out from Atlanta a notice to the druggists throughout Georgia. This notice was signed by Fred King of Atlanta, L. W. Hunt of Macon, and perhaps others. The notice was published in the *Atlanta Herald* and *The Macon Telegraph*, as well as in two or three journals, the medical journals and others, to the effect that the druggists of the State were to assemble in Macon on October 20, 1875 "to consider the organization of a pharmaceutical association, binding each other with closer ties of friendship and to promote interest in the junior members of the fraternity and exciting the spirit of emulation and ambition; the interchange and dissemination of scientific researches; the framing of laws to be enacted that will result not only in the protection of the profession but the public in general."

This notice just referred to was carried by the newspapers without charge, due to the fact that the formation of this association was considered of sufficient importance to justify any publicity that might be obtained through the columns of the newspapers. The railroads of the State had agreed to give reduced rates from any point in the State to Macon to any of those who might attend this meeting.

As a result of this notice—no doubt aided and abetted by letters and by personal contact—the meeting was held in Macon in Freeman's Hall at eight o'clock on the evening of the twentieth of October, 1875. At least 20 druggists of the State were reported as being present for that first meeting. Unfortunately, no minutes were kept of this meeting, but it did develop that some of the persons present did retain and publish some of the facts.

℞ PUBLIC HEALTH, ORGANIZATION, EDUCATION

John M. Clarke, of Milledgeville, was called to the Chair; and Fred King, of Atlanta, was requested to act as Secretary. The list of officers chosen to head the Association included the following: John M. Clarke, Milledgeville, President; John Ingalls, Macon, First Vice-President; Theodore Schuman, Atlanta, Second Vice-President; J. R. Jaynes, Dalton, Third Vice-President; Fred King, Atlanta, Secretary; L. W. Hunt, Macon, Treasurer.

Indicating an interest in pharmaceutical organization on the part of the medical profession and the State Board of Health, Dr. C. D. Nottingham, of Macon, a member of the State Board of Health, appeared before the body and offered the cooperation of the Board of Health in all matters affecting the welfare of the pharmacists of the State, particularly in the matter of legislation. At the moment, deliberations in the body were concerned with the matter of poisons. Dr. Nottingham congratulated the Association and prophesied a vast field of benefits for the profession of medicine and of pharmacy in their broader sense by such a move. (Author's Note: It was approximately 60 years following this first meeting, and this offer of cooperation between the Board of Health and the Pharmaceutical Association, before pharmacists were placed on the State Board of Health as full-fledged members.)

Following the withdrawal of Dr. Nottingham, a committee of three physicians of the Macon Medical Society appeared, and through their chairman expressed a desire "to cooperate with the Association in the accomplishment of any work for the procurement of any laws that would redound to the future benefit of medicine and pharmacy."

A Constitution was adopted at this first meeting which seems to be a copy of the Constitution of the Tennessee Pharmaceutical Association. One of the objectives expressed in the Constitution was the bringing together of "the reputable druggists of the State" in an Association in the interests of the profession at large, specifying that every druggist and apothecary of good moral and professional standing whether in business, or in retirement from business, or employed by another, and the teachers of pharmacy, chemistry, materia medica, and botany, who may be professors in any college of pharmacy, should constitute the membership of this Association.

At the First Annual Meeting following the organizational meeting, in 1876, it was specified that the Georgia Association would always be represented by delegates to the American

Pharmaceutical Association, in recognition of their appreciation of the national body. The first delegates named from the Georgia Association were John Ingalls, John M. Clarke, and Fred King.

At the Second Annual Meeting of the Association, held in Atlanta, in 1877, President L. W. Hunt gave the following figures: "Georgia has over 300 druggists and apothecaries, and out of this number, 112 were licensed October, 1874, with the license fee being $25.00." No explanation is given of this statement, but it is supposed that licensure of pharmacists by the Medical Board had been somewhat careless. It is then supposed that in 1874 all those individuals who were practicing pharmacy or could secure a license on application must have done so. Just who secured License Number 1 has been a matter of controversy in Georgia for a number of years. The two claimants to this honor were Mr. George S. Vardeman, of Sparta, and Mr. John Polhill, of Louisville.

At this Second Annual Meeting it was reported that 88 pharmacists of Georgia were now dues-paid members of this Association. This included a number of physicians who were practicing pharmacy as well as medicine. This list will appear as a part of the Supplement previously referred to. It represented a very distinguished group of Georgia pharmacists, the names of many of them being intimately and definitely associated with the steps that were taken at that time tending towards modern pharmacy, particularly as regards the laws having to do with the practice of pharmacy. Most, or perhaps all, of these men who were physically fit had passed through the Civil War and the tragic era of the Reconstruction days which followed, and were therefore mature in years, in thinking, and in experience, and had had some contact with the outside world beyond the State of Georgia as far as pharmaceutical matters were concerned.

The Poison Law previously referred to had been agreed upon and was introduced in the Legislature in 1876. With the support that was given it by the physicians, the State Board of Health, and the pharmacists of the State, the Law was enacted, and it has remained as originally introduced, with only minor amendments through the years.

Several of those individuals mentioned in the above list were to be recognized nationally. Among them was John Ingalls, of Macon, who was to be President of the American Pharmaceutical Association in 1884, the first Georgian to be so honored.

It is extremely fortunate that Dr. Henry R. Slack was active in the State at that time. He it was who, acting in his capacity as Secretary of the Georgia Pharmaceutical Association for a number of years, began the preservation and publication of any Minutes taken of the Proceedings of the Association during those years.

But, unfortunately, the publication of Minutes of the annual meetings was not uniform over a period of years, and at times there have been skips of some ten or fifteen years. A few copies have been collected here and there in these cases, and, fortunately, these are preserved in the Archives of the Library of the University of Georgia. It is from these sources that any historical data concerning the Georgia Pharmaceutical Association has come.

It was the custom in 1877 that on most important occasions someone was selected to be "Orator of the Day." Mr. T. A. Cheatham was chosen to be "Orator of the Day" at this Second Annual Meeting of the Georgia Association. His main stress in the course of his oration was an argument for educational standards for the practice of pharmacy. But it was thirty years after this oration before any real step was actually taken for establishing reasonable, or even any, educational requirements for licensure. He paid due respect to the apprenticeship system, which had prevailed, and which had proved of value in the training of young pharmacists. He argued that in the event the apprenticeship system continued for any additional length of time, it, too, would have to be standardized and safeguarded.

This argument of Dr. Cheatham was, so far as the records advise us, the first step taken toward introducing a program of education for pharmacists in Georgia. However, in 1880 a committee of the Association authorized to draw up the proposed Pharmacy Act reported progress, and in 1881 this Law was enacted giving us the first real Pharmacy Law sponsored entirely by the pharmacists of the State. In this Act of the General Assembly a Board of "Pharmaceutic Examiners" was established. This basic law, amended many times, is still on the statute books of Georgia.

On December 17, 1881, this new "Board of Pharmaceutic Examiners" held its first meeting, and the following presented themselves for examination: T. D. Dodson, Columbus; M. G. Little and T. C. Jones, Albany; C. O. Tyner, Atlanta; B. P. Reed, Savannah; R. P. Johnson, Smithville; B. E. Roughton, Sandersville; J. E. Jones, Fort Valley; J. H. Harper, Covington.

The Minutes of this first Board Meeting indicate that some of those applying for license failed the examination but were given a temporary license, good until the next meeting of the Board, when they were to take a re-examination. Also at this first Board Meeting, honorary licenses were issued to the following gentlemen: W. A. Taylor, Atlanta; W. W. Lincoln, Savannah; A. A. Solomons, Savannah; Wm. Rook, Marietta. All of these men had previously been licensed by the Medical Board of Examiners.

At the Ninth Annual Meeting of the Georgia Pharmaceutical Association held in Macon, April, 1884, President J. W. Rankin of the Association made some significant comments in which he used the following expressions: "Our Pharmacy Law, as far as I know, or have heard, is operating very well. It is a good law as far as it goes, and it is probably as desirable as any we could hope to obtain. It has protected the public in a large degree from incompetent or careless compounding of prescriptions, and has limited the sale of poisons to legitimate pharmacists."

He is critical of the fact that, "strange to say, the greatest and most determined opposition to a better pharmacy law came from a quarter which was least expected; namely, the medical profession," but he states that this must have been due to a total misapprehension of the purposes of the law. He argues further that sooner or later, in his opinion, the people will see the need for more stringent laws regulating the practice of pharmacy, and laws to prevent the "adulteration" of drugs, ("particularly in the cities"), and that when that time comes a statute will be enacted which will not only protect the public but will elevate and dignify pharmacy.

Mr. Rankin was one of those people who at that time were fighting the Revenue Tax on Alcohol. He makes this statement, "The whole revenue system is oppressive to the poor, unjust to the druggist, and not necessary to the support of the Government."

At the time Mr. Rankin was speaking, alcohol was selling for approximately two dollars ($2.00) a gallon, including the Government tax, the tax being $1.50 per gallon for 95% alcohol. It is interesting to speculate what Mr. Rankin's opinion would have been if he could have known that in 1959 the price of alcohol had risen to around $30.00 per gallon, even though the cost of the manufacture of the alcohol in 1959 is approximately the same as in 1884.

℞ PUBLIC HEALTH, ORGANIZATION, EDUCATION

At this same meeting in 1884, Mr. N. I. Brunner, of Macon, is critical of the fact that so many of the pharmacists are buying ready-made products rather than manufacture them in their own places of business. He argues that to save the profession the pharmacist must learn to manufacture his own products, including many chemicals.

The age-old problem of price-cutting was brought up for discussion and bitterly condemned by the Association as being not only unwise from an economic standpoint but unprofessional and unethical. Certain members were driven out of the Association on account of the fact that they followed the practice of the cutting of prices.

At the meeting of the Association in 1885 Dr. R. H. Land, of Augusta, presented a paper on the subject, "What Plants Indigenous to Our State Can Be Gathered or Cultivated Profitably"? He makes the statement that "in our gardens the mints all grow luxuriantly, as do hops, belladonna, hyoscyamus, digitalis, chamomile, ricinus, and a thousand other useful plants which it would take too much time to enumerate." He states that there is not an acre of land in Georgia which would not produce some plant of medicinal value, and he lists a large number of plants which have been identified as growing in Georgia.

In 1885 the terms "disinfectant" and "antiseptic" were comparatively new, and Mr. Butler of Savannah discusses the meaning of those words when he states: "Disinfection means any process by which the contagium of any given disease may be destroyed, or be rendered inert." He cautions against the confounding of the term "disinfectant" and the term "deodorant." He states further: "Antiseptics are 'fatal to the growth and multiplication of microzymes.'"

Mr. W. A. Loyless takes a shot at price-cutting when he says: "The price-cutter is a wrecker who is both unwilling to make a fair, legitimate profit himself and determined no one else shall."

At this meeting in 1885 a committee on legislation was instructed to use cooperation with the National Wholesale Druggists Association in an effort to repeal the Internal Revenue Tax on alcohol for the use of druggists.

For the first time there appears on record a discussion of the sale of medicines by general merchants, who are not only selling medicines but in some instances are also compounding medicines without a license. The Board of Pharmacy is directed to prosecute such violators.

At the 1885 meeting Mr. R. H. Land puts into words his picture of what pharmacy is or should be when he states the following: "Pharmacy embraces much that is good, much that is true, and much that is beautiful. In its everyday relations to the community in which we live it brings us in contact with human nature in every phase; in its scientific relations it unfolds the wonders of botany, chemistry, and mineralogy, and the kindred sciences, as well as the laws of physics. As an art or practice either in preparing, compounding, or preserving substances for the purposes of medicine, it brings to light the simple arrangements and the grand results that arise from the union and disunion of nature's own trades and treasures."

At the 1886 meeting the President complains about the "seduction of the average physician who is induced to prescribe ready-made prescriptions."

The Secretary of the Association read a paper on the subject, "Is a Mixture of Nitric and Carbolic Acid Explosive?" It must not have taken him long to find the answer to this question! He said that it "is equal in violence or exceeds that caused by mixing iodine and turpentine."

At this meeting in 1886 Dr. J. S. Pemberton (who was later to evolve the formula for Coca-Cola) read an "Essay on Guarana, Caffeine, and Coca."

At the 1887 meeting of the Association the President was very critical of the fact that incompetent persons in many instances were operating drug stores who were not licensed, but depended for the operation of their store on some licensed person who, as he said, sometimes was a "broken-down physician" who had gotten a license to practice pharmacy simply because the law at that time stated that anyone with a medical license could secure a license to practice pharmacy without examination, and who could not by any stretch of the imagination pass the rigid examination given by the Pharmaceutic Examining Board. He was critical also of the ownership of drug stores by a non-licensed pharmacist.

At the meeting in 1887 a very important matter was discussed. It appears that prior to that time appointment to the State Board of Pharmaceutic Examiners was left entirely to the Governor. This soon developed into a political setup, and at this meeting it was proposed that a law should be drafted stating that the names for membership should be persons recommended to the Governor by the Association, so as to remove as far as possible the political influences in these appointments.

℞ PUBLIC HEALTH, ORGANIZATION, EDUCATION

Bearing in mind that prior to this time there had been no educational requirements whatever for the practice of pharmacy in Georgia, a proposal was now offered to locate a school of pharmacy supported by the State at the Georgia School of Technology in Atlanta, which had just then been established and activated.

At the Thirteenth Annual Meeting in 1888 President Case made some terse remarks in which he stated: "Thirteen years ago our profession was bound tight and fast to the doctors. Every sensible person knows, or ought to know, that the two are separate and distinct professions. Formerly, a druggist license was to be obtained in Georgia only from the Medical Examining Board. We had no professional recognition at that time, while today we have our own Board of Pharmacy. With no pharmacy school in our midst with which to gauge a respectable professional standard, our pharmacy board was a necessity, and is now no longer an appendage to the medical profession."

The names of the Board of Pharmacy (whose names were submitted to the Governor by the Pharmaceutical Association, constituting the first all-pharmacy Board) were the following: Theo Schuman, Atlanta; J. W. Goodwyn; S. C. Durban, Augusta; George D. Case, Milledgeville; and Henry R. Slack, LaGrange. This Board was appointed by "His Excellency, Governor John B. Gordon, November 12, 1887."

President Case argued that a well-organized and well-conducted educational program for the pharmacists of Georgia would constitute an answer to many of their problems. This appears to have been the first time that the possibility of introducing education as a requirement for the practice of pharmacy in the State was really put forward.

In 1889 it is pointed out that there was a Bill in the Legislature to incorporate the Georgia Pharmaceutical Association, and that as a corporate body it might achieve some objectives that were not attainable otherwise.

In this same year an important step was taken to provide that the Board of Pharmacy members should have their terms arranged on a staggered basis, so as to have a nucleus of men of experience on the Board at all times. It was also proposed that the terms should run as follows: One should serve for a period of one year, one for two years, one for three years, one for four, and one for five. Thereafter, the term of one of them only should expire each year. For the first time this year it was proposed that samples of drugs for analysis by the state chemist should be taken up, to determine the matter of adulteration or of low standards.

It was reported in 1889 by Secretary Slack that there were now "440 drug stores in operation in Georgia, and 600 licensed pharmacists."

It was pointed out at this meeting that a very peculiar legal situation had arisen. The Attorney-General of the State had claimed that a man could not be prosecuted for selling adulterated drugs, as it was not a penal offense, but that the charge would have to be brought for "cheating and swindling." The person against whom the adulteration charge was brought was an active member of the Association at the time, but he was expelled from the Association on such a charge.

At the 1891 meeting, President Durban is very critical of the fact that physicians are still allowed to obtain license without examination. He argues that, "They have none of the heritage of pharmacy." Further, he states that "it is a gross injustice for the public as well as for the bona fide pharmaceutically trained people." He points out that as a matter of record it has been found that in a number of instances physicians had found it simpler and more economical to go and get a degree in medicine than it was to prepare themselves to take the rigid examination for the Board of Pharmacy. On graduation from a medical school, physicians would automatically be issued license to practice pharmacy.

The year 1891 marked the first establishment of a school of pharmacy in this State. The Atlanta College of Medicine had instituted a college of pharmacy under the Deanship of Dr. George F. Payne, who in addition to the deanship and teaching duties was State Chemist and also a newly elected member of the State Board of Pharmacy.

It was also pointed out at this 1891 meeting that the Law had been changed now to the extent that physicians no longer would be granted license to practice pharmacy simply on the basis of graduation from a medical college or on the basis of a license to practice medicine. But a physician desiring to practice pharmacy would be required to take the Pharmacy State Board examination. In order to avoid any confusion or controversy that might occur, however, the Law stated that any physician who had been graduated prior to 1887 and could prove continuous practice for five years was entitled to registration as a pharmacist without examination.

℞ PUBLIC HEALTH, ORGANIZATION, EDUCATION

The period 1892 to 1903 appears to be one of those periods when no Proceedings of the Georgia Pharmaceutical Association were published, or, if so, no record of their existence can be found at the present time.

At the 1903 meeting, President Polhill congratulates the pharmacists of the State, noting the pharmaceutical advance in education. In that year the Southern College of Pharmacy was organized, and Mercer University and the University of Georgia announced the addition of Schools of Pharmacy. These three new schools were in addition to the Atlanta College of Pharmacy, which had been in existence since 1891.

It is interesting to point out that as late as 1903, and for some years thereafter, the State Board of Pharmacy issued three types of license based on various grades made by the applicants on examination. The lowest grade was given a druggist license (which involved an average of 75), the next highest grade was given an apothecary's license (85), and the highest grade was given a pharmacist's license (90 and above). These differentiations were honorary in character only, meaning that all or any of them carried the same rights and privileges under the law as licensed persons.

In 1904, attention is called to the fact that for the first time in Georgia's history Negroes were granted licenses to practice pharmacy.

At the 1906 meeting, attention is called to the fact that even though there is a good pharmacy law, there are no efficient enforcement regulations possible under this law, and in order to perfect this law in service to the people of the State, a Drug Inspector is necessary. His duties would be to inspect every drug store in the State at least once a year.

It is interesting to note that at this meeting in 1906 Mr. Thad Rice, former practicing pharmacist but now associated with the Southern Bell Telephone Company, "announces that free long-distance service from the long-distance lines of the Company, before 10:00 o'clock in the morning and after 4:00 o'clock in the afternoon, will be provided for those attending the meeting, but that the calls may be made from the Kimball House booth only."

In 1907 the Georgia Pharmaceutical Association introduced in the Legislature a Bill to control the sale of Opium and its products along with all other narcotics, holding that the indiscriminate use and sale of these items was growing in Georgia, and that they should be placed under the restriction of a prescription prior to their sale. This proposed law, when it was introduced into the Legislature, was opposed by some of the country doctors who were members of the Legislature. Yet it was passed, constituting probably the first, or among the first, state laws having to do with the control of the sale of narcotics. This law preceded the Harrison Anti-Narcotic Law (the Federal law) by seven years, and was to be followed over the years by other laws that circumstances seemed to justify to restrict the sale of all drugs which could be interpreted as dangerous for indiscriminate use on the part of the public.

In the passage of educational requirements and in the passage of laws prohibiting the indiscriminate sale of dangerous drugs of every description, the Georgia Pharmaceutical Association has assumed its full responsibilities in safeguarding the public against improper and dangerous uses of drugs, and other practices.

A full, rather complete, and detailed story of the activities of the Georgia Pharmaceutical Association from 1875 to 1959 is appended as Supplement D of this volume. To this Supplement the reader is referred for further information.

A list of officers of the Georgia Pharmaceutical Association (1875-1959) appears on page 403.

Also, a list of all State Board of Pharmacy members (1881-1959) appears in the Appendix.

Professional Education in Georgia

The reader will understand that the preceptorship-apprentice system for the training of pharmacists, physicians, preachers, teachers, lawyers, and others, prevailed in Georgia from the beginning of the Colony and State. It is interesting to note at this point, however, that with the advancing program of education which has occurred in practically all the professional fields, the value of the preceptorship system is still recognized; for, in the case of pharmacy, medicine, and dentistry, a certain amount of preceptorship training is required by law for license under what is known as one year or more of "internship." In pharmacy the requirement is that, following college training, the applicant for license must have had at least one year of internship in a place (drug store, hospital, or other place) where drugs and medicines and poisons are sold or compounded under the supervision of a licensed pharmacist. In the case of medicine the requirement is that the applicant for license must, following graduation from a recognized medical school, spend one or more years in internship in a hospital under the direction of someone who serves as a preceptor there. A similar situation prevails as regards dentistry. Even as regards general education, applicants for license to teach in the public schools of Georgia are required to have gone through a preliminary teaching experience under the guidance of an experienced teacher. In the case of law, most young lawyers upon graduation from college go into an office which is operated by some one or more experienced lawyers, where the young person receives some guidance in the conduct of the legal practice.

MEDICAL EDUCATION IN GEORGIA

So far as medical education in Georgia is concerned, there were no educational facilities for the training of physicians prior to the passage of a legislative Act on December 20, 1828, establishing what was known as the Medical Academy of Georgia, which was to be located in Augusta with the following doctors named as Trustees: Drs. Wm. H. Waring, John Carter, Lewis D. Ford, Ignatius P. Garvin, Benjamin A. White, Samuel A. Boykin, Wm. T. McConnell, Walter H. Weems, Wm. Graham, Thomas P. Gorman, Alexander Jones, Milton Antony, John J. Boswell, Thomas Hoxey, J. P. Scriven, Wm. C. Daniel, Richard Banks, Henry Hull, John Dent, Thomas Hamilton, Tomlinson Fort, Nathan Crawford, O. C. Fort, and John Walker.

This Medical Academy in Augusta, established in 1828, was to undergo a change of name from time to time over the years. Finally, it was to become the "Medical College of Georgia, being the Medical Department of the University of Georgia."

The Faculty of the Academy was composed of medical practitioners of Augusta, who were serving as instructors in the Academy on a part-time basis. One of these instructors gave instruction in pharmacy, not for the purpose of granting a degree in pharmacy but for instructing the medical practitioners who would eventually purchase and dispense their own drugs. Following the custom prevailing in medical education throughout the country, the curriculum covered a period of two terms of four months each. But over the years this period of instruction was increased to two terms of six months each, then to three terms of six months, then four terms of six months each, and finally four terms of nine months each.

Like most professional schools of that period, this medical academy, which later was to be called a "medical college," was operated on a proprietary basis; that is, it was to be financed by the fees of the students.

In 1839 the Savannah Medical College was chartered, and shortly thereafter the Oglethorpe Medical College in Savannah was chartered. But neither of these medical schools was very long-lived.

It is well to note that in 1894 a Nurses Training School was organized at the Medical College in Augusta, and this was one of the first such schools to be organized in Georgia.

In 1853 a medical college was established in Atlanta under the title, "The Atlanta Medical College," and, like the Medical College in Augusta, it was operated on a proprietary basis with a similar curriculum, including instruction in pharmacy and with the same length of term. This school was closed during the Civil War, and following the War a division in the Faculty resulted in the formation of a competitive medical college, known as "The Southern Medical College." These two schools, however, eventually merged to form "The Atlanta College of Physicians and Surgeons."

Again a difference in opinion in the Faculty resulted in the formation of a new college, "The Atlanta Medical College." In the meantime a Dental College had been organized in Atlanta in 1891, which shared the building with a school of medicine then operating under the name, "The Atlanta School of Medicine." This school of dentistry operated under the name, "The Southern Dental College," which later came to be an independent institution, and, along with the Atlanta School of Medicine, was absorbed by Emory University.

The Allopathic system of medical practice (or the Regular system) was challenged in 1839 by the existence in Georgia of a group of medical practitioners who were known as the "Botanic" or Thomsonian or "Eclectic" practitioners. They became rather influential in the political affairs of the State, and eventually obtained an appropriation from the State for a Charter for the creation of a medical college to be located at Forsyth, Georgia, in 1839. A number of students entered this school and graduated, increasing the number of these "Botanic" practitioners in Georgia very rapidly. Their system of training was the administration of vegetable drugs to the exclusion of all mineral drugs, and even of all surgical operations. This "Botanic" or "Eclectic" or "Thomsonian" medical school was moved eventually to Macon, and served there for a number of years, licensing a large number of physicians in the State who were to practice under that system.

Also, this system eventually set up its own Board of Medical Examiners for examining applicants for license to practice under this "Botanic" system. Even pharmacists were directed to be licensed to practice by this "Botanic Medical Board," and no pharmacy was permitted to handle eclectic remedies without obtaining a license from this "Botanic" or "Eclectic" Board.

But the "Eclectic" school of medical thought in Georgia gradually disappeared and, following the Civil War, their college was closed. Since that time we have had only one recognized system of medical thought and practice in the State; i.e., the Regular or Allopathic system.

Thus there were several medical colleges operating in the State during the years between 1840 and the Civil War: one in Macon, one in Augusta, two in Savannah, one or perhaps two schools in Atlanta. In 1866 an additional school was granted a Charter to be opened at Dalton, Georgia.

Details of the program for medical education in Georgia are given in full in Supplement A of this volume.

PHARMACEUTICAL EDUCATION IN GEORGIA

Even though the apothecaries of the days of the settlement of the Colony were considered the scientifically trained persons, (as witnessed by the fact that Patrick Graham was sent to Georgia as "Apothecary" to General Oglethorpe and later Hawkins came as "Apothecary" to the Army, and Patrick Hunter came as "Apothecary" to the Orphans House at Bethesda, these men being medical officers as well as trained apothecaries), a hundred years intervened before there was anything like a program of medical education in the State. But it should be noted here that the term "Apothecary" as used here by the British implied a very broad base of training, and far outranked the terms "medico" or "surgeon," which terms were in use in the early 1700's. It is interesting to note how the term "Apothecary" has over the years been down-graded, as compared with the terms "medicine" and "medical" and "surgical" training.

During this long period (1733-1881) pharmacists (at least those who were interested specifically in the retail drug business, as well as those individuals who were practicing both medicine and pharmacy at the same time) were trained through the process of the preceptorship-apprentice system. No doubt, many individuals trained through this system in the State rendered a very great service to the public in the early days of the Colony and

State. It was argued then—and even now—that preceptorship training for pharmacists had certain advantages which did not apply in the case of medicine, and that the preceptorship system was capable of turning out well-rounded, practical pharmacists who could serve the public of their communities. That sentiment on the part of the people of the era was responsible for the lack of interest in providing a program of education for pharmacists for many years. But, after the formation of the Georgia Pharmaceutical Association in 1875, they began to compare themselves with members of other professional fields, educationally speaking, and found themselves lacking, so far as educational requirements were concerned. But it took yet another long period before any real step toward progressive pharmaceutical education was adopted by the State.

The first serious thinking about pharmaceutical education in Georgia came about the time of the creation of the Georgia School of Technology in Atlanta in 1887, for it was planned at one time for a school of pharmacy to be located in that institution. In fact, the Trustees of the University of Georgia, with Henry Grady as spokesman for the Trustees, had agreed that this would be done. But some internal politics in the Association as to the location of the school developed, making it a controversial issue, so that the plan for locating a school of pharmacy at Georgia Tech was eliminated.

Nearly every drug store in Georgia had one or more employees in the store who were serving their apprenticeship. In certain instances the work which they were doing was not of a pharmaceutical nature at all but comprised simple clerk duties around the store. However, the law at the time specified that a person who had served three years in a drug store could appear for licensing by the State Board of Pharmacy. A number of these young men coming up for the examination were lacking in educational background; and many of them, even after three years of experience in a drug store, had had no real preceptorship training and therefore were ill-prepared to take an examination before the State Board. Many of them failed.

To offset this situation, a few people located at different points in the State took it upon themselves to give to these prospective applicants for license some coaching as to the questions and answers which the Board of Pharmacy might require. These came to be known as "Quiz Schools" and several of such schools existed in the State at one time or another. At first, they served a real purpose in helping those deserving young men and boys.

℞ PUBLIC HEALTH, ORGANIZATION, EDUCATION

But when it came to a point when large numbers of persons were being brought in to the State from other sections of the United States to take the Georgia Board examination, and then reciprocate back into their own states, the situation caused the State to become a place for the dumping of large numbers of ill-prepared, uneducated people to be competitors of the legitimate practitioners of pharmacy here in Georgia.

Yet, even in the face of this development in the State, there came about in 1903 the establishment of three schools of pharmacy, in addition to the one already in operation at the Atlanta College of Medicine. Mercer University at Macon added a school of pharmacy. The Southern College of Pharmacy opened in Atlanta as an independent institution, and the University of Georgia instituted a School of Pharmacy in Athens. All these three schools opened in that year, 1903, and in competition with the "quiz" schools which later developed over the State.

The presence of the "quiz" schools dissuaded students from going to college, for, under this system, they could get a job in a drug store, work for a period of years, and then obtain a license by attending one of the "quiz" schools, rather than attending college for 2 years.

The college entrance requirements at that time were nil, a condition which prevailed in medical schools for many years. But, gradually, the entrance requirements were raised, even though the law had never been changed to specify that educational requirements were either desirable or necessary. At last, most of the pharmacy schools required certain preliminary education for entrance into the school or college. Later, this was raised to graduation from high school; finally, in 1933, graduation from a recognized school or college became the prerequisite for licensure.

In the meantime the curriculum in the schools extended over a period of two terms of nine months each. But, beginning with the new era, and following a precedent established at the University of Georgia, all the pharmacy schools went to a minimum of four college years with the present prospect that by 1960 there will be required five college years of training plus a year of internship in a drug store or hospital pharmacy.

A complete story of pharmaceutical education will be found in Supplement B of this volume.

Laws Governing Medicine and Pharmacy (1825-1958)

Supplement C of this volume carries a full account of the laws governing medicine and pharmacy in Georgia. But at this point attention will be called to the fact that it was early recognized in professional practice involving the health of the people of the State that laws were necessary. The laws which were adopted in the State are given here in chronological order. It should be borne in mind that all the laws that were passed between 1825 and 1881 were directed toward the governing of both pharmacy and medicine, since pharmacy was controlled by the Medical Board until that date.

In 1825 came the first law which was known as the "Physicians Bill." It was simply an Act to regulate the licensing of physicians to practice in the State and to set up a Board of Examiners who were to examine not only physicians but pharmacists for license to practice in this State.

In 1835 there was passed an Act to prohibit the employment of slaves and "free persons of color" from compounding or dispensing medicines in doctors' offices or drug stores, and to compel druggists and physicians to keep arsenic and other dangerous poisons under lock and key.

Attention has already been called to the formation of the Georgia Medical Society. This organization was incorporated by Act of the Legislature in 1836.

In 1847 an Act was passed to establish a "Botanic Medical Board of Physicians" to examine applicants for license to practice medicine or pharmacy under the Thomsonian system.

In 1850 some novel legislation is recorded whereby licenses were granted by the General Assembly to various individuals to practice medicine or pharmacy without examination. The names of these individuals are given in Supplement C of this volume.

In 1860 a law was passed which exempted Elbert County from having to be governed by the laws regulating the licensing of physicians or apothecaries whereby they could practice in Elbert County without license or any educational background.

During the Civil War period of 1861, provision was made for temporary license to be given. Whether these licenses were ever revoked, or whether they were continued, is not recorded.

Also in 1861 a law was passed making it possible for physicians who were in practice prior to the 24th of December, 1847, to be exempted from all educational and licensing requirements.

That same year an Act was passed which provided that no person should "vend or expose to sale any drug or medicine without first obtaining a license therefor from one of said examining Boards."

In 1872 appears the first legislation having to do with the practice of dentistry in the State. This Act was passed to "regulate the practice of dentistry" and to "protect the people against empiricism in relation thereto in the State of Georgia."

In 1873 came a law prescribing punishment for keeping a drug or apothecary store without first acquiring a license.

In 1876 attention has already been called to the formulation and enactment of a Poison Law, which came in that year.

In 1881 the Board of Pharmaceutic Examiners was created, with this noteworthy Preamble to the bill:

Whereas in all civilized countries it has been found necessary to restrict the traffic in medicines and poisons, and to provide by law for the regulation of the delicate and responsible business of compounding and dispensing the powerful agents used in medicine, and

Whereas the safety and welfare of the public are endangered by the sale of poisons by unqualified or ignorant persons, and

Whereas the power of physicians to overcome disease depends greatly upon their ability to obtain good and unadulterated drugs and skillfully prepared medicines, and the sophistication and adulteration of drugs and medicines is a species of fraud which should be prevented and suitably punished;

Therefore, the General Assembly of the State of Georgia do enact this Pharmacy Bill.

In 1884-85 there was passed an Act prescribing the manner of the selling of the sulphate and other preparations of morphine in the State. This law covered purely the matter of labelling, and did not prohibit the sale of these items.

In 1904 an Act was passed amending the Pharmacy Law to specify that members on the Board of Pharmacy must be "actively engaged in the retail drug business."

Attention has already been called to the passage in 1907 of the Narcotic Law here in Georgia on the state level as being the first, or among the first, state narcotic legislation. It prohibited the sale and distribution of narcotics except under a doctor's prescription.

In 1908 an Act was passed setting up rules and regulations for the inspection of food and drugs, and creating the position of Chief Drug Inspector in the State of Georgia.

In 1913 a law specified that if any product contains any "alcohol, morphine, cocaine, heroine, alpha or beta ucaine," or various other items, it should be so stated on the label.

In 1927 a law was passed specifying that an applicant for license must "be 21 years of age, shall have at least a high school education," and shall have served at least 36 months in a drug store under the supervision of a licensed pharmacist.

In 1933, the existing law was amended to provide that each applicant for registration as a pharmacist should be not less than 21 years of age, and shall be a graduate of a generally recognized school or college of pharmacy.

In 1935, the Uniform State Narcotic Act was passed.

In 1939 an Act was passed providing for the regulation of the sale or possession of certain so-called *dangerous drugs*.

In 1947 a law provided that the Board of Pharmacy shall have the authority to make such rules and regulations as it deems desirable for the enforcement of the Pharmacy Laws of the State, and that such rules and regulations shall have the full intent of law.

In Supplement C of this volume the reader will find a rather complete listing of all laws having to do with the practice of medicine and pharmacy from 1825 to 1958.

Chapter VII

THE RETAIL DRUG STORE IN GEORGIA—
PAST AND PRESENT

THE first apothecary shop to be opened in Georgia was located in Savannah. It was founded and operated by Dr. Samuel Nunez, who came to Georgia in 1733 and promptly opened his shop. Dr. Nunez was a native of Spain and was said to have been highly trained in medical and pharmaceutical practices. In his professional capacities he proved to be quite an asset to the Colony of Georgia. His arrival in the Colony (July, 1733) is recorded in Chapter Two of this volume, the story of the founding fathers.

No one has recorded the location of Dr. Nunez' office and shop, and one has to draw on his imagination to picture the appearance of this, the first apothecary shop in the Colony. It was probably modeled in a modest form after the apothecary shops of the European Continent from whence Dr. Nunez had come, and where he had received his instruction.

The chances are that this shop was located as part of Dr. Nunez' office, since, in addition to his pharmaceutical practice, he was actively engaged in the general practice of medicine. But, unfortunately, Dr. Nunez remained in the Colony only a short while, and, following his departure, his apothecary shop was either abandoned or conceivably was taken over by one of the others who had come to Georgia as apothecaries or surgeons; notably, Patrick Graham, who came as Apothecary to Secretary Stephens; Patrick Hunter, who came as Apothecary to the Orphans House; or Thomas Hawkins, who came as Apothecary and Surgeon to General Oglethorpe. Any one of these men may have taken over Dr. Nunez' shop, but there is no record of this having been done. There is record of the fact that Apothecary-Surgeons Patrick Graham, Patrick Hunter, Thomas Hawkins, and perhaps the others, were engaged from time to time in manufacturing various pharmaceutical preparations (some of which involved the process of distillation), and in the sale of drugs, as well as in the prescribing of drugs in connection with their general practice of medicine.

The stock of drugs handled by these apothecaries of Colonial Georgia was modest in comparison to present-day inventories, but most of these drugs were imported and were considered necessary for the life of the Colony. In making excavations at Sunbury, on the Coast of Georgia, an inventory of drugs belonging to Dr. Allan Stuart, dated 27th February, 1777, was discovered.

Various other lists of the drugs being handled by importers, as well as by the apothecaries, physicians, or surgeons themselves, will be found in Chapter Five of the present volume (where such long drug lists are advertised for sale). It would be mere repetition to insert these lists of medicinal agents at this point. It may be said that since there were no educational requirements or legislative restrictions regulating the sale or quality of drugs, many dealers importing other merchandise from abroad took on the business of the importation of drugs. Among the dealers was Button Gwinnett, previously referred to in Chapter Two of this volume.

Whereas Patrick Hunter, Patrick Graham, Thomas Hawkins, and others of that early period were definitely pharmaceutically and/or medically trained individuals, the possibility is that the operation of drug stores by others who were not professionally trained, or the sale of drugs, was loosely handled for many years, thus making it possible for that group of persons who were neither apothecaries nor physicians to deal in drugs.

But in the early 1760's, when newspapers first came into existence in the Colony, advertisements began to appear signed by individuals who were operating various kinds of drug businesses. The number of places of this kind is not definitely known, except as judged by a count of those who were advertising. Most of such men were persons who were practicing both pharmacy and medicine, since the income from either one of these sources was not sufficient to maintain the individual.

In the days of the Colony, there was no occasion for drug stores to appear in the country districts where the doctors traveled by horse-back through the wilds. This development was to wait until civilization had advanced to the point where newer

Inventory and Appraisem. of Medicines belonging to
the Estate of Doctr Allan McLean late of Sunbury in the
State of Georgia Practitioner in Physic deceased, produced
to the Appraisers by Miss Ann Stuart Administratrix

Pulv. Cort. Pemv. ℥i   R. Senn ℥ſs
Tinct. Rhei ℥ss   Balsam Traumat. ℥i
Elixir Salut. ℥i   Spt. Vitriol. d. ℥ſs
Spt. Nitr. D. ℥ij   Elix Vitriol. ℥iij
R. Ipec. ℥ij   Spt. Vin. R. ℥ij
Spt. CC. ℥x   — Lavnd. C. ℥iv
R. Cort. Peruv. ℥ij   Elix. paregoric. ℥i
Ol. Amygdal. Dulc. ℥iij   19 Pint glass stop'd bottles
— Vitriol. ℥iv   Ol. Lin. d. Zyn. ℥vi
R. Ipecac. ℥iv   Bacc. Juniper ℥iv
Consew. Rosar ℥iv   Empt. ex Althae. ℥vi
3 Syrup pots   5 large doz. green glass bottles
1 lar. & 4 small jugs   Ol. Succin. ℥ii
Ol. Lavend. ℥iij   — Menth. ℥ſs
— Juniper ℥ſs   — Sapafras ℥ſs
— Cariophyll. ℥vij   Spirit Limon. ℥iij
Tinct. Castor. ℥i   Tinct. Aromat. ℥iij
— Cantharid. ℥i   — Antimon. ℥i
Extract Saturn. ℥iſs   Balsam Peruv. ℥ſs
Sal Tartar. ℥ſs   Sal Absynth. ℥ii
Mosch. Chin. ℥i   Arg. Viv. ℥i
Turbith Miner. ℥ij   Caust. Lunar ℥ij
14 doz. glass stopt pint bottles — —
Sal Prunelle ℥ſs   Rad. Gentian. ℥v
Ichthyocoll. ℥iv   Gum Myrrh ℥iv
Pulv. Contrayerv. ℥i   Crem Tartar ℥xij
Rad. Jalap. ℥x   Rad. Seneck ℥xij
Crocus Antim. ℥ſs   Rad. Columb. ℥iſs

SUNBURY INVENTORY

modes of travel had been adopted other than water travel up the rivers of the State.

But it can be safely said of the drug stores or apothecary shops of that period that they were *drug stores* or *apothecary shops* in fact as well as in name, for these stores were handling nothing but drugs and simple surgical apparatus. As late as the late 1760's or early 1770's the drug stores of the Colony were located primarily in Savannah or Augusta, since these were the larger and earlier settled towns. Medicines were dispensed by physicians or from the "Medicine Chests" which were in the hands of most laymen.

As the population grew, however, *drug stores* were opened in the larger settlements of the State. These early places of business were also *drug stores in fact,* but were probably not long to remain so. Many of them, perhaps most of them, were associated with some doctor as a part of his business, as witnessed by the advertisements which occur in a previous chapter.

The reader will bear in mind—as previously called to his attention—the fact that most of the drugs commonly used during Colonial days and the early days of the State were vegetable drugs; that is, roots, barks, flowers, fruits, and other parts of a plant, in crude state, were carried in the drug store. These plant products gave rise to various odors, mixtures of which are still fresh in the memories of many persons who were familiar with those old drug stores where the drug merchandise in the store was made up of Asafoetida, Camphor, Peppermint, Spearmint, Catnip, Valerian, Ginger, Bay Leaves, Perfumes, Spices, Cinnamon, Cloves, Nutmeg. Those odors, blended together, gave to each drug store its characteristic odor, which was identifiable even by blind-folded persons, so familiar were they with these distinctive drug-store aromas.

But, with a pitifully small business available to the operators of these earliest drug stores, the necessity arose for the addition of merchandise side lines. These were to vary with conditions in the particular areas of the State.

Among the early merchandise items taken on as side-line products were garden seed and some field seed. Herb gardens were popular on the plantations and some of the larger homes of the State, and a demand arose for propagating various items which the early settlers had known abroad and were preparing to grow in their present homes in Georgia.

℞ THE DRUG STORE IN GEORGIA 167

Next on the list of side-line merchandise items outside the field of pharmacy were house paints and window glass, which were handled in most smaller towns through the drug stores. Except in a few isolated cases, the handling of paints and window glass has long since been abandoned. But in earlier times the cutting of glass to fit various openings or window frames was considered quite an art, and was one of the skills in which the apprentice was taught to become proficient. Most of the drug stores where glass was handled carried a diamond cutter as a device for scratching or etching the glass for breaking along the proper line.

Perfumes, cosmetics, and dental preparations of every kind were all originally pharmaceutical products prepared by the pharmacist and sold entirely through the retail drug stores. Most pharmacists had secret, and jealously guarded, formulas for the preparation of these items. Some name was coined for the product, and this name in many instances was copyrighted. Some of these original products, now more than a hundred years old, are still for sale at the cosmetic counters of drug stores.

Spices of all kinds, and flavoring agents—vanilla, lemon, orange, peppermint, pineapple, strawberry and cherry—were considered pharmaceutical products and therefore legitimate and ethical side lines to be prepared in the store.

The drug store, with its increasing line of merchandise products, was not restricted to those operators who were pharmacists, for it was often advertised as being owned and operated by outstanding medical men such as Dr. Crawford W. Long and his brother, who operated a retail drug business in Athens for many years. A photostatic copy of one of Long's advertisements is shown in the illustration, p. 114.

During the greater part of the 19th century, most of the *preparations of medicinal agents* were manufactured or prepared in the drug store, and the ability of the pharmacist to prepare these products set the standard by which he was judged as to efficiency.

The apothecary or physician or proprietor, with the assistance of his apprentice, was confronted with the necessity of manufacturing various classes of "preparations" involving the mixture of two or more medicinal agents. These classes of preparations could be logically divided into certain categories, as shown herewith.

TABLE

I. All Those For Internal Administration
   A. Powdered Drugs
      1. In Substance
      2. Charts or Papers
      3. Pills or Boli
      4. Capsules
      5. Tablets
      6. Lozenges or Troches
   B. Liquid Preparations
      1. Waters
      2. Spirits
      3. Syrups
      4. Elixirs
      5. Tinctures
      6. Wines
      7. Vinegars
      8. Emulsions
      9. Mixtures

II. Those For External Application
   A. Liquids
      1. Lotions
      2. Liniments
      3. Antiseptics
   B. Semi-Solids
      1. Ointments
      2. Cerates
      3. Plasters or Cataplasms

Powdered drugs could be dispensed "in substance", where the dose could be measured out by the teaspoonful; or as "charts" or "papers", each containing one dose; or as "pills" or "boli", "capsules", "tablets", "lozenges", or "troches".

The "pills" of the 19th century were prepared in the drug store with the use of a so-called "pill machine." This device is still among the museum items of the old drug store. Prescriptions for pills were written to be prepared extemporaneously, all of them varying in composition, size, and dosage forms. No coating methods existed for pills in those early days, nor were capsules available. Formed as they were by hand, pills were rather crude affairs as judged by the "elegant" present-day standards for pharmaceuticals. The "bolus" was a very large pill. Being large, it was sometimes very difficult to swallow; therefore it was usually prepared much softer than a pill so that the mass could conform to the shape and size of the throat.

The choice of massing or binding agent (the "excipient") was left to the judgment of the pharmacist, who would make the choice according to the nature or character of the medicinal ingredients of the pill. The character of medicinal materials called for varied widely, and the number of ingredients for a pill varied from one to five or more.

A physician sometimes had a formula for a given pill, and the druggist would prepare these pills in convenient quantities so as to be able to dispense any number of them which might be ordered on prescription. The doctor might also carry them in his medicine bag. Or, individuals might buy them in quantity to maintain their "medicine chest" or "medicine cabinet."

The manufacture of pills on a quantity scale by the druggist was a plan of his to provide occupation and instruction for the apprentice in his store. Many an apprentice received his certificate of apprenticeship on the basis of his ability to manufacture pills in quantity in a reasonable length of time, of uniform size, consistency, and quality.

The "pill" has been a popular means of administering medicine orally. Today pills are made by the thousands by the pharmaceutical manufacturer. They are coated to mask the taste, keep well, and are easily swallowed, as well as reasonably priced.

Powdered drugs were not always prepared into "pills." Sometimes they were directed to be divided into parts for dosage effect, each part to be folded in a "paper" or "chart" containing the proper amount for *one dose*.

This method of preparing powders was employed especially for children who could not swallow a pill, capsule, or tablet.

The dividing of powders to be dispensed in "papers" or "charts" was, and is, a "pretty" but time-consuming operation.

Gelatine "capsules" were patented in France in 1833, but did not come into general use in America for some years later because of the cost. They were intended for the administration of disagreeable-tasting substances, such as quinine.

"Tablets" began to come into use about 1880, thereby precipitating a revolution in the storage and administration of drugs "in substance." They constituted a boon to the pharmacist, eliminating to some extent the necessity of making "charts" and "papers", and were handy also for the physician, who could carry his medication in proper and convenient dosage form.

Today, of necessity and for economic reasons, tablets are prepared by machinery by large-scale manufacturers. They are much more readily and cheaply made than pills, and they may be coated with various coating agents.

"Lozenges" or "Troches" are in fact nothing but tablets. They are not intended to be swallowed in mass, but rather to be dissolved slowly in the mouth, releasing the medicinal agent (or agents) gradually for the local or systemic effect. They were manufactured extemporaneously in the drug store for many years, but today are entirely in the hands of the large-scale manufacturer.

An example of a large and popular class of liquid preparations was "tinctures." Primarily they were prepared from vegetable drugs, some of which were collected locally. It was considered highly unethical to prepare tinctures by any method other than that prescribed by the U.S.P. The process of percolation was generally employed and directed. A few tinctures were prepared from mineral products; for example, "Tincture of Iron and Iodine." A very few were prepared from animal products, for example, "Cantharides and Musk." Today, due to the high cost of alcohol, the manufacture of tinctures is almost entirely in the hands of the pharmaceutical manufacturer.

A second class of liquid preparations for internal administration is "emulsions." The preparation of these products constituted another example of the testing of a pharmacist's skill. Prescriptions for emulsions varied widely, Cod Liver Oil and Turpentine Emulsion being the most popular. The term "to homogenize" is given to the mechanical process for producing an emulsion. It represents the oil or fat in a very finely divided state.

Of the various liquid preparations for external application two classes came to be quite popular. "Liniments" were prepared in the retail drug store and usually contained one or more agents classified as counter-irritants: Chloroform, Ammonia, Turpentine, Camphor. Liniments may be rediscovered for it is instinctive *to rub* when and where it hurts. "Lotions", like liniments, were to be applied externally. But, whereas liniments were to be applied to unbroken skin surfaces, lotions were intended to be soothing, antiseptic, and healing in nature, and to be applied to broken skin surfaces.

Also for external application, "Ointments" (or "Unguents") of various kinds have been extensively used from the beginning of time to produce local or systemic effect. Arguments as to various types of ointment bases have continued through the years. It was contended by some that "petrolatum" was an *epi*dermatic base, thus holding the action of the drug to the exterior of the skin; that lard and similar fats were *en*dermatic in character, in that they penetrate and enter into the skin, thus being valuable as an anti-parasitic carrier of medicinal agents; that woolfat ("lanolin") was *dia*dermatic in character, thus promoting absorption of drugs into the circulation. "Petrolatum", however, has one advantage over animal and vegetable fats, in that it does not rancidify and is more economical. Most of the Official or Special ointments are now prepared in large quantities by machinery by manufacturers.

"Cerates", a related class of preparations, differ from ointments in that they have a higher melting point.

"Plasters" or "Cataplasms" constituted a popular medium of external medication, whereby the medicating agents were made into a semi-solid condition and spread on cloth for application to the desired part. This produced anodyne, astringent, or stimulant action. Cantharidal plaster was used to produce a blister of the desired size and location. As a class of preparations, plasters are now almost extinct, except for non-medicated adhesive plaster, which is used for mechanical support.

These classes of preparations constituted convenient products for which the physician might write a prescription.

Most of the prescriptions of the early period—not only throughout the 19th century but well into the 20th century—were written in Latin, and abbreviated, so that to the average layman the prescription was absolutely unintelligible. And, in the handwriting of the older doctors, the reading of the prescription was considered to be quite an art, and evidence of the pharmacist's professional knowledge and skill.

These prescriptions usually contained more than one ingredient and frequently contained a substantial number of ingredients, necessitating the process of being "compounded" by the pharmacist.

In the medical schools where physicians were being trained, the subject of "materia medica" came to be quite important, and the writing of prescriptions was considered one of the important phases of a young physician's training. Since polypharmacy was being generally practiced, prescriptions of the era were frequently complex in character, and the ingenuity of the pharmacist was taxed to the limit in filling them. Dangerous incompatibilities were frequently involved. But, under all circumstances, the prescription was a dignified and ethical instrument, though not necessarily scientific.

For some thirty or forty years during the 19th century, there

Prescriptions

Prescriptions

existed in Georgia a group of practitioners known as the "Botanic" or "Thomsonian" or "Eclectic" practitioners. These practitioners used vegetable drugs almost exclusively—sometimes in the powdered state, sometimes in substance, but also in the liquid state (in the form of tinctures or fluidextracts). They were distinguished from the "Regular" practitioners, who were known as "Allopaths." This system of medicine persisted well into the 20th century.

The prescription part of the store of the 19th and early 20th centuries was considered the heart of the drug store because here it was that the professional knowledge, skill, or art of pharmacy was practiced. This being true, it is incomprehensible that no educational requirement existed in the training of pharmacists for some two hundred years after the establishment of the Colony, but that all training for pharmacy was confined to the preceptorship-apprentice type of training. But even so, the pharmacists, as well as their helpers, or apprentices, occupied a very unique place in the life of the State, particularly in the small communities. For it was here that the people could come for information in regard to drugs, and the druggist became the "confidante" of the community and was accepted as a professional man even though he may have had only a limited general education or no formal (college) technical education.

It is interesting to note that through the years various organs of the body have been charged with being the chief offenders in their responsibility for ill health. A wide variety of medicinal agents or compounds for prescription usage, as well as for self-medication, were made available.

During the 19th century, so far as ill health was concerned, the chief offender was the liver. Hundreds of preparations appeared on the market which were intended to be liver remedies, and these were sold under various proprietary names. Mercury in some form was considered the most desirable liver remedy of that period. Calomel was the most convenient and most commonly used mercurial, though metallic mercury in the form of "Blue Mass" or "Gray Powder" was used in the treatment of liver conditions. Calomel was valuable in many respects, and, whereas it has come into unfavorable reputation in recent years, *it may be rediscovered* for the treatment of some intestinal and general conditions. Due to its popularity and extensive use, Calomel was the target of advertisers of those liver preparations which did not contain it, and this gave rise here in Georgia to the popularity of a preparation sold here very profitably by its manufacturer—a product which made its reputation by fighting Calomel. Later, however, the curious fact is that the same manufacturer put out another product containing Calomel which, after extensive advertising, made another fortune for its promoter.

During this period when the Liver was being attacked from all angles, there came on the market various mineral preparations—salts known as "Liver Salts"—some of which products are still advertised on radio and television, or otherwise, and are still in extensive use.

The vegetable liver medicines on the market today are also a hang-over of the old days, most of them containing senna and other purgatives of one kind or another but said to be "liver stimulants." It may be safely said that more drugs, so far as tonnage is concerned, have been used as laxatives or purgatives than all other drugs put together.

Rheumatism was another popular enemy, and hundreds of preparations have existed during the years for its treatment, some of them to be taken internally and some of them to be applied externally—and some to be consumed "eternally."

The Kidney has been considered another offender, and various remedies have been sold under the promising name "Kidney Cure" or "Kidney Remedy." These products flourished particularly during the 19th century and even well into the 20th century.

The Venereal Diseases were on a progressive program of expansion during the 19th century and into the 20th century. Mercury in some form was the primary agent used in the treatment of syphilis. Thousands of prescriptions are on file in the older drug stores of Georgia showing that mercury in some form (associated usually with iodides and sometimes with arsenic) was used in treating syphilis. However, there were a number of vegetable preparations which were believed to have some antisyphilitic or alterative properties: sarsaparilla, stillingia, burdock, pipsissewa, poke root, prickly ash; and various other vegetable products including red clover (trifolium) were popular in this connection.

Recognizing that there were other disease conditions to which the people were generally subject, advertisers extensively claimed certain medicinal agents as "cures" for "Cancer," "Consumption," "Catarrh," and others.

The Physical Appearance of the Drug Store

The average drug store or apothecary shop of the early days was probably a very small institution, when physician-owned and operated or when operated by a pharmacist or apothecary. If the store were physician-owned and operated, it was a part of his office or an adjunct to his office, and the office and store frequently were located in his home or on the premises of his home.

If the apothecary shop were located in the business district of the town or city, the building would of necessity be very small, since the stock of merchandise was limited. The building was usually of wooden construction, poorly lighted and ventilated, and, as judged by modern standards, was unsanitary and unsightly.

These conditions extended well into the 19th century, but they were gradually to improve with the increase in population, an increase of volume of business due to a larger demand for drugs, and the addition of many side lines. A contemporary observer in 1850 stated that, "Pharmacy in Georgia is in a sad state." Fortunately, it was not long to remain so, for changes were on the way.

The changes in the appearance of the store, in volume of business as well as in the conduct of the business, appeared first in the cities of Georgia and gradually spread to the smaller towns and settlements. These changes probably began imperceptibly, but continued on a definitely progressive basis, dependent upon existing local conditions.

More and more of the drug stores ceased to be identified with physician ownership and came to be operated by licensed pharmacists who had come along under the preceptorship-apprentice system and who were impressed with their responsibilities as members of a dignified profession. They demanded for themselves and the public whom they served more attractive and convenient surroundings, a more prominent location, a larger storeroom, more attractive fronts, buildings of better construction, better lighting, more ventilation, *and more paint*.

Many of the apothecary or chemist's shops of England and the Continent had been equipped with glass-stoppered and glass-labeled bottles for the storage of liquids as well as solids. This custom naturally found its way into the drug stores of Georgia as the drug business expanded and proper storage facilities became increasingly available.

It was routine in most of the drug stores of the State—even in the small towns—to equip the stores with these very attractive bottles. Usually, one entire wall of the store-room, from the front to the rear, was equipped with proper shelving to handle these bottles, frequently numbering several hundred.

The glass label on the bottle carried the name of the drug, usually printed in Latin and abbreviated; i. e., Tr. Op. Camph. These bottles constituted a trade-mark or insignia of the drug store, comparable to the mortar and pestle, and they were usually kept in sparkling condition at the hands of the apprentice, whose responsibility it was not only to keep them clean and sparkling but also to begin the study of Latin names for drugs in this manner. The bottles also constituted an advertisement which attracted the attention, interest, and curiosity of the layman.

The installation of the glass-stoppered, glass-labeled bottle was probably the first attempt to break the monotony and drabness of the drug store shelves, which up to that time were loaded with packages of varying size and condition of storage. These bottles began to disappear from the drug store shelves about 1890, those few still to be found in Georgia being retained as antiques, or as sentimental reminders of the past.

This first break in monotony was to be followed by such features as the soda fountain, show cases, and other furnishings of an attractive nature, as well as certain installations which were to change the "old" drug store into the "modern" store of the 20th century.

The Soda Fountain Enters the Picture—1890

The advent of the soda fountain in the life of the Georgia drug store is probably more responsible than any other influence for the revolution that was to take place in the physical appearance of the store, as well as in its operation, and these changes, once begun, came thick and fast.

The fountain grew in popularity from year to year, thus bringing into the store an increasing number of patrons who were to suggest—and probably demand—additional items of merchandise. Thus began the expansion in the number of side-line items of merchandise which the drug stores were to take on.

The drug business in Georgia was now about 160 years old and had not changed much over the years in the physical appearance of the store or in its operation. The proprietors had grown old in the traditions absorbed from the preceptorship system under which they had been trained, and they were not happy over the changes which they grudgingly but eventually recognized as a necessity to attract and hold more and more patrons, and to meet the competition of the chain drug store and those others outside the drug field who were potential competitors in some merchandise items which had hitherto been claimed by the drug store.

The soda fountain of the 1890 period was usually an ornate and highly decorated piece of drug-store furnishing and seemed out of place in the setting in which it found itself in the average drug store of the period,—all of which demanded physical changes to conform, in some degree at least, to the fountain.

CHAIN DRUG STORES

Though resented and resisted by the individual druggist of Georgia, as well as by the Georgia Pharmaceutical Association, as being unethical and un-businesslike in establishing the practice of cutting prices, the first chain drug store came to Georgia via Atlanta about 1890. This chain was locally owned and operated under the name, "Jacobs Pharmacy Company." The number of units in the chain has increased over the years.

The chain drug store brought to Georgia a type of competition with which the average Georgia pharmacist was unfamiliar and unprepared to meet. The original chain has been followed by many others, large and small, foreign-owned as well as locally owned.

The merchandising of drug and related products under "chain" practices was to take precedence over the "normal" or "professional" phases of the drug store with which the Georgia pharmacist was familiar and which he had been taught to revere. This change in the operation of a drug store meant to the average pharmacist the loss of a way of life which was to him worthy of the long, bitter, but losing fight to preserve.

Apparently, the advanced theories and practices introduced by the chain drug stores proved popular with the public, for to meet the competition as a means towards self-preservation, the independent drug stores of Georgia—or most of them, at least—began to follow "chain" ideas and practices.

There is today, however, a trend to return to the so-called "ethical" type drug store, and the reader may live long enough to see the old "apothecary shop" again in operation in most of the cities and in some of the smaller towns of Georgia.

The changes in physical appearance and accommodations in the store, once initiated, began the process of evolution which has given us the attractive drug store of today.

Depending on the location of the store and conditions (i. e., whether located in an urban or a rural area), there was no generally accepted order in which improvements in the form of many changes were to come. But there are listed below some observations as to an approximate order in which physical changes came to the drug store:

1. Free use of paint on walls, shelving, and ceiling of store. (This is a continuing "must".)
2. More glass in fronts.
3. Tables and chairs to accommodate fountain customers.
4. Glass-doored wall fixtures. (Now, display shelves.)
5. Show cases. (Now, replaced by self-serve, open display cases.)
6. Covering for the crude wooden floors, with paint or linoleum. (Now, tile or terrazzo.)
7. Screens at windows and doors to repel insects.
8. Electric ceiling fans for cooling in summer, and "pot-bellied" stoves for warmth in winter. (Now, airconditioning.)
9. Electric lighting, as soon as electricity became available.) (Now, replaced by fluorescent or neon lighting day and night.)
10. Neat and hygienic conditions throughout the store.
11. Neat attire of all store personnel. (Now, uniforms for fountain operators and for other store personnel.)
12. New "dress" donned by the prescription department.

The net result of the many changes in the physical appearance of the drug store, and the larger number of merchandise items added, and the impetus given to the professional phases by the telephone and a modernized prescription service, is reflected in the change in the volume of business. In 1890 the average annual volume of drug business in Georgia was estimated at $10,000, whereas the average annual volume in 1959 is estimated at $100,000.

But the increase in patronage and in dollar volume of business done is negligible as an estimate of the value of the drug store to the community, in comparison to the quantity and quality of health service offered by the average drug store.

The attractive and comfortable store encouraged the public to consider it a desirable meeting-place for social and business engagements, so that as a result the small-town or community drug store has come to be recognized as a social and business center, conveniently located, open for long hours, popular with all ages and classes of people, and a place where all of the gossip and news of the town is distributed—along with discussion of local, state, and world problems, as witnessed by the famous Scopes trial in Tennessee of several years ago. In short, the drug store has come to be recognized as a "community" institution in hundreds of the towns of the State, comparable in importance in the citizen's mind with churches, schools, hospitals, and other public institutions.

Even at the risk of repetition, it is pardonable to point out that there are approximately 1100 drug stores in Georgia (1959), so strategically located that one of them is available within a short time and distance to every person in the State for advice and counsel in those health matters in which a pharmacist of the present era is trained.

It may be pardonable to point out again also that on an average basis the entire population of the State passes through the drug stores of Georgia every ten days, placing a responsibility on the pharmacists of the State to qualify themselves—intellectually and professionally—to advise and counsel those who may need and seek information regarding drugs.

Chapter VIII

SPECIALIZED FIELDS OF PHARMACY—WHOLESALE AND MANUFACTURING, THE PROFESSIONAL STORE (THE APOTHECARY SHOP), HOSPITAL PHARMACY, EDUCATION AND RESEARCH

THE author has long believed and taught that the interests of the wholesale and retail drug businesses are identical—that there is such a close interdependency between the two that all problems confronting either or both should be recognized by the other, and that, together, a solution to the problems could and should be arrived at.

The author also believes that the pharmaceutical manufacturing industry should be recognized as the third member of what should become a triumvirate. In such a union could be realized the principle of interdependency and of the mutuality of the business, as well as the professional features of all phases of the manufacture, distribution, sale, and dispensing of medicinal and related products.

Wholesale Drugs.

With these thoughts of interdependency of pharmaceutical interests in mind, it was the plan to have a full chapter covering the "History of the Wholesale Drug Business in Georgia." But when the search for historical data revealed that very little information has been recorded and preserved whereby the complete history of the wholesale drug business might be told, the plan and hope for such a full chapter was of necessity abandoned. However, a brief statement covering the establishment of the existing wholesale businesses is given here in the hope that the wholesale interests involved will eventually compile complete data for preservation for posterity.

During the early life of the drug business in Georgia, as a Colony and as a State, the records reveal a number of individuals who, as importers of general merchandise from abroad, also brought in drugs which were advertised and sold at retail and/or wholesale.

With no legal restrictions as to the quality or standardization of drugs or as to the technical training of those who were to sell or dispense them, the majority of these importers and dealers were non-professional in character—one of these being Button Gwinnett, who in later years became one of the singers of the Declaration of Independence and, for a brief period, Governor of Georgia.

The historical records of retail pharmacy in Georgia are far from complete; but, fortunately, some history-conscious individuals did record some historical data, and it is hoped that other individuals of both the retail and wholesale field will be stimulated to bring all historical data together to make a clear picture of their origins, their problems, their contributions to the life of the State, and their struggles to become a profession in fact as well as in name.

To pin-point the year when the first strictly wholesale drug business began in Georgia is apparently impossible, for it seems to have been customary in the early years for any retail business having achieved an appreciable volume of business to advertise under the title, "Wholesale and Retail."

This was true not only of the apothecary or pharmacist-owned stores, but of the physician - pharmacist - owned - and - operated stores, as witnessed by the advertisements of both types of stores. Among physician-pharmacist owned stores were those of the following: in Athens, Dr. Crawford W. Long; in Rome, Dr. Robert W. Battey; in Augusta, Drs. Cunningham and Dunn (1817), Dr. Dysart (1797), and Dr. Ulmo (1800); in Savannah, Dr. George Harral (1797), and others.

In nearly every town of any size in the State, there was at one time or another one or more pharmacists who advertised as wholesale and retail dealers. Among them are the following: in Atlanta, Asa G. Candler, John B. Daniel, and John S. Pemberton; in Macon, H. J. Lamar, and others; in Rome, Curry and Arrington; in Columbus, Brannon and Carson; in Savannah, A. A. Solomons; in Athens, Palmer and Kinnebrew, and E. S. Lyndon; in Augusta, Land Drug Company, and others; in Gainesville, Brown Drug Company.

As the number of retail drug outlets increased in the State, there was a corresponding increase in the number of distinctly wholesale outlets; and, with the increase in numbers, competition became sharper during periods when the price of cotton and other farm products was low, and the purchasing power of the retailer, and his ability to pay, was naturally curtailed. For a period of years during depression and keen competition, it became the practice of some wholesalers to finance or help to finance the opening of new stores, with the result that for many of these years a large percentage of the retail stores of Georgia were mortgaged to some wholesaler. The average annual volume of business in the average retail drug store during the period (about 1890) approximated $10,000 per year. This practice of financing the opening of new retail stores on the part of the wholesalers was eventually discontinued to the advantage of both the retail and the wholesale interests, the public in Georgia, however, being assured of a complete and efficient system of distribution of medicinal agents in the interest of the public health and welfare.

The wholesale distributors of Georgia in 1959 are so located that prompt delivery of drug products may be made to any area of the State. They are situated as follows: in Atlanta, John B. Daniel Drug Company and Economy Drug Company; in Augusta, McKesson and Robbins (Murray Division); in Columbus, McKesson and Robbins (Columbus Division); in Macon, McKesson and Robbins (Riley Division), and Coleman, Meadows, Pate Drug Company; in Savannah, Solomons Drug Company and Columbia Drug Company; in Valdosta, Valdosta Drug Company.

There follows a brief statement covering the establishment of each of these wholesale companies from data supplied by them.

THE SOLOMONS DRUG COMPANY AT SAVANNAH

Whereas the Solomons Drug Company is not by any means the first of the wholesale establishments in Georgia, it does carry the distinction of being the oldest wholesale drug business under the same name in the State at this time (1959), and is representative of those wholesale businesses which were originally retail in character as well as wholesale.

Abraham A. Solomons, the founder of the business, was born in Georgetown, South Carolina, in 1816. He evidently served the usual apprenticeship period, and was licensed by the Medical Society of South Carolina as an apothecary on December 15, 1835.

He opened an apothecary shop in Savannah at Whitaker Street and Bay Lane in 1845. There being no large pharmaceutical manufacturing establishments in the area of Savannah, he, like most other retail pharmacists, apothecaries and druggists of that period, manufactured most of his pharmaceuticals from the crude vegetable drugs of the region or from imported crude drugs, and promptly began to supply other shops and stores with his manufactured products.

This was probably the stimulus which influenced him and those who were to follow to enter more and more into the wholesale business, and, the business volume growing apace, various changes in location were made necessary to supply needed additional space. However, the retail store was maintained as such until 1940.

During the life and activities of the retail business, many notables patronized the store, two of whom the Company is especially proud and whose identity as patrons has been documented by the Company.

On the 14th of August, 1869, Alexander H. Stephens, Vice President of the Confederacy, writing from his home at Liberty Hall, Crawfordville, Georgia, ordered "half a dozen bottles of your 'bitters' to be sent via express C.O.D."

On the 20th of April, 1870, General Robert E. Lee, on a visit to Savannah, addressed a communication to the Company as follows: "Please prepare for me the enclosed prescriptions and return them with the medicine and oblige, Yours, Robert E. Lee."

Presidents of the Company over the years are as follows:
- 1845 - 1899   Abraham A. Solomons
- 1899 - 1921   Joseph M. Solomons, brother of the founder
- 1921 - 1940   Isaiah A. Solomons, son of the founder
- 1940 -   Isaiah A. Solomons, Jr., grandson of the founder

Over the years, the Company has continued to prosper and to serve druggists and people of Savannah and Southeast Georgia even though called upon to face many difficulties and vicissitudes: financial depressions; epidemics of diseases; the Reconstruction

℞ WHOLESALE DRUGS 185

period following the Civil War; and last, but by no means least, the tragedies and problems of two world wars.

The Solomons Company is one of Savannah's oldest and most highly honored institutions.

COLEMAN, MEADOWS, PATE DRUG COMPANY, MACON, GEORGIA

"This Company was organized in 1919 and began business in July of that year. Sam Coleman, a prominent and successful business man of Macon, seeing the need for an additional wholesale drug house in Macon, associated with himself Messrs. Martin Meadows and Jesse H. Pate in the formation of the Company.

"At the time the Company was in process of organizing, many of the successful retail pharmacists of the State were given the opportunity to purchase stock in the Company, and, in every instance where the stock was so issued, the entire issue was subscribed for.

"During Sam Coleman's life, he served as Chairman of the Board, and, following his death, this office was assumed by his son, J. D. S. Coleman."

Martin Meadows was a licensed pharmacist and had previously traveled over the State as a representative of one of the large pharmaceutical manufacturing houses. He was greatly loved by the pharmacists with whom he had business relations. As Director of Sales of the Company, he lived to see it expand from infancy to the full stature of a large and successful business.

Jesse Pate was General Manager of the business until within five years of his death, having retired in 1950. His interest in the business was acquired by J. D. S. Coleman.

Following the death of Martin Meadows, James T. Riley was elected Sales Manager of the Company, and was later elected President, in which capacity he served until his retirement in 1954.

Following Mr. Riley's retirement, T. D. Fitzgerald was elected President and is now (1959) serving in this capacity.

For 36 years, the Company occupied the same building, which housed 28,000 square feet, but in 1957 a new building covering 52,000 square feet was occupied.

The territory of the business embraces Central, Southern, Southeastern and Southwestern Georgia.

VALDOSTA DRUG COMPANY, VALDOSTA, GEORGIA

In 1890 Dr. J. M. Harvey established a business in Valdosta under the name, "The J. M. Harvey Medicine Company," which eventually grew into a wholesale drug business.

In 1902, the business was bought by James Stewart Plowden, and incorporated under the name, "Valdosta Drug Company," and was owned and operated by him until his death in 1924. At that time his widow assumed the ownership and operation of the business and she continued operation of the business until her death in 1937. (Author's Note: So far as can be determined, this is the first and only instance in Georgia, and perhaps in America, where a woman owned and successfully operated a *wholesale* drug business.)

Following Mrs. Plowden's death in 1937, and for the next eight years, the Plowden sisters—Hyta, Matilda and Russell—owned and operated the business with Hyta as General Manager.

On Hyta's marriage to Leonard J. Mederer in 1945, the interest of the other sisters was purchased by Mr. and Mrs. Mederer, and Mr. Mederer became President and General Manager, the business now being owned and operated by them.

The Company serves a large area covering Southern Georgia and Northern Florida.

McKESSON AND ROBBINS MURRAY DIVISION, AUGUSTA, GEORGIA

Looking over the names of apothecaries, druggists, physicians and dealers in Augusta who advertised as "Wholesale and Retail" outlets, there seems to be no direct link between any one of these from 1740 to 1900 and the present wholesale business of 1959.

Listing some of these early dealers in drugs who advertised as Augusta wholesalers—Prior to 1800: Drs. Dysart, Payne, Lauder, Ulmo, Montgomery, Casey, Ewell, Todd, Burke, Murry, Smelt, Hull, Cocke. Additional physicians who were also wholesale and retail dealers from 1800 - 1814: Drs. Gantt, Harris, Childers, L'Homme, Watkins, Fendall, Wray, Howard, McWhorter, Meigs, Cunningham, Dunn, Pew et al. In 1820, W. H. Turpin, Druggist; 1824, L. Rossegnol, Druggist; 1825, Thomas Lang; 1852, Philip A. Moise, Importer and Dealer; 1870, W. H. Barrett Drug Company; 1852, D. B. Blumb, Drug Dealer, and W. H. Tutt, Wholesale and Retail Druggist; 1877, R. H. Land, Sr.; T. A. Beall, and W. H. Alexander; 1884, S. C.

℞ WHOLESALE DRUGS 187

Durban; E. Berry; D. E. McMasters; H. P. Tarrant; W. H. Barrett; 1885, J. B. Davenport; T. A. Cheatham; J. N. Horsly; 1886, H. C. Baker, F. J. Moses; 1887, George Perrin, Jas. P. Smith; 1889, R. L. Bradfield, George Crouch, Dan Crouch, P. O. Clark, Chas. A. Morgan, J. M. Posey, et al.

W. T. Edmunds, retail pharmacist of Augusta, gives the following as background for the present (1959) wholesale house in Augusta:

"Howard Willett owned and operated a business known as a 'seed and drug store' prior to 1900, and about 1900 took in as partners N. L. Willett, and Dr. W. B. Marks. Marks later acquired the wholesale drug interest of the other partners, and was joined in partnership and ownership by John Phinizy and the business was operated for a number of years under the name, 'Augusta Drug Company.' About 1930, the business was sold to the Murray Drug Company of Columbia, S. C., which shortly thereafter was sold to the McKesson and Robbins Company, the business now operating under the name, 'McKesson and Robbins, Murray Division.' The territory covers portions of South Carolina and Georgia."

MCKESSON AND ROBBINS, COLUMBUS DIVISION

In addition to several other wholesale drug establishments in Georgia, the Brannon and Carson Wholesale Drug Company originated in a retail business, under the name, "A. M. Brannon's Drug Store," which gradually grew into a wholesale business following the formation of the partnership with Mr. Carson.

Mr. W. T. Hendry of the McKesson Columbus Division has compiled a brief but interesting history of this business which is quoted in full in order that it may be preserved for all time.

"Brannon and Carson Company began business in 1859, and the business was therefore eighty five years old when it was sold to McKesson and Robbins, Incorporated, in 1944. It was started as a retail drugstore, and, in the beginning, was known as A. M. Brannon's Drug Store, founded by A. M. Brannon. Later on, Mr. Brannon took into partnership with him his son-in-law R. A. Carson and Mr. Sam H. Williams; the firm's name was changed to Brannon, Carson and Williams. Then the firm began, in a small way, to do some wholesale business in addition to their retail business. For a number of years, they had on the road only one salesman, Mr. L. B. McKee, who remained with the firm until he died. In 1903, the partnership business was incorporated and the name was changed to Brannon and Carson Company; their wholesale business began to grow and they gradually discontinued their retail business.

"In the eighty five years this firm had only three Presidents: A. M. Brannon until 1903; R. A. Carson until 1914, and Mr. H. E. Weathers from 1914 until 1944 when it was sold to McKesson and Robbins, Inc. It was never one of the biggest drug firms but always one of the best. It had the reputation of being one of the best known firms, both by the manufacturers and by the retailers. They sold only the best quality of goods known to the trade.

"One thing happened when the President of the Company went to New York to sell it to McKesson and Robbins, Inc., in 1944. Our lawyers said that we would have to go home and comply with the bulk-sales-law; however, the President of McKesson and Robbins, Inc., Mr. W. J. Murray, said that that was not necessary as he knew about Brannon and Carson Company, and when their President told him that all they owed was that month's current bills, he felt satisfied. However, the lawyer for Brannon and Carson Company insisted that we must do it and so he made us go through all that detail for nothing. Our merchandise was so clean and our accounts were so good that McKesson and Robbins, Inc., paid us in cash—without Brannon and Carson Company giving any discounts—for all of it, and after one year's operation, they had not lost one dollar on the accounts.

"Brannon and Carson Company prided itself as a service jobber, and they rendered a service second to none.

"After all, it matters little how big you are or how old you are—but rather how good you are and what advice you have rendered."

The territory covered by the present Company covers Western and Southwestern Georgia and Eastern and Southeastern Alabama, and portions of Western Florida.

JOHN B. DANIEL, INC., ATLANTA, 1867-1958

"John B. Daniel, Inc., was founded in 1867 by John Benning Daniel* who opened a small retail drug store just one block from

―――――――
*John B. Daniel was one of the early and very active members of the Georgia Pharmaceutical Association.

Five Points in Atlanta. From this small start, the Company branched out into manufacturing and wholesale distribution of pharmaceuticals and moved its operation to larger quarters at 34 Wall Street across from the old Union Station."

"Mr. Daniel remained at the head of the firm until his death in 1914 at which time the Company was incorporated. At this time, Paul L. Fleming, a nephew of Mr. Daniel who had been with the Company since 1894, was made President of the Company. Frank L. Fleming, another nephew of Mr. Daniel, was made Vice-President, and Lucien L. Knight, a third nephew, was also made a Vice-President. A few years later, the Flemings acquired Mr. Knight's interest."

"After Frank L. Fleming passed away in 1950, Paul L. Fleming was elected as Chairman of the Board and Fred L. Lewis was elected as the third President of the Company."

"Mr. Lewis served as operating head of the firm for two years until the day he passed away, at which time Mr. Fleming again assumed the position as both Chairman and President."

"In July 1956 the following officers were elected by the Board:
Robert L. Garges, President
Frank L. Fleming, Jr., Vice-President
V. Carlton Henderson, Vice-President and General Manager
Henry B. Sacre, Vice-President and Treasurer

"The present location of the Company is 80 Central Avenue, but plans are under way to build a new warehouse on Lidell Drive."

"Grier's Almanac, founded in 1806, is owned by the Company. George M. Kohn, Jr., is General Manager."

(Author's Note: The above material was supplied by Robert L. Garges, President.)

THE ATLANTA ECONOMY DRUG COMPANY

The Atlanta Economy Drug Company is one of three establishments which operate under the general title, "Economy Drug Company," the parent Company being located in Cincinnati, Ohio, and a branch at Dayton, Ohio. The slogan of the three businesses has been, for a number of years: "Three Houses —One Service."

"The Atlanta branch was opened for business in Atlanta January 1923 occupying a small building on West Cain Street, and, as late as 1951," says *Retail Drug Trade News*, July, 1951, "three of the five original employees of the Company are still with the firm:—W. A. Volk, Manager; A. W. Duke, Sales Manager; J. C. Brown, Buyer."

With the rapid increase in the volume of business, the Company purchased property at 199 Jackson Street, N. E. and erected a building providing 16,000 square feet of floor space. The building has expanded over the years to cover 50,000 square feet of floor space.

Most of the original wholesale houses in the South had developed from retail establishments, which, like Topsy, had just "growed." Most of them manufactured many of the pharmaceutical products they sold or repackaged many items which had been bought in bulk volume, and, therefore, usually occupied buildings with a basement and several additional floors.

When Economy erected their first building in Atlanta, the principle was adopted of a one-story building since no manufacturing was contemplated nor repackaging of drug items.

Manufacturing on the part of the wholesaler and repackaging of drug items in general has gradually faded from the picture so far as the service jobber business is concerned and most modern wholesale houses are now constructed on the one-floor principle.

In addition to the Atlanta area which is covered by city salesmen, Economy has other salesmen and the business covers most of the Central and Northern sections of Georgia.

COLUMBIA DRUG COMPANY, SAVANNAH, GEORGIA

In 1949, Columbia Drug Company, in celebration of the 50th year of its existence as a wholesale drug business, published a booklet entitled, "50 Years of Fashions In Drugs," from which booklet the facts are taken for this brief historical statement covering the life of this popular and valuable business.

The cover page of the booklet carries a drawing of a young lady and gentleman in the typical dress of the 1900 period, and on the left of the drawing, there are photostats of some popular proprietary drug products of the period: Lydia E. Pinkham's Vegetable Compound; Sloan's Liniment; Mother's Friend, and Smith Brothers Cough Drops. On the right of the drawing, four modern drug packages are displayed: Cremo-Suxidine; Pyrobenzamine; Streptomycin; and Penicillin. The title of the page is "The Gay Nineties."

℞ WHOLESALE DRUGS

"The Gay Nineties of the world's social development became the prosperous Nineties of Savannah's commercial progress. The founding of the Naval Stores Exchange established Savannah's rank as the leading naval stores port in the world while tremendous exports of cotton, lumber and tobacco brought wide-spread prosperity. A new process for refining cottonseed oil was developed in Savannah and led to the erection of a large plant for its production. (Wesson.) At the turn of the century, the Savannah Sugar Refinery was founded. Into this world of expanding activity, Columbia Drug Company was born on December 28th 1899.

"Abraham E. Smith had come to America from Bavaria (about 1880) when he was a boy of sixteen and settled in Bainbridge, Georgia. He had but little money and less knowledge of English to smooth his way. After establishing himself in business, he brought over two brothers, Emanuel and Henry. In 1883 the family moved from Bainbridge to Savannah and the three brothers established a wholesale grocery business, Smith Brothers, of which business, Abraham was President."

In 1899, the wholesale grocery business was converted to a wholesale drug business with Abraham Smith as President of the new business, to be known as Columbia Drug Company.

Following the death of Abraham Smith in 1924, the son, Jacob Smith, who had served as Vice President since 1903, was elected President; and, under his leadership, Columbia Drug Company experienced rapid expansion. He served as President until his death in 1946.

Kayton Smith, the son of Jacob Smith, and grandson of the founder Abraham Smith, came to the Presidency of the Company following the death of his father. Following his graduation from Williams College in 1928, he had come to work under his father, and, after an apprenticeship of several years, was elected Treasurer and Assistant to the President in 1946.

"Through changing fashions in costumes, customs and in drugs, through eras of prosperity and depression, through two world wars and days of peace, Columbia Drug Company can trace an unbroken continuity achieved through the unchanging loyalty of its friends and the integrity of its staff. As this Company looks back with pride on the fifty years since its organization, it can mark a steady growth with an ever enlarging circle of friends."

The traveling salesmen of Columbia Drug Company cover

MCKESSON AND ROBBINS, RILEY DIVISION, MACON

Even though Macon was the meeting place of the first gathering of pharmacists to consider the organization of the Georgia Pharmaceutical Association in 1875, and the home city of many of the prominent retail pharmacies of the State, there is but little of record which has to do with the wholesale drug activities prior to 1880.

From the Proceedings of the American Pharmaceutical Association 1852 and from Proceedings of the Georgia Pharmaceutical Association 1875, there are found some names of the retail pharmacists of Macon of the period indicated: 1859, J. Henry Zeilin; 1870, J. B. Huddart; 1871, L. W. Hunt; 1875, John Ingalls and J. J. Pinckard; 1876, E. R. Beckwith; 1877, R. B. Hall, A. A. Maynard, G. F. Payne, F. K. Peacock; 1879, T. L. Massenberg, H. W. Ellwood; 1880, T. A. Cheatham, H. J. Lamar, Sr., H. J. Lamar, Jr., J. W. Rankin (also listed as of Atlanta).

Of this number of retail pharmacists, the Lamars and the Rankins are or seem to be the only ones definitely identified with the wholesale business.

From data supplied by Mr. T. A. Davis of McKesson and Robbins and from personal recollections of the author, the following facts are gleaned: Henry J. Lamar, Sr. was born in 1825 and died in 1896. Just when and how he became identified with the drug business is not of record, but, at various times, the name "Lamar" appears in the publications of the 1870-period usually identified with the retail drug business; but the first instance where the name occurs as identified with the wholesale business with which the author is acquainted is an advertisement in the Proceedings of the Georgia Pharmaceutical Association (1877) under the name, "Lamar, Rankin and Lamar," later to be known as Lamar and Rankin. The Macon business wholesale and retail was operated under the name, H. J. Lamar and Sons.

During the 1880's and later, the firm operated a total of five retail drug stores in Macon, in addition to the Atlanta wholesale house and a business in Albany, Georgia, both wholesale and retail, the Albany Drug Company.

℞ WHOLESALE DRUGS

J. B. Riley became identified with the Lamars in 1882-84. Though never a licensed pharmacist, Mr. Riley came to be greatly loved by the retail pharmacists of Georgia, and, at one time, he served as Secretary of the Georgia Pharmaceutical Association though engaged in the wholesale business at the time.

In 1899, the wholesale drug house, Taylor-Peek Drug Company, was organized in Macon by R. J. Taylor; but in 1902 this business was merged with H. J. Lamar and Sons to form the Lamar, Taylor, Riley Drug Company with J. B. Riley as Vice President and General Manager.

The Lamar family continued to own the Lamar and Rankin business in Atlanta. But in 1908 the new Company of (Lamar, Taylor, Riley) purchased the business, and it was later sold to R. J. Taylor.

In 1920, Mr. Riley and his son-in-law J. D. Crump and their associates purchased the Lamar, Taylor, Riley Company, and re-established the business under the name, J. B. Riley Drug Company.

In 1929, the J. B. Riley Drug Company was merged with McKesson and Robbins, Inc., with Mr. Riley and Mr. Crump serving as Vice Presidents. Mr. Riley remained with the Company as General Manager until his death in 1933, and Mr. Crump remained with the Company until his retirement in 1954, having followed Mr. Riley as General Manager. Following Mr. Crump's retirement, T. Alton Davis succeeded him as General Manager.

Through all the mergers and/or consolidations which occurred during the years, the business, regardless of the name under which it operated, has enjoyed a large volume of business, and has maintained a close and intimate contact with the retail business in the State. The territory covered through the years includes large areas of the State.

Pharmaceutical Manufacturing

As was true of the wholesale drug business as distinguished from the retail, pharmaceutical manufacturing was likewise an offshoot of the retail drug store.

Since there has never been any large pharmaceutical manufacturing plant located in Georgia, there is no historical data to record so far as pharmaceutical manufacturing in Georgia is concerned. But pharmaceutical manufacturing—even though the plants have been located in areas other than Georgia—has been of increasing importance and advantage to the retail drug business of the State, thereby enabling the pharmacists of Georgia to render a higher quality of service to the patrons of their stores, and at a cost far below what it might have been, had the product been prepared by the time-consuming process of the earlier years.

Pharmaceutical manufacturing on a large scale began with the manufacture of the early classes of preparations—pills, tablets, tinctures, fluidextracts, elixirs, syrups, ointments—and has expanded with the passage of time into wider and still wider fields.

The manufacturer of the earlier years was usually one who had passed through the apprenticeship of a retail store, who knew the problems of the retail store and recognized the possible opportunities in a manufacturing enterprise. He probably started his business on a shoe-string basis, and peddled his wares to a skeptical retailer who was loath to give up the old for the sake of the new, even though the evidence was all in favor of the new.

There is no evidence to offer as proof, but, basing his decision on his long experience and perhaps his efficiency in the process, this manufacturer used the pill as the first item of production since the pill was the most commonly used medium of medication at that time, and he saw that the pill could be improved in appearance, made more stable in character, and made to offer medication in a more readily active form.

To distinguish them from the hand-formed pills made in the retail store, he probably coated them in a crude sort of way, gradually improving this process through experience and research until the final result of his efforts are the beautiful pills of this era (1959), sometimes coated with gelatine, sometimes with sugar, chocolate, or some other suitable material, and colored to suit the prescriber or purchaser.

It would be educational and historically interesting to have been a "fly on the wall," and to have watched his reactions—in his failures of investigation as well as in his successes. For one can be sure that he failed as often as he succeeded, and—but for his failures—might not have succeeded.

If his work had not been so well done, pills might never have reached their high degree of popularity and efficiency, which has enabled them to live through the years as media for administration of medicinal agents.

When tablets showed their head, this manufacturer was well-equipped with experience in dealing with drugs "in substance" to see the possibilities in this new and attractive mode of medication. He was quick to improve the product and the process of its manufacture, and as a result of his effort participated in bringing the tablet to this generation.

The "tablet triturate" was, of course, the pioneer of all tablets, but was soon to find a competitor in the "compressed tablet" of this era. The manufacture of the "compressed tablet" has suggested the possibility of compressing pill materials, which has resulted finally in the making of a "compressed pill" which may be coated with any of the acceptable coating materials.

The manufacture of tinctures of vegetable drugs, formulas for which appeared in the Formularies and the Pharmacopoeias of the period, usually involved the process of "percolation" with alcoholic or hydro-alcoholic menstrua.

In the retail drug store where relatively small quantities of tinctures were needed, the process of percolation consumed so much time in some instances—frequently running into several days—that this manufacturer realized the possibilities in the manufacture of tinctures on a large scale.

He knew from experience that the products prepared in a small way were rarely uniform as to "color" and activity. He further saw that no more time would be consumed in making multiple gallons of the tinctures than in making a few fluid ounces, and that the product prepared on the large scale would be more nearly uniform as to color, stability, and activity.

When his tinctures, prepared on a large scale, were then offered to the druggist who had suffered through the period of the manufacture of tinctures in a small way, he not only did not find resistance to this new idea, but was welcomed with enthusiasm.

When fluidextracts were first admitted to the U.S.P. in 1850, they likewise involved the process of "percolation." But in addition they involved the process of "concentration by evaporation" and, eventually, "vacuum evaporation," a process which the retail drug store was not equipped with proper apparatus to carry out.

So this manufacturer promptly equipped himself with the proper apparatus to produce fluidextracts in quantity at a price which not only was not prohibitive but actually cheaper than the retailer could possibly have prepared them himself.

During the years when "Botanic," "Eclectic," or "Thomsonian" medicinal products prevailed, the number of fluidextracts in common use by these practitioners ran into the hundreds.

These preliminary manufactured products necessarily suggested expansion into the manufacture of other pharmaceutical products. This manufacturer then found himself called upon to produce Plasters, Ointments, Cerates, Liniments, Syrups, Elixirs, Spirits, and other U.S.P., N.F. or Special Formula products.

With the advent of biological pharmaceutical products—Sera, Antitoxins, Toxoids, Vaccines, et al—the manufacture of which was not conceivable on a small scale, the manufacturer was called upon by the medical profession, the pharmaceutical profession, governmental, and all other health agencies, to provide the risk capital and the know-how for the manufacture of these items. What a job they have done!

When vitamins came into recognition as essential agents for maintaining life processes, the manufacturer again was called upon to isolate and concentrate vitamins and to standardize them. Under the impact of long and expensive research, the manufacturer has again provided millions of dollars of risk capital and years of experience in the know-how of pharmaceutical manufacturing to give to America these essential agents, of the highest degree of uniformity and purity and at a price which has steadily decreased over the years.

When sulfa drugs—the first of the so-called "wonder drugs" —were introduced into extensive medical usage, the manufacturer was called upon once more to provide the risk capital and the know-how of manufacture, and to produce them in such quantity and of such quality, and at such a price, as to make them available to the people of America.

When penicillin—the forerunner of the antibiotics—was announced, the manufacturers of America did not hesitate to risk multi-millions of dollars in equipment and experiment for its manufacture and distribution. It is difficult to picture what disease conditions in America may have been but for penicillin and other antibiotic products.

The pharmaceutical manufacturing industry is solely responsible for the production of the tools with which disease can be successfully treated, and all branches of the pharmaceutical profession, including retailers and wholesalers, can claim a stake in the production and distribution of these and most other medicinal products.

The Atomic Medical Era is now upon us, with all its possibilities and potentialities for a broader and more efficient medication, not only for the treatment of disease but for its detection and prevention as well. There is the possibility and probability that through atomic agencies some of the heretofore unconquered diseases may be added to the list of those now labeled as "conquered."

The pharmaceutical manufacturers are already active in research in this field, and their millions of dollars of risk capital await the opportunity to produce new products as they are revealed by research.

Other Specialized Fields of Pharmacy

It is not only safe but true to say that the modern era, so far as drugs are concerned, and the practice of pharmacy and medicine, begins at the turn of the 20th century. The progress that has come in these fields, both in quantity and quality as judged by modern standards, far excels that of any other similar period of history.

The progress that has come in the practice of medicine and surgery in this century is astounding, and in 1900 would have been considered unbelievable. In the opinion of this writer, this progress has come as a result of the higher and higher standards of education and the high degree of specialization that has followed. The story of this achievement at the hands of medical and surgical practitioners has already been told by others. But it should be pointed out that this progress and this achievement could not have been possible but for the tools that have been provided by pharmaceutical industry, and their storage and distribution by wholesale and retail pharmaceutical institutions.

Pharmacy in Georgia, though far behind medicine in developing a program of education and specialization, has come forward rapidly—professionally as well as economically—since a higher plane of educational development has not only been adopted but is now in process of being improved by the addition of another year to the present four-year requirement for graduation from college, and for licensure.

In previous chapters, attention has been called to the fact that (first) wholesale and (second) manufacturing industries constituted the first movement toward specialization in pharmacy. However, economic features rather than professional ones probably prompted this development. Yet wholesaling and manufacturing came into existence by way of the retail drug store, thus establishing a tie between the three which should never be broken but strengthened and broadened.

The retail pharmacist is, of course, acquainted with the various specialized fields in which pharmacy makes its many contributions to the life of the State. But, for the instruction and benefit of non-pharmacists who may scan this volume, it is deemed desirable to record some of this data here.

The Professional Store - Apothecary Shop

In England and on the Continent of Europe pharmacy was for many years purely professional in character, and the store was known in England, and possibly on the Continent, as the "Chemist's Shop." In more recent years some commercialism has penetrated the profession in England and on the Continent.

The American drug stores—especially those in rural areas where self-medication was practiced for a long period—were rarely purely professional, even when owned and operated by physicians, as for many years a large number of them were.

In recent years there has been a growing tendency toward the "professional" type of store. For some years this type of store was confined to the cities, but in the present period (1959) they are appearing in small towns as well, and are proving successful economically as well as professionally, with some 50 such stores in operation in Georgia.

So popular has been the movement toward the "professional" type store or shop that a sufficient number of such stores are operating throughout America to justify the organization of "The American College of Apothecaries," affiliated with the American Pharmaceutical Association.

Hospital Pharmacy and Women in Pharmacy

For a number of years the larger hospitals of America have operated dispensaries or hospital pharmacies, where prescriptions for patients were filled, and from which places medicines for these patients were supplied.

In those cases where the dispensary or pharmacy was operated by a licensed pharmacist, the service was of value to the patient, the physician, and the hospital management.

The building of new general hospitals in America in recent years has been phenomenal. The impetus began with the inaugu-

℞   WHOLESALE DRUGS   199

ration of the Hill-Burton program whereby federal and state governments participate with the local government in the cost of such buildings.

Georgia has played a part in this hospital growth to the extent that, for the year 1957, the State Board of Health reported 231 hospitals, large and small, in operation in the State, divided as follows:

2-10 Beds 59	60- 99 Beds 24
11-24 " 34	100-199 " 21
25-39 " 50	200- " 12
40-59 " 31	

Only a small percentage of these hospitals had hospital pharmacies *operated by a licensed pharmacist.*

In those cases where a hospital dispensary repackages or compounds medicinal products for patients, it should be obvious that the hospital patient is entitled to the same legal protection provided by law to people of the State when the law specifies that a drug store, apothecary shop, or dispensary, or wherever drugs are dispensed, shall be *under the direct supervision and direction of a licensed pharmacist.*

The demand for more hospital pharmacists has resulted in special curriculum additions for those students who are registered in a school of pharmacy and contemplate practicing in the field of hospital pharmacy. The hospitals of Georgia can use to advantage the scientific service the trained pharmacists of Georgia are prepared to render.

The number of hospital pharmacies and pharmacists in the United States has increased to such an extent that it has justified the formation of a national body, "The American Society of Hospital Pharmacists," which is affiliated with the American Pharmaceutical Association, as is also "The Georgia Society of Hospital Pharmacists."

This specialized field of Hospital Pharmacy has proved to be very attractive to women, and increasing numbers of them are entering this field as well as the general drug store or "professional shop or store" in Georgia, as evidenced by the ever increasing number of women licensed to practice as pharmacists during the past several years, as shown in the table below.

Beginning in 1904, there was one woman applying for license in Georgia, and from time to time a small number of women operating drug stores have appeared for license. But, until the year 1946, no official report was given concerning the actual number of women licensed and engaged in the active practice of pharmacy. Since that date the number has increased steadily as shown in the table.

Women in Pharmacy in Georgia

1946	 31	1956	 100
1950	 52	1957	 110
1951	 70	1958	 130
1955	 97		

Following a custom in the Eastern (Oriental) countries where many or most of the drug stores are operated by women, more and more American women are becoming interested in entering some phase of pharmaceutical practice. Over the years an increasing number of retail drug stores in Georgia have been owned and successfully operated by women.

OTHER SPECIALIZED FIELDS OF PHARMACY

The table given below, taken from Chief Drug Inspector P. D. Horkan's Report to the Georgia Pharmaceutical Association and the Georgia State Board of Pharmacy for the year 1957-58, illustrates the various capacities in which the licensed pharmacists of Georgia are engaged.

1957-1958

Number of Retail Drug Stores in Georgia	1,091
Number of Licensed Pharmacists Registered with Secretary	2,262
(This number includes some out-of-state, some retired or temporarily inactive pharmacists.)	
Number of Pharmacists Actually Engaged in Drug Stores	1,644
As Owners 781	
As Partners 252	
As Employees 611	
Number Employed in Hospital Pharmacies	69
Number Employed in Wholesale and Pharmaceutical Houses	75
Number Employed as Manufacturers Field Representatives	102

℞ WHOLESALE DRUGS   201

Number Employed as Teachers or in
    Government Positions   42
Miscellaneous   40

Pharmacists in Government Service

Higher educational standards for the licensure of pharmacists has encouraged and enabled state and federal governmental agencies to utilize the services of pharmaceutically trained and educated men and women in such varied capacities as:
Drug Inspectors on federal and state levels
Narcotics Inspectors on federal and state levels
Hospital Pharmacists in Army, Navy, Veterans Administration and Public Health Hospitals

Education

The field of pharmaceutical education—for teaching and research—is absorbing a larger number of those who have acquired the Master's or the Doctor's degree.

Journalism and Art

The fields of Journalism and of Art can be profitably explored by pharmaceutically trained men and women who have interest in and the qualifications for writing or art. These fields are almost virgin territory so far as pharmacy is concerned and therefore offer opportunities for the properly trained and qualified pharmacist.

Research

Since it has been the function of pharmacy through the years to provide proper medicinal materials for the treatment and prevention of disease, research in the field of drugs has come to be the responsibility of pharmaceutically trained people—whether the drugs come from the vegetable kingdom, or the animal or mineral kingdom, or from some phase of synthetic chemistry, and whether these drugs may be used for human diseases, animal diseases, fowl diseases, or plant diseases.

As workers in a specialized field of pharmacy, pharmaceutical researchers are carefully chosen from those who have been selected from the undergraduate student body, and who have demonstrated their ability and their interest in research, and have proceeded to qualify for the highest graduate degrees.

Public Health

Attention has been called to the fact that the entire population of Georgia passes through our drug stores on an average of once every 10 days. The drug stores of Georgia are therefore on the frontiers so far as the health of the people is concerned, and the pharmacists of the State have functioned in the health interest of the public, being prompted by their interest and desire to be of service. Laws have been enacted whereby two pharmacists hold membership on the Georgia State Board of Health.

With the advancement of the program of education now in operation, in which a broad basis of general as well as technical education is pursued in the schools of pharmacy, the students are more definitely fitted for their places of service in the matter of advice and counsel to the people with whom they come in contact. For it happens perhaps thousands of times each day that the public seeks some advice and counsel from the druggists of the State regarding their own health or that of their families.

It is therefore the aim and the objective and the hope of pharmaceutical educators today that practitioners of pharmacy, in view of their many close contacts with the people of Georgia, may be utilized as a definite part of the Public Health program of the State.

Chapter IX

THE SODA FOUNTAIN—SODA WATER: AT FIRST A MEDICINAL AGENT, BECOMES A BEVERAGE

A LONG evolutionary process is involved in the development of the modern soda fountain, and those of us who came into the profession of pharmacy via the soda fountain feel that, in view of the important part it has played in the creation of the modern drug store and in improving the financial status of drug stores, some permanent record should be made of the historical data involved in the process of its development, and that this historical data should find a proper place in the history of pharmacy in the State.

The soda fountain was designed, of course, to dispense the solution of carbon dioxide in water (otherwise known as "soda water" or carbonated water), and it is therefore the history of the gas, carbon dioxide, which deserves first consideration.

Carbon dioxide has existed, of course, from the beginning of time; but the product probably was never recognized and identified as a specific agent until well into the 16th century, apparently, when Paracelsus reported the presence of an "unknown effluvium" which many years later was tentatively identified as carbon dioxide, a gas which had been known to exist in caves and grottoes, to be formed from the combustion of charcoal and to be liberated from carbonates when decomposed with acids, as well as from the fermentation of vegetable matter.

Through the years the product has been known by different names, being called "carbonic acid" or "fixed air" or "aerial acid" and later, of course, by its correct name, "carbon *di*oxide," which name distinguishes it from the poisonous and combustible product, "carbon *mon*oxide."

In 1767 Priestley, the discoverer of oxygen, became interested in a gas which he found escaping from brewery vats, and which later was identified as carbon dioxide. By pouring water from one glass to another in the presence of the gas, he established the fact that this gas was soluble in water. And, finding that the gas in solution was drinkable, the name "carbonated water" was given to it.

This apparently simple discovery proved to be the focal point from which came the carbonated beverage industry which has long since reached world-wide prominence, proportions, and importance as an industrial product.

Inorganic or mineral carbonates such as chalk and marble were abundant throughout the earth, and no doubt had been studied in the laboratories of the time. It is difficult to pinpoint the date when it was first recognized that these carbonates could be decomposed by acids to produce the gas, carbon dioxide. This was probably in the early part of the 17th century when Van Helmont coined the word "gas" to describe it.

The name "soda water" was given to carbonated water because of the fact that ordinary cooking soda was available in all drug stores or chemists' shops, and was economical enough to prepare the gas carbon dioxide in small quantities, by treatment of the carbonate with any acid. The solution of the gas in water was to be used for medicinal purposes only. There being no soda in soda water, the title is a misnomer, but its usage through the years has given this term a permanent place in our vocabulary.

The word "fountain" is derived from the Latin word "fons," which name was given to any stream of water issuing from the earth, such as a spring. The term "fountain," then, has been applied to sprays of water being delivered into the air under pressure. It is therefore logical that the apparatus which delivered "soda water" or carbonated water under pressure should be called a "fountain." And, since the name "soda water" had attached itself to carbonated water, the apparatus could not avoid being called a "soda fountain."

Spring waters have attracted the attention and interest of people from the beginning of time. And, if there happened to be any unusual quality to the appearance or taste or odor, the spring was designated as a "mineral spring" and therefore thought to have valuable medicinal properties, perhaps attributable in part at least to the presence of carbon dioxide in the water.

We people of Georgia have not been immune to this interest in mineral springs since there is scarcely a community in the State that has not claimed one or more "mineral springs." Among the better known of Georgia's "mineral springs" are the following: Indian Springs, Warm Springs, Lithia Springs, Franklin Springs, Madison Springs, Watson's Springs, White Sulphur Springs, Blue Springs, and Radium Springs.

Carbonated water has been reputed over the years to have many medicinal qualities. In 1806 Professor Silliman, a teacher in Yale University, advertised carbonated water as being made up according to "correct chemical principles." In 1807 Dr. Physic of Philadelphia had Pharmacist Speakman prepare for him carbonated water for use with his patients. By 1808 a public establishment was opened in Hartford, Connecticut, for the sale of carbonated water and certain mineral waters, also carbonated. In the same year one or more similar establishments were opened in New York. Because the carbonated waters were deemed to be "an aid to health," outlets were established in drug stores, and the waters were first distributed in bottles or in glasses at the fountain or store.[1]

As evidence of the increasing popularity of "soda water," the following advertisement appeared in *The Augusta Chronicle*, Augusta, Georgia, dated June 9, 1815:

Soda Water

The subscriber three doors above Mr. Fox's corner has commenced the manufacturing of this healthy beverage, where it can be had in the best order till nine o'clock P.M.   Signed—John Pew.

In *The Augusta Chronicle* for December 18, 1820 appeared the following advertisement:

A new spring of health at the Hygeian Fount, the product Ginger Beer. This pleasant and truly delightful beverage has the two-fold advantage of combining the carbonic acid gas, which corrects the bile, strengthens and warms the stomach so as to cause a general perspiration. This being in great use in the winter season in most of the Northern cities and very highly approved of by the best physicians as a great restorative.

Families can be supplied by sending "at the fountain," where it will be put up in bottles for use. Soda water will be furnished as usual.

Signed—Joseph LaFitte

The *U. S. Dispensatory* of 1843 (Fifth Edition) shows the following discussion under the heading "Carbon Dioxide":

---

[1]. Palmer, Carl J., *History of the Soda Fountain Industry*. Publication of the Soda Fountain Manufacturers Association (Glencoe, Illinois).

Carbonic acid water is diaphoretic, diuretic and anti-emetic. It forms a very grateful drink to febrile patients, allaying thirst, lessening nausea and gastric distress, and promoting the secretion of urine.

Dr. T. Sollmann, in the fifth edition of his textbook on Pharmacology (1936),[2] states under the heading "Carbon Dioxide (Carbonic Acid)":

In the stomach, carbonated water ("soda water") hastens absorption, increases the secretion of acid gastric juice, and acts as a carminative. It is useful against nausea, and valuable for disguising the taste of medicines. It produces marked augmentation of the gastric contractions and of the pyloric discharge.

The *U. S. Dispensatory* of 1947 (24th edition) gives the following notation:

Carbon Dioxide. (Carbonated Water). McClellan and his associates (American Heart Journal, 1945, 29, 44) have studied the physiologic effect of baths in carbonated water, or carbon dioxide-charged waters; they reported a decrease in pulse rate and diastolic blood pressure, better return of venous blood to the heart, hyperemia of the skin, a slight increase in cardiac output, an increase in respiratory minute volume, and an increase of from five to ten percent in pulmonary excretion of carbon dioxide; these findings suggest absorption through the skin.

Since there was no commercial source for procuring carbon dioxide prior to 1888, each fountain operator manufactured the gas in his store or laboratory by the usual method of decomposing some carbonate with *sulphuric acid*. This particular acid was preferred for two reasons. First, it was the most economical; and second, it was non-volatile.

Up to 1832 no apparatus had been designed for the specific purpose of manufacturing carbon dioxide in large or small quantities. Each person had his own small crude outfit for its manufacture. Even so, he had no means of accumulating the gas under pressure. So, one John Matthews of Massachusetts manufactured for sale the first carbon dioxide generator. Modifications of this generator, using calcium carbonate or marble dust and sulphuric acid, were used by independent and retail dealers until the discovery that carbon dioxide gas could be manufactured on a large scale, liquefied under high pressure (about 1000 pounds), and transported in steel cylinders any distance, to be released through a valve as needed.

2. Sollmann, Thorald, M.D., *A Manual of Pharmacology*, 5th ed., 1936, p. 745.

One of Matthews' advertisements of those days is as follows:[3]

1 upright generator	$115.00
1 four-gallon fountain frame	25.00
1 draught apparatus for counter	40.00
6 patent soda tumblers	1.25
1 case extracts for syrups	6.00
1 barrel Matthews' ground marble	2.00
165 lbs. sulphuric acid with carboy	6.53
	$195.78

John Matthews' effort constituted the beginning of the manufacture of apparatus for the production of carbon dioxide and for dispensing the product from what was called a "fountain." Matthews referred to carbonated water as "aerated water." He resented its being called "soda water." When the gas was manufactured, it was passed into a container of water (usually a metal container) which was rocked during the process. This was done in order to saturate the water as nearly as possible with the gas. If a mineral water was to be manufactured, all that was necessary was to add the proper mineral to the carbonated water, and dissolve it by shaking. This would constitute the artificial Vichy, Kissingen, Carlsbad, Hunyadi, or other water.

Up to 1838 carbonated water had been used simply as a medicinal agent in itself, or for the manufacture of "mineral waters," and used therein not only to disguise the disagreeable taste of the salts but to give its own medicinal effect. But in 1838 a Frenchman, who operated a perfumery shop in Philadelphia and who dispensed mineral waters and plain aerated water from a so-called "soda fountain," conceived the idea of adding a flavor to make the carbonated drink more palatable. One of his products, a lemon soda, was so successful that he bottled the product and shipped it over the country, even as far as New York. Within a few years thereafter there were said to be half a dozen or more bottlers of soda water in Philadelphia, and the number of flavors of "soda" offered had constantly increased. It was noted that when carbonated water was added to the fruit products, or to the flavored products, it enhanced the taste of the product and brought out certain of the aromatic principals present in the fruit juice or flavoring agent.

3. Palmer, Carl J., *op. cit.*

It was not until somewhat late in the manufacture and use of carbon dioxide that temperature was noted as having anything to do with the retention of the gas in solution in water. So, in these early founts, even though there was no machinery such as we know today, soda water was passed through refrigerated coils made of lead or block tin or stainless steel, and these delivered the carbonated water at such temperature that it retained more of the gas and was therefore more pleasant to the taste and more refreshing.

Dr. Charles LaWall of Philadelphia makes the comment that "carbonated water plus the addition of fruit juice gave us what we now know as soda water," except for the fact that apparently it was not sweetened then. In an article written for the American Journal of Pharmacy, he states: "The first soda water was dispensed regularly to patients from fountains at a dollar and a half per month for one gallon per day."

During the 1830's, and as the demand for carbonated products increased, crude soda fountains began to appear on the market. The first ones were probably by Matthews.

Soda water and soda fountains were becoming more popular from day to day and from year to year, and evidently there was profit in the sale of soda water apparatus as well as in the sale of the beverage itself. Following Matthews as a manufacturer of carbon dioxide generators and fountains, there came a number of others: Puffer, Tufts, Lippincott, Green, Walrus, Liquid Carbonic, Bishop-Babcock, Becker, Knight, Lipman, and various others, with the result that the competition became so keen that when a depression period came along, consolidations took place among various of these manufacturers. Over the years, the price of the fountains and fountain apparatus gradually increased, the manufacturers vying with each other in the ornateness of the fountains. Fountains were built representing villas and castles and various other types of buildings, under such names as "The France," "The Pontiac," or "The Borealis." These adornments added to the expense of the apparatus and tended to dissuade the small operator from the purchase of a fountain where his volume of business would not justify it.

But the development of the manufacture of liquefied carbon dioxide and its transportation in steel cylinders was responsible for a great impetus in the soda fountain industry because it relieved the small operator from manufacturing his own carbon dioxide. This liquefying process was begun in 1888 in Chicago by Jacob Baur, who was managing a drug store for his father. Following his discovery of a practical process for converting carbon dioxide gas into a liquid, the product was prepared shortly thereafter in all sections of the country, including Atlanta.

In Atlanta, it seems that the first (or at least among the first) plant to manufacture liquid carbon dioxide in commercial quantities for sale was the Pratt Laboratory. Originally, this company used marble dust and sulphuric acid in the manufacture of the gas, liquefying it under pressure, and shipping it out to other parts of the State in steel cylinders. A number of drug stores which had not previously installed soda fountains were now interested in taking up this sideline because of their ability to get carbon dioxide without the expense of machinery for its manufacture.

The Pratt Laboratory found that instead of using marble dust, dolomite (which is a mixture of the carbonates of magnesium and calcium) could be used. Treating this product with sulphuric acid resulted in the formation of calcium sulphate and magnesium sulphate, with the liberation of carbon dioxide. The magnesium sulphate, being soluble in water, was dissolved and filtered out from the calcium sulphate, carried through one or more processes of re-crystallization and purification, and sold as Epsom Salt of U.S.P. quality. The resulting volume of Epsom Salt was great enough to supply all of the Southeast, and shipments of it went to other parts of the country.

In the fountains of the early 1880's and on into the 90's—and even in some instances for many years thereafter—refrigeration of the carbonated water and the syrups was carried out by the use of ice, since mechanized refrigeration had not yet been developed.

James W. Tufts, one of the early fountain manufacturers, was also a pharmacist. He made enough money out of the sale of soda fountains to buy about 5,000 acres of land in North Carolina, which he converted into a summer and winter resort, known as Pinehurst.

As a pharmacist, Tufts published a book of formulas for various drinks, and also gave some advice about the operation of soda fountains. Among other items he advised: "Keep the ice box well supplied. The ice should be broken very small. A convenient way is to place it in a stout bag and beat it up with a mallet made of oak with a long handle in the end; or use an ice dealer's chisel."[4] Then Tufts says of "impulse buying," a term we use today, "the chair is a good thing. For when resting, the customers drink slowly. This means an opportunity to look about, seeing other things to buy." An admonition of Tufts to operators is: "If a man has a prejudice against any fountain beverage, coax him into trying it just once. If your fountain is irreproachable in cleanliness, and your beverage good, you have won him over. He will no longer hesitate to allow his children to patronize your fountain and will sing its praises to everyone."[5]

Matthews as a manufacturer vied with Tufts, publishing in his 1870 catalogue various statements, among them the following item: "An unfortunate name or misnomer is a constant bar to progress. This is well illustrated in the old name of 'soda water,' as 'soda water' does not contain any soda or other alkali. It is simply pure water charged with carbonic acid."[6] He then explains that carbonic acid is harmless, is found in the air we breathe. And he continues by saying, "Nearly all physicians are consumers of this beverage. Among the most civilized and cultivated of mankind, its consumption is rapidly increasing." Then, in a flight of fantasy he exclaims: "Youth as it sips the first glass [of 'soda water'] experiences sensations which, like the first sensations of love, cannot be forgotten and are cherished to the last."[7]

Matthews also reported in this 1870 catalogue that there was some question about the drinking of soda water, as to whether to allow children or even adults to drink it. The matter was presented to the Metropolitan Board of Health of New York, which body on studying the matter declared that soda water is an "innocent beverage." Matthews claimed that, "We ourselves conduct the most extensive business devoted to the supply of stores in the world, employing over 4,000 ten-gallon fountains, and furnishing 1,000 stores daily with 'aerated beverages.'"

One of Matthews' advertisements puts forward the following claims: "We offer this season our patented steel fountain and wagons for transporting the same, and exclusive rights in accordance with our printed agreement to wholesale dealers."[8] It would appear that Matthews sold everything connected with soda

4. Palmer, *op. cit.*
5. *Ibid.*
6. *Ibid.*
7. *Ibid.*
8. *Ibid.*

fountains except the horse to draw these wagons which he mentions!

Credit for introducing the ice cream soda is generally given to Robert M. Green of Philadelphia. It is said that in the 1870's the popular soda fountain drink was a concoction made up of sweet cream, syrup and carbonated water (probably also flavored). But on one occasion at Green's fountain the sweet cream was exhausted. So in desperation he used ice cream as a substitute for the sweet cream, and that was the beginning of the ice cream soda. This incident happened at the Centennial celebration of the Franklin Institute in Philadelphia in 1874, where Green had a concession. His sales there on the first day amounted to $8.00; but before the Exhibition closed, his sales amounted to $400.00 per day. Ice cream soda was the main factor in that increase.

Palmer[9] uses an allegory to describe this new development of the year 1874: "The marriage of the 23 year old Miss Ice Cream and the 66 year old Mr. Soda Fountain, was not headlined in the newspapers, but it 'turned out well.' Despite the disparity in the ages of the contracting parties, the union prospered and its progeny enveloped the United States."

As previously indicated, the manufacturers of soda fountains were giving advice and counsel in their catalogues as to how to conduct a soda fountain. In 1875 Tufts gave the following advice:

"Cleanliness is the capstone." Fountain operators are admonished to "use thin glasses" and to "keep attendants neat and clean." "See that attendants are courteous. Serve highly charged carbonated water. Use the best flavors." Tufts was especially critical of what he called "specialty drinks" or "patent drinks," to which he was very much opposed. He referred to them as "an octopus that is fastening itself on the soda fountain trade." Evidently the days of advertising on a national scale were not in existence at that time, for he said that "rum, port wine, prune juice, raspberry syrup, orange syrup, are generally the basis of these patent drinks, and *it is easier and much more profitable to concoct your own specialty than to push somebody else's.*"[10]

His advice on the subject of "ice cream soda water" is as follows: "Ice cream soda water is very popular, and some dealers have increased their business to a remarkable degree by its sale.

9. *Ibid.*
10. *Ibid.*

The ice cream should be kept in a large can and packed in ice, and placed under the counter within convenient reach. Draw the syrup required, less than for ordinary soda, put the ice cream into the tumbler with a large spoon, fill it up with soda water, and give the customer an ice cream soda water spoon to stir and eat the ice cream with."[11]

The growth of the soda fountain industry during the 60's, 70's, 80's and 90's was phenomenal. The number of fountains in operation increased annually; the number of fountain customers increased even more rapidly; the drug stores operating fountains were increasingly popular and prosperous; the volume of merchandise business brought to the drug store through the soda fountain was growing from year to year; and the prospect for further and more profitable years was self-evident.

During the early 90's the soda fountain had developed to such an extent that it was recognized as an important and almost imperative feature of the retail drug store and as a potential financial adjunct of such magnitude that the installation of a fountain became a must in the average retail drug store.

The stimulus responsible for this rather sudden new interest in the fountain was due in large part to the appearance on the market of a new drink under the name of Coca-Cola. This product was being manufactured in Atlanta, and its promoters were, for the first time in the soda water industry, using newspaper and other advertising media in its promotion. Furthermore, this advertising was designed to direct the public into the drug store since at that time the drug store was the only establishment to install soda fountains.

One of the first and unique methods of advertising used by The Coca-Cola Company was to mail tickets to a selected list of residents of a community with the instruction that the drug store in the community would accept the ticket as cash for a glass of Coca-Cola. Except perhaps for some proprietary medicine advertising, this was the first generally advertised product which directed the public to the drug store. As a result of this and other advertising, most of which was original and unique, more and more people were being directed into the drug stores of the State.

Recognizing this fact, many or most of those stores which had not previously installed fountains now became interested in tak-

---

11. In *loc. cit.*

ing this progressive step, to the end that by 1900 most of the drug stores of the State were operating fountains and on a profitable basis.

Prior to 1900, many or perhaps most of the soda fountain operators in the small towns of Georgia closed their fountains in the early Fall and opened them again in the Spring, on which occasions it was usually the custom to invite the school children to come in a body for a free drink of the suds type of soda water then popular, especially among children, who at that time were the principal customers of the fountain. It was not until Coca-Cola had interested adults in fountain drinks that the adult population was thought of as potential customers of the fountain. But when adults became regular soda fountain customers most of the fountains were kept open during the entire year.

To realize the great progress that has come in the evolution of the soda fountain, it is necessary to visualize the type of fountain and the type and variety of drinks served, and the conditions under which the fountains operated in the "Gay Nineties" in the average small town of Georgia.

The fountain of that period usually occupied a place on the counter between the customer and the operator. It was made by one of the popular manufacturers of that period—Matthews, Tufts, or Puffer. The body of the fountain was constructed of colored marble, the draught arms of highly polished metal, and decorations extending in quantity and quality to cost an amount which the purchaser felt able to pay. For that period this ornate fountain was considered a thing of beauty. The coils through which the carbonated water passed from the tank to the draught arm were refrigerated with crushed ice and at that time were made of lead, which was, of course, subject to chemical action by the carbonated water and required frequent attention by a plumber. These lead coils were later supplanted by block tin or stainless steel.

The carbonated water was stored under pressure in ten-gallon steel drums which were located under the counter and attached to the pipes leading to the coils.

One or more of these ten-gallon drums or tanks were always kept in reserve. To fill these tanks or drums the water was placed in the drum and carbon dioxide gas under pressure was passed into the water, the drum being shaken on the "rocker" during the process until the water was saturated and the proper pressure was established.

The draught arms on the fountain were so constructed as to give either a fine stream or a coarse stream of water, the fine stream being used to produce the "suds" or "foam" in the glass which was considered so desirable. The coarse stream was used for the non-suds type of drink such as Coca-Cola and the phosphates or "solid drinks."

Each fountain was equipped with six or more syrup jars, and the six most popular syrups of the suds type were lemon, vanilla, strawberry, pineapple, chocolate, and orange (ginger or raspberry or sarsaparilla). And, since there were no means of preserving the syrups against souring, they were made up according to daily needs. Simple syrup was either made up in quantity on the basis of 7½ pounds of sugar to the gallon, or bought in quantities of a barrel (which was usually labeled Rock Candy Syrup) and the flavoring agent added in proper quantity. The quality of the finished drink was usually determined not only by the taste and temperature, but by the amount and relative stability of the suds. To produce the latter quality a small amount of solution of Quillaja (or soap bark) was added to the syrup. In drawing the suds type of drink, about two ounces of the syrup was drawn into a ten or twelve ounce glass, one or two ounces of milk added, the fine stream then being used to fill the glass. All of this mixture was served for the price of 5 cents.

There being no running water available in the average small town of Georgia, it was utterly impossible to apply ordinary sanitary measures in the washing of the utensils around the fountain.

Door and window fly screens had not been made available at that time, and the problem of flies and other insects around the fountain was not only a nuisance but a health menace as well. The volatile oils such as Sassafras or Pennyroyal, applied to the counter and tables, had some repellent effects on the insects and sometimes on the customers, who frequently objected to these odors.

Electricity not being available, there was no practical way by which fans could be employed to meet the insect problem or to furnish power to the ice crushers or ice cream freezers or other utensils.

The alert fountain operator of 1900 realized that ice cream might prove a desirable adjunct to his soda fountain business, since it was not available for purchase elsewhere. But since there was no commercial source for its purchase, he proceeded to

℞ THE SODA FOUNTAIN   215

manufacture his own ice cream by the old "ice-salt" process, in such quantities and of such flavors as might be disposed of that day. This was a necessity for there were no means by which ice cream might be refrigerated from one day to the next.

The demand for ice cream increased rapidly, and this small beginning toward popularizing the product was the foundation upon which the ice cream industry has eventually arisen, thus constituting a contribution by the drug store not only to the ice cream industry but to the dairy industry in the State as well.

Ice cream and the soda fountain thus became complements one of the other, the fountain being the medium through which ice cream and the customer were to meet, and ice cream the agency for bringing customers to the fountain.

But the full benefits to be derived for either the fountain or the ice cream industry could not be realized until ice cream could be manufactured in quantity, preserved in frozen state, and transported from manufacturing plant to fountain distributor.

With the advent of mechanical refrigeration in 1923-1930, the stage was all set for the development of an industry which was to stabilize and make profitable the dairy industry, and which was to increase the volume of its manufactured product from year to year in rapid strides, as evidenced by the gallonage figures given by the U.S.D.A. Agricultural Marketing Service Bulletin for November, 1956, Number 199, for the United States as a whole.

Year	Type	Gallons
1900	Hard Ice Cream	5,000,000 Gallons
1914	" " "	72,000,000 "
1930	" " "	240,000,000 "
1945	" " "	471,000,000 "
1954	" " "	596,000,000 "
1956	" " "	628,559,000 "

The soda fountains in Georgia's 1,100 drug stores claim a stake in the remarkable progress and profits of the Ice Cream Industry and the Dairy Industry it has supported in the State. It is an interesting question as to whether the increased consumption of dairy products including ice cream may have been a factor in raising the health standards in Georgia.

But the soda fountain industry could not reach its full development of efficiency, service and popularity until progress along other lines had come into existence.

The *first* of these factors necessary for the proper operation of the soda fountain was the matter of running water of a high degree of purity, which now prevails even in the smallest communities where soda fountains are operated.

The *second* development involved the bringing of electricity into the drug store for the operation of fans, lights, pumps, cooling systems, and other appliances.

The *third* development involved the introduction of the first practical mechanical refrigeration, the Nizer Ice Cream Cabinet in 1923, which revolutionized the entire operation of the soda fountain, including the freezing and preservation of ice cream. Following the success of the first mechanical ice cream cabinet, mechanical refrigeration began to appear for the refrigeration of all soda fountain products, as well as for the shipment of food products and ice cream.

The *fourth* item was the matter of sanitation, and this was perhaps the most important and far-reaching of all the conditions that had to do with the progress in the development of the soda fountain. By this time fly screens had come into general use, and milk products were being standardized on the basis of their bacterial count, and the public was becoming sanitation conscious, largely influenced by the principles and practices they observed in public eating and drinking places. Thus, today, most soda fountains and most eating and drinking places are operated at a high degree of efficiency so far as sanitary principles are concerned. The soda fountain, therefore, visited as it is by almost the entire population in the course of time, has been a prominent factor in the teaching of the principles, practices, advantages and necessity of sanitation, this being particularly true of the soda fountains operated in the drug stores, where they are operated under the guidance and direction of a licensed pharmacist.

The soda fountain has thus played an important part in the evolution of the modern drug store, which, in turn—particularly in the average small town—has come to be a community center where all the issues of the day are discussed, be they political, social, economic, educational, or some other; and those who come to the drug store for any reason represent the old and the young, the male and the female, the rich and the poor, the sick and the well.

CHAPTER X

ETHER ANAESTHESIA, 1842, AND COCA-COLA, 1886: BORN IN GEORGIA DRUG STORES. A STORY WHEREBY COCA-COLA BECOMES THE COMPLEMENT OF ETHER ANAESTHESIA

BORN AS they were in Georgia drug stores, ether anaesthesia and Coca-Cola were destined to be known in the far corners of the world. Ether anaesthesia came from the drug store, and at the hands of Physician-Pharmacist Crawford W. Long in the small town of Jefferson, Georgia, in 1842. The formula for Coca-Cola came from the drug store of Pharmacist John S. Pemberton of Atlanta, in 1886, and it was first dispensed in the drug store of Pharmacist Joe Jacobs of Atlanta. The breath of life was breathed into this new product by Pharmacist Asa G. Candler of Atlanta, promoter-extraordinary.

Crawford W. Long was born in Danielsville, Georgia, November 1, 1815, and at the age of 14 he entered the University of Georgia, where he was assigned to room with Alexander H. Stephens in a dormitory which had been erected in 1810 as the first building on the campus. These two boys were destined to become famous: Stephens as the Vice-President of the Confederacy and Long as the discoverer of ether anaesthesia. A bronze plaque now marks the room they occupied as students in 1829, and for all time they will continue to be roommates as Georgia's representatives in the National Hall of Fame where their statues rest.

Following graduation from the University of Georgia in 1835, Dr. Long read medicine for a time with Dr. Grant of Jefferson, a town within a few miles of the place of his birth.

After spending a year in the Medical Department of Transylvania University in Lexington, Kentucky, he matriculated in the Medical Department of the University of Pennsylvania in 1838, from which institution he was graduated in 1839. Following his internship in hospitals of New York City, he returned to Jefferson and purchased the business (including the drug store) of his old preceptor, Dr. Grant.

Then, as now, the drug store in a small town was the meetingplace of the young people of the community. The young people of Jefferson, having read about "laughing gas," asked Dr. Long to administer it to them. But, having none, he persuaded them to inhale "ether." His observations of these young people under the influence of ether led him to the discovery that complete and safe anaesthesia could be produced with ether, and that a surgical operation could be performed without pain.

In 1842, James M. Venable submitted to an operation for the removal of a wen on the back of his neck while under ether anaesthesia. This operation by Dr. Long was a complete success and became the precedent for all other surgical operations under anaesthesia, however produced, from 1842 to this good day. This marked one of the greatest, or perhaps the greatest, advance in the history of medicine up to that time.

Ether as a chemical or pharmaceutical product had been known for 300 years prior to Dr. Long's birth, for Valerius Cordus described the product in the 16th century and named it "Oleum Vitriolo Dulce" or "Spiritus Vini Aetherius" or "Ether Sulphuricus." A mixture of ether and alcohol known as Hoffman's Anodyne or Drops is one of the old reliable and safe internal agents for colic and is still a drug store product. It is therefore evident that Dr. Long's pharmaceutical acquaintance with ether made his discovery of anaesthesia possible.

In 1852, Dr. Long moved to Athens and promptly bought a drug store there from a pharmacist-physician owner, which business grew to large proportions under the guidance of Dr. Long and his brother, Dr. H. R. J. Long, both of whom continued the active practice of medicine and pharmacy until Dr. Long's death.

While operating this drug store, Dr. Long, on his own initiative, became the pharmaceutical preceptor of Joseph Jacobs, in whose drug store in Atlanta, some years later, the first glass of Coca-Cola as a soda fountain product was to be dispensed. In still later years Mr. Jacobs actively supported the efforts of Dr. Frank Boland and other citizens of Georgia in establishing without question Dr. Long's priority in the use of ether as an anaesthetic. He was also instrumental in the placement of the statue of his beloved preceptor in the National Hall of Fame in Washington.

Note: In another chapter of the present volume, the reader may find a photostatic copy of an advertisement of Dr. Long's drug store in Athens.

Thus Joseph Jacobs constitutes a connecting link between Dr. Long and the development of the formula of Coca-Cola by Pharmacist Pemberton, its first sale by Pharmacist Jacobs, and its promotion by Pharmacist Asa G. Candler.

Joseph Jacobs was the oldest of fourteen children to be born of immigrant parents who had escaped from Germany during a period of persecution of Jewish people. They came to Jefferson, Georgia, where Joseph was born in 1859. As a child he attended Martin Institute in Jefferson. This school was considered then, and for many years thereafter, to be of the highest quality.

Given to reminiscing, Mr. Jacobs was a frequent contributor to various pharmaceutical journals, including *Drug Topics, American Journal of Pharmacy, Southeastern Drug Journal,* and others, from which sources most of his biographical data is drawn.

Speaking of his childhood in Jefferson, Mr. Jacobs tells of the first drug store with which he was familiar, which belonged to "old Dr. Doster," and how he was intrigued by the skeleton and by the pharmaceutical equipment in the old doctor's drug store. Of him Mr. Jacobs states: "The doctor was of the Thomsonian school (Eclectic or Herbalist), and there was displayed in the drug store the legend (of that school of medicine), 'No implements of death used here', (meaning that no medicines of mineral origin had a place on his shelves)."

In Mr. Jacobs' own words: "At the age of 13, my family moved from Jefferson to Athens, a distance of about twenty miles, and I became an apprentice in the drug store of Dr. Crawford W. Long. For the first six months my salary was zero, after which my salary was fixed at ten dollars per month." His chief responsibility was the operation of the soda fountain and the manufacture of carbon dioxide gas for the fountain, from bicarbonate of soda and sulphuric acid. The soda fountain was of the "Puffer" manufacture.

During his apprenticeship under Dr. Long (a period of approximately three years), he attended lectures in chemistry at the University of Georgia, and received at the same time pharmaceutical instruction from Dr. Long, his preceptor. Mr. Jacobs recalls that ice for the fountain was brought from Augusta, a distance of 125 miles by rail, at a cost of 10 cents per pound.

At about the age of 17, he entered the Philadelphia College of Pharmacy in 1877. Following his graduation from that school in 1879, he returned to Athens and opened a business under the title, "The Athens Pharmaceutical Company." He manufactured pharmaceuticals for sale to country doctors, including his old friend, Dr. Doster, of Jefferson, most of his fluid extracts and tinctures being manufactured from locally growing drugs which he collected. He also manufactured a line of household remedies for sale to country merchants.

This business proving profitable, Jacobs moved to Atlanta in 1884 and purchased the drug store of his former classmate, Walter H. Taylor, which business had been established by Walter Taylor's father, James A. Taylor, in 1854.

Jacobs remodeled the interior of the store, moving all of the glass-labelled bottles which adorned the shelves to the rear, and substituted therefor merchandise items of an assorted nature. He then changed the name to Jacobs Pharmacy.

At that period the standard prices of patent or proprietary medicines ranged as follows: 25 cents, 50 cents, or one dollar. And, to cut these prices by even as small an amount as one cent was considered by organized pharmaceutical bodies as highly unethical. Jacobs Pharmacy, much to the annoyance of other retail drug stores and manufacturers, began to cut the prices of advertised patent medicines, thus becoming the first cut-rate drug store in the South. This proved to be a bombshell in the ranks of organized pharmacy in the State, and all legal attempts to curb price-cutting were exhausted, but leaving in their wake much bitterness in the hearts and minds of the "full-price" group of pharmacists. By cutting prices to the odd cent, Mr. Jacobs claims that he brought the copper penny to Atlanta.

Jacobs pharmacy was the first outlet to establish branch stores in Atlanta. This movement was also bitterly condemned and opposed by the other pharmacists in Atlanta.

Speaking years later of his purchase of the Taylor store, Mr. Jacobs gives a "historic statement" when he says: "When I moved to Atlanta in January, 1884, to take possession of my purchase of Walter Taylor's store, which was located at the corner of Peachtree and Marietta Streets (known then as the Norcross Corner), on the right hand side of the entrance was the soda fountain conducted by Willis Venable, who was assisted in the operation of the soda fountain by his brother John Venable and his son Edward Venable." The "historic statement" has reference to this soda fountain, from which the first glass of Coca-Cola as a carbonated beverage was dispensed.

It is an interesting coincidence that James Venable was the first person in world history to be operated on while under ether anaesthesia, and that Willis Venable should dispense the first glass of Coca-Cola, and that the drug store in which the fountain was located should belong to Joseph Jacobs, who had served his apprenticeship at the soda fountain of Dr. Crawford W. Long, the man who had performed that first operation under ether anaesthesia some forty years previously.

On coming to Atlanta to operate a drug store, Joseph Jacobs found two other pharmacists there who were to be his competitors but also his intimate friends, with whom he was to cooperate in the early days of the life of Coca-Cola. These two pharmacists were John S. Pemberton, who originated the formula for Coca-Cola, and Asa G. Candler, who, as its promoter, was to make of Coca-Cola a product destined to be universally known.

Pharmacist John Styth Pemberton was one of the triumvirate of contemporary pharmacists in Atlanta (the other two being Joseph Jacobs and Asa G. Candler) all of whom were to play a definite and distinctive part in the birth, nurture, and promotion of Coca-Cola.

He was born in Knoxville, Georgia, in 1833, and as a child moved with his family to Columbus, Georgia, where he received his basic education.

The historical or biographical records are not clear as to when or how he became interested in the profession of pharmacy, or when he was licensed as a pharmacist.

There is a story, however, to the effect that "he obtained a degree in pharmacy at Macon, Georgia," but no dates are given and the name of the institution from which he is supposed to have received a degree is not mentioned.

The date must have been about 1850, -51, or -52, for he was then approximately 20 years of age. "He returned to Columbus, and in 1853 married Miss Clifford Day Lewis of that city, and operated a wholesale and retail drug business there."

According to pharmaceutical records there was no institution in Georgia authorized to grant a degree in pharmacy prior to and until 1891, when the Atlanta College of Pharmacy was established in connection with the Atlanta Medical College.

There was in existence in Macon during the 1850's an Eclectic or Thomsonian School of Medicine. And it is possible that Dr. Pemberton may have obtained a degree in medicine from that institution, for it is reported by some of his family that he actually did have a degree in medicine. This may explain why, during his years of residence in Atlanta, and following his death, he was almost universally referred to as "Dr. Pemberton," and for the purposes of this story he will be referred to as "Dr. Pemberton."

The law in Georgia at that time provided that any person graduating from any medical school could, by presenting evidence of graduation to the Medical Board of Examiners, be licensed to practice pharmacy. And most physicians of that time held such a license. This may be helpful in setting the date as to when Dr. Pemberton was licensed as a pharmacist, though the license may, on the other hand, have been granted after a period of apprenticeship and examination by the Medical Board, there having been no Pharmaceutical Examining Board until much later.

In the early years of the Civil War, Dr. Pemberton was probably exempted from military service because of the need for him in the community as a physician or pharmacist. But in the latter months of the War, he organized a company of volunteers known as "Pemberton's Cavalry" and served for the remainder of the War as the captain of this company under General Joseph Wheeler.

Following the War and the movement to rebuild the City of Atlanta, which had been virtually destroyed by Sherman's Army, Dr. Pemberton came to Atlanta in 1869 to continue in the drug business and to promote some of the medicinal products he had created, of which there was a considerable number. His promotional policies, however, did not keep pace with his creative abilities, with the result that he was never considered a successful business man, though highly esteemed as a citizen and as a pharmacist.

Almost concurrent with Dr. Pemberton's arrival in Atlanta in 1869 there was introduced into England and the European Continent in 1870 a medicinal product which had been used by the natives of South America for centuries, known by them as the "Divine Plant of the Incas." This product was very promptly to become world famous under the name of "Coca" or "Coca Leaves" as a delightful cerebral stimulant, and its fame was to spread to North America in due time.

Dr. Pemberton became interested in this new product and described its properties in glowing terms in an address before the Georgia Pharmaceutical Association. Had it been the present era, it probably would have been referred to as a "wonder drug."

In 1885, Dr. Pemberton prepared a medicinal product which was copyrighted under the name, "French Wine of Coca, Ideal Tonic." This product proving popular and salable, somewhat later he conceived the idea of combining Coca with Kola Nut as a remedy for headache and "quick pick-up," Kola itself being a new and highly publicized product similar in properties to coffee or tea. As a headache remedy, in the concentrations he was using, this combination was all Dr. Pemberton claimed for it.

To make this combination more palatable than his "Wine of Coca," he aromatized it and combined it with syrup. This product was intended to be advertised for domestic and general use, but was lacking a suitable name until one of his business associates, Frank Robinson, an accomplished penman, changed the spelling of "kola" to "Cola" and created the trademark name "Coca-Cola."

Having some difficulty in creating a demand for the new product, even after an advertising extravagance of $46.00 in one year, Dr. Pemberton conceived the idea of introducing it at the soda fountains in the drug stores of his friends and fellow pharmacists. There were said to be only three soda fountains in Atlanta in the drug stores at that time (1886), one of which was in Jacobs Pharmacy, the most modern and most progressive store in Atlanta. The fountain in this store was also considered the most popular soda fountain in the city, and was under lease to Willis Venable, who was the acknowledged "soda water king" of Atlanta.

There seems to be no evidence that Dr. Pemberton had thought of the product as a carbonated beverage. Mr. Venable contributed this important and valuable idea, therefore becoming the first individual in the world to dispense Coca-Cola as a carbonated beverage.

Dr. Pemberton, being of frail health and lacking proper financial resources to promote the sale of Coca-Cola, sold a two-thirds interest to George S. Lowndes for $1200, who in turn chose Mr. Venable in Jacobs Pharmacy as his associate in ownership, believing that he (Venable) might or could supply the spark to start the product on its way. This partnership was agreeable to Dr. Pemberton, who still retained a one-third interest. But this agreement between Mr. Lowndes and Mr. Venable did not prove satisfactory, and the partnership was dissolved. The two-thirds interest in Coca-Cola changed hands again, and Coca-Cola was to await the magic touch of promoter Asa G. Candler, who later acquired all fractional interests in the product, including Dr. Pemberton's remaining one-third (1888), thus promptly starting it on its way to a fabulous success.

Asa Griggs Candler was the third member of the triumvirate of Atlanta pharmacists who played a part in the creation and promotion of Coca-Cola. He was born in Villa Rica, Georgia, December 30, 1851, and it was he who supplied the spark which carried Coca-Cola to fame.

His father was a merchant in the town of Villa Rica and owned large acreage of land in that section. He was also interested in politics in the State, serving in both branches of the General Assembly from Carroll County.

Following the Civil War the fortunes of the Candler family suffered greatly, Villa Rica being in the line of march of Sherman's Army. In addition to the many readjustments made necessary, the education of the Candler children became a pressing problem. It had been the plan of his father that Asa Candler should study medicine. But financial difficulties made this impossible, and Asa himself said: "My hopes never ventured further than an apothecary shop, and a prescription clerk in a drug store near my boyhood home was greater in my estimation than the President or the world's greatest ball-player."

At the age of 19, in 1870, he apprenticed himself to two fine physicians, Doctors Best and Kirkpatrick in Cartersville. As was the almost universal custom then, the doctors operated a drug store as an adjunct to their practice. Candler was a man of all work in the drug store, and slept on a cot in a room in the rear of the store. His apprenticeship there covered a period of three years. It is interesting to note that in all of Mr. Candler's experience in drug stores there is no mention of his having any soda fountain experience.

Asa Candler, hoping for a broader opportunity than afforded itself at Cartersville, came to Atlanta in 1873, and his biographer, Charles H. Candler, tells this story:

> Seven days after the expiration of his service as an apprentice in Cartersville, on Monday, July 5th, he had left Cartersville for Atlanta. All he had when he came to Atlanta were the homemade clothes he wore and exactly $1.75 in his pocket. He began to walk the city streets looking for work. Until nine o'clock that night he carried on a systematic search, going

into every drug store as he came to it asking for a chance to make a start. One of the places he tried was a store called the Pemberton-Pulliam Drug Company, located off the lobby of the Kimball House. He had no way of knowing that the senior partner in this enterprise, who had no place on his staff for an enterprising young druggist from Cartersville, was to have a profound influence upon the whole course of his life.

Finally, at nine o'clock, weary from his journey to the city and the daylong search, he found an opening. George J. Howard, who owned a popular drug store around the corner from the Kimball House on Peachtree Street, agreed to try out the young pharmacist. No salary was promised until he could prove himself worthy of compensation. Nor was there to be any waiting period. As soon as the young man had reached an agreement with Mr. Howard, he went to work, and stayed until midnight that night when the store was closed.

It seems that Mr. Candler occupied a tiny room on the ground floor at the rear of the three-story building, such as he had in Cartersville. But he soon made for himself a permanent trial job with Howard Drug Company, and was soon made Chief Drug Clerk. He was then 21 years of age.

He was out of Atlanta for a year, when he returned to Villa Rica to settle his father's estate. But at the end of the year, he returned to Howard's drug store as Chief Clerk, and remained there for two years.

He was now (1877) 25 years old, and he formed a partnership with M. B. Hallman under the firm name of "Hallman & Candler, Wholesale and Retail Druggists," to operate a store in close proximity to Mr. Howard's. It is a coincidence of note to find Dr. Pemberton, who had refused to give Candler a job, now working at Howard's drug store in the vacancy created by Candler's resignation.

In 1878 Mr. Candler married the daughter of Mr. Howard, to which marriage Mr. Howard was most bitterly opposed. But reconciliation came within a short time, as evidenced by the fact that later Mr. Candler and Mr. Howard were to become partners in the drug business, following Candler's purchase of Mr. Hallman's interest in the H. & C. drug business in 1881, and then selling one-half interest in the business to Mr. Howard in 1882, only to buy it back in 1886.

Dr. Pemberton, it seems, left Howard's drug store and formed a partnership under the firm name of "Pemberton, Iverson & Denison," which business was sold to Howard and Candler following a disastrous fire in their store in 1883. Dr. Pemberton then formed the Pemberton Chemical Company with his son, Charles, as partner, and it was this company which was to originate and control for a time the new product, Coca-Cola, of which product Mr. Candler came to be sole owner in 1888 at a total cost to him of $2300. The assets of the company included the valuable formula, all of the manufacturing apparatus, all special ingredients for the manufacture of the drink, the trademark "Coca-Cola," and all advertising materials then on hand. At this point Mr. Candler observed that by some refinements in the formula the product could be converted into a beverage rather than as a headache remedy, and from this point on in its history Coca-Cola was to be known as a beverage and not as a pharmaceutical product.

There came into the Candler organization just at this time (1888) two men who were to participate actively in the development of Coca-Cola and remain in The Company as associates in high positions as long as they lived. One of these was F. M. Robinson, who had created the trademark name "Coca-Cola" and fervently believed in its future; and the other was Samuel C. Dobbs, Mr. Candler's nephew.

Without any coordinated or sustained advertising program the gallonage sales of Coca-Cola in 1890 had reached 9,000 gallons, much of which increase came from sales from Venable's fountain in Jacobs Pharmacy.

This increase in gallonage must have been a persuasive influence in Mr. Candler's and his associates' minds that the future of Coca-Cola, with sustained and coordinated advertising, could be assured and would therefore justify the sale of the wholesale and retail drug business so as to enable them to give all of their time to promotional and sales activities.

The sale of the Candler drug business came in 1891, thereby furnishing the initial capital with which to expand all promotional activities, and in 1892 The Coca-Cola Company was incorporated in Georgia, with a capital stock of $100,000. The advertising budget for that year was set at $11,401.78.

Fortunate indeed were those few outsiders who availed themselves of the opportunity to purchase some of this original stock. Sad to relate, the author was not one of these. If every pharmacist in Georgia had invested $1000 in that original stock, there would never have been cause for the financial failure of any drug business in Georgia, or for hunger in any druggist's home.

Before continuing the story of Coca-Cola, it is interesting to review some incidents and coincidents which resulted in the birth of Coca-Cola and which give a preview of what followed.

The Coca-Cola idea was born in the mind and in the retail and manufacturing drug store of Dr. John S. Pemberton, with no thought of it other than as a "tonic" or "headache remedy," but never as a carbonated beverage. He did know that people frequently call at the soda fountain for "something for the headache," and that the product might thus be introduced via the soda fountain. It was therefore logical that he should find a proper fountain for this experiment.

His friend of the years, Joseph Jacobs, was operating a progressive and popular retail drug store in the heart of downtown Atlanta. And his soda fountain was being operated under lease to Mr. Venable, the popular "soda fountain king of Atlanta," who was, for a time at least, the key man in the life of Coca-Cola for he it was who kept it alive. It was he who first dispensed it under his own initiative as a carbonated beverage and was the guiding influence, perhaps, in persuading other fountain operators to recommend and dispense it as such.

It is interesting to speculate as to whether Mr. Jacobs might never have operated a drug store had it not been that Dr. Crawford W. Long, his preceptor, influenced him to complete his education for the practice of the profession of pharmacy. And if there had not been a Jacobs Pharmacy, would there have been any Coca-Cola?

Messrs. Candler, Pemberton, and Jacobs had all been members at one time in the American and the Georgia Pharmaceutical Associations, and were friendly competitors all during the years.

Mr. Candler had operated a wholesale, as well as a retail, drug business and as a wholesaler had relations not only with the Atlanta druggists, but with others in the Atlanta shipping area. As an astute business man, he was aware of all developments in the drug field, and was fully acquainted with the result of the experiment of popularizing Coca-Cola at the soda fountain in Jacobs Pharmacy. He was the first person to visualize the vast opportunity for popularizing a product through the medium of the soda fountains in the drug stores of the world, and, particularly, if that product was pleasing to the taste and could be sold at a price all persons, rich and poor alike, could afford.

The drug store, the home of practically one hundred per cent of the soda fountains of that time, was therefore to play a most important, and probably the most important, role as a medium of distribution of Coca-Cola.

Mr. Candler, as a pharmacist himself, realized that he must

have the confidence, influence and intelligent cooperation of retail pharmacists. As a wholesaler, he was in position to know that the volume of business in the average retail drug store needed the stimulus of a profitable sideline.

The program of the Company was therefore so ordered as to insure a proper and profitable relationship with retail pharmacists to include the following items: (1) The price of syrup was to be such as to insure a profit to the dealer. (2) The syrup was to be of uniform quality. (3) It was to be packaged in convenient quantities. (4) There must be a differential in price for quantity lots to encourage distributors to push the product. (5) Prompt deliveries must be assured. (6) An advertising program was to be developed which would bring people into the store for the purchase of Coca-Cola.

When Mr. Candler began advertising Coca-Cola in the other towns and cities of the State, the druggists over the State began to install soda fountains, and they shared in the development and the profits of the new product, Coca-Cola, the author being one of those who promoted its sale as early as 1898, at the soda fountain of Rozier and Middlebrooks at Sparta, Georgia. Always profitable in that respect, Coca-Cola had been the first item to come into general popularity which actually brought people into the drug store for trade at the soda fountain, because it was the first product to be advertised as being sold exclusively over the soda fountain. Mr. Candler, among other activities in promoting the sale of Coca-Cola, mailed out tickets for the drink, whereby people would take the ticket into the store and get a drink of Coca-Cola, and The Coca-Cola Company would redeem the tickets from the druggists for the full price of five cents. Another advertising item much sought after was the large Coca-Cola wall clock, given to those proprietors who evidenced a spirit of cooperation and showed an increase in volume.

Then, as now, Coca-Cola was advertised extensively. And since it was sold strictly and solely from the soda fountain of the drug store in those early days, it was a profitable venture on the part of the drug stores; and the economic status of the drug stores of Georgia, and of America eventually, began to improve with the increase in volume and profits in the sales of Coca-Cola. It has always been a profitable item for the drug store, not only in the profit that comes directly from its sale, but from the number of people the product has brought into the drug store who purchase other items.

Over the years, with the profits from Coca-Cola increasing rapidly both from the standpoint of the retail druggist and for The Coca-Cola Company itself, the accumulation of profits derived from Coca-Cola grew to such a point that Mr. Candler, out of his generosity, gave several million dollars for the establishment of Emory University to carry into perpetuity the values of denominational (Methodist) education.

However, the concept of the creation of Emory University was born in the mind of Bishop Warren A. Candler, who was the devoted brother of Asa G. Candler, and was President of Emory College located at Oxford, Georgia, from 1888 to 1898. This institution at Oxford at that time was a small, struggling denominational college of arts and sciences which was devoted to the objective of carrying forward the principles and practices of the Christian religion.

It was the dream of President (later Bishop) Candler that Emory College could and should be expanded into a university to provide for an expanded program of arts and science training for undergraduates and for the establishment of a theological school for the training of ministers. His brother Asa G. Candler caught the vision of President Candler, and on July 16, 1914, he directed a communication addressed to Bishop Warren A. Candler, Chairman of the Educational Commission of the General Conference of the Methodist Episcopal Church, South, which included this paragraph:

> In this I do not seek a sectarian end; for I gratefully acknowledge that I have received benefits and blessings from all the churches of our land. I rejoice in the work of all the denominations who love our Lord Jesus Christ in sincerity and are seeking to do most good to men; but to some one church I must commit my contribution to Christian education, and I see no reason to hesitate to trust money to that church to which I look for spiritual guidance; to that church at whose altars I receive the Christian Gospel and sacraments and upon which surely I depend, I safely entrust the things I possess—to this end I offer the sum of one million dollars for the endowment of sound learning and pure religion. . . . The faith, the love, the prayers and the zeal of good people must supply the force to do that which money cannot accomplish. . . . In humble trust in that God to whom I look for Salvation, I dedicate the means with which Providence has blessed me to the upbuilding of the Divine Kingdom.

Following the gift of $1,000,000, it was decided to build Emory University on the campus it now occupies. During the remainder of his life Mr. Candler continued to donate liberally to the building and expansion of the University, and his son Howard Candler, a former President and Chairman of the Board of The Coca-Cola Company, and his brothers and sisters, have since made further and many liberal donations.

It is an intriguing thought and fact that the sons of Mr. Candler were students at Emory College when it was located at Oxford and that Robert Winship Woodruff was also a student there, and later came to add his extensive contributions to the building and maintenance of Emory University.

With the assurance that the University would be properly supported, the Candler Theological School (in memory of Bishop Candler) was added, and shortly thereafter the Lamar School of Law. The Atlanta College of Physicians and Surgeons and the Atlanta Dental College, both of which institutions had been operated for a number of years under private ownership, were absorbed in toto into Emory University, and hospital facilities became a natural adjunct of the Emory Medical School.

In 1919 Asa Candler sold The Coca-Cola Company to a syndicate headed by Ernest Woodruff of Atlanta, who was recognized as one of the leading financiers of the South. Under the new management the advertising and promotional plans of the Company took on new impetus, with the result that the Company has grown into a world-wide enterprise with an ever increasing volume of sales and profits. Its product is now sold in more than one hundred countries, territories and possessions throughout the world.

The Emily and Ernest Woodruff Foundation was created in 1938 by Mr. and Mrs. Ernest Woodruff. Mr. Robert Woodruff, a son, is Chairman of the Board of Trustees and Mr. George Woodruff, also a son, is Vice-Chairman of the Board; other Trustees are Messrs. Hughes Spalding, John A. Sibley and Arthur A. Acklin. Mr. L. L. McCullough is Secretary and Treasurer.

Mr. Robert Woodruff, a former President, Chairman of the Board and Chairman of the Executive Committee, and now Chairman of the Finance Committee of The Coca-Cola Company, has personally made large donations to Emory University, and the Woodruff Foundation contributions have been largely centered in building up the School of Medicine and expanding the facilities of Emory University Hospital, and in promoting research in medical and health fields.

As further evidence of Mr. Woodruff's interest in health matters, he has, in addition to his contributions to Emory University, made substantial contributions for research to the School of Pharmacy of the University of Georgia.

The establishment in 1937 of the Joseph B. Whitehead Foundation was provided for in the will of Joseph B. Whitehead, the Foundation receiving the residue of his estate. The income thus received by the Foundation is used for charitable and educational purposes in the territory of Atlanta, Georgia. Mr. Robert Woodruff is Chairman of the Board of Trustees; other Trustees are Dr. F. Phinizy Calhoun, Vice-Chairman, and Mr. James F. Alexander. Mr. Samuel L. Jones is Secretary and Managing Director.

The financial and moral support, reinforced by virile leadership on the part of the Candlers, the Woodruffs, and the Whiteheads, is responsible for enabling Emory University and its Medical School and Hospital to occupy one of the highest places among similar institutions of the world, which will continue on into perpetuity as an agency of service to the people of the South and as a monument to these families. Robert W. Woodruff, the son of Ernest Woodruff, has served as one of the Trustees of Emory University, and Charles Howard Candler, the son of Asa Candler, was at the time of his death (1957) Chairman of the Board of Trustees of Emory University.

It is an intriguing story that these products, Coca-Cola and sulphuric ether for anaesthesia, should come to be complements one of the other in the building and maintenance of a hospital for service to a suffering humanity. Both products, born as they were in retail drug stores of Georgia, were nurtured there, the one, Coca-Cola, contributing to the economic development of the drug stores of Georgia, and the other, anaesthesia, contributing to the saving of human life. It is a coincidence that they should be thus associated in the operation of Emory Hospital and Emory University School of Medicine.

But out of the profits derived from Coca-Cola by many others in addition to the Candlers and the Woodruffs and the Whiteheads, including the bottlers of Coca-Cola in various parts of the State and the world, many other educational and religious institutions along with Emory University have been beneficiaries.

Since John S. Pemberton, Joseph Jacobs, and Asa Candler were themselves retail pharmacists, and, since the drug stores of Georgia constituted the springboard from which Coca-Cola achieved its fabulous success, they can justly claim a stake in the fortunes and in the institutions Coca-Cola has built for service to mankind.

Chapter XI

DRUGS IN THE MODERN ERA

TWO HUNDRED and thirty-six years have elapsed since the first apothecary and physician, in the person of Dr. Riberio Nunez, came into the Colony of Georgia, July 11, 1733.

In a previous chapter, the reader has been made acquainted with the disease and medical problems of the early years of the Colony; with the theories of disease and treatment as proposed by Dr. Tennent (1734), John Wesley (1747), Dr. George Harral (1807), and Dr. Ewell (1807); and with the wide variety of treatments recommended by them all of which constituted encouragement in self-diagnosis and treatment. For several decades thereafter, other physicians were writing books of similar nature, but all of them with encouragement and instruction in self-diagnosis and medication.

For the first hundred years of the life of the Colony there were no educational or legal requirements applying to those who entered the practice of pharmacy and/or medicine. Progress was therefore necessarily slow in developing along either educational, legal, or ethical lines. As a substitute for formal educational and professional training, the apprenticeship-preceptor system was of necessity utilized.

In the meanwhile, the practice of self-diagnosis and treatment had become so firmly entrenched in the life of the average layman that the physician was forced to augment his meager income by adopting some sideline—and the one nearest in line with his medical practice was the sale of drugs.

This practice became so common that the business of the apothecary, druggist, or pharmacist was absorbed to a large extent by the medical practitioner; and as a matter of self-preservation and finding no restrictions in the matter, many of those who were practicing pharmacy adopted the practice of medicine as a sideline. These steps taken on the part of physicians and apothecaries laid the foundation for the controversy which extends into the present era; namely, the dispensing physician and the prescribing pharmacist.

This centralization of all knowledge of drugs *in one individual* militated against the possibility of the expansion of knowledge in any one scientific field or direction. Any observation in the matter of diagnosis or treatment—if successful—was usually carefully guarded in the interest of the practitioner, thus preventing the expansion of knowledge.

There were some gestures from time to time to indicate that a separation of pharmacy and medicine into their respective fields of specialization might be possible. But the first evidence of such thought is illustrated in the Fee Bills of a previous Chapter, when, after a ten-year period, the price of drugs was discontinued in the advertisements announcing the adoption of a schedule of fees and prices. Actually, however, this proved to be merely a gesture, for the practice of the sale of drugs by the physician had been generally followed, and has never entirely disappeared.

For the remainder of the 18th century, and well into the 19th century, since there was no educational or other stimulus to a broader knowledge of diagnosis or treatment, there is but little evidence of any progress that can be pointed to as of value in medicine and pharmacy.

Education, both general and technical, for pharmacists and physicians was making some slow but definite progress, and organization of each group was instrumental in developing a code of ethics and in concentrating thinking toward some definite objectives.

Thus it is that pharmacy and medicine approached the opening of the 20th century with the recognized responsibility that the function of diagnosis and prescribing should be restricted to those who were medically trained and licensed and that those who were pharmaceutically trained and licensed would be charged with the responsibility of discovering, standardizing, storing, compounding, and dispensing drugs and medicines.

Drugs and/or medicines, therefore, constitute the tools with which the physician is to treat disease, or to prevent it, his function being to supply the "know-how" of their use.

The pharmacist who supplies the tools, the physician who supplies the "know-how" of their use, and the patient who is to profit by such orderly process should recognize that the pharmacist-physician relationship constitutes not only the best, but the only agency which functions in the general health interest under free enterprise. The "teamship" of the pharmacist and the physician must therefore be maintained on the highest possible level to best insure the health interest of the public.

Those pharmacists and physicians, most of whom had come into practice via the preceptorship system and who had come through the hardships and professional uncertainties of the 19th century, were now entering the 20th century with full recognition, on the basis of past failures, that a new order of medical-pharmaceutical practice must be evolved.

They recognized the weaknesses of their system of education, organization, and legislation, which had prevailed through the years, and then set about strengthening them, thereby initiating a system which was to bring more progress in diagnosis—and drugs of higher standards of purity and efficacy—in the first half of the 20th century than probably had been developed in all the preceding years of history.

Volumes could be written on the progress in diagnosis and the development of new drugs and their uses this half-century has seen come into practice; but a summation of the highlights of pharmaceutical and medical progress should find a place in this volume.

No attempt will be made to follow the exact chronological order in which new drugs—or new methods of diagnosis and treatment, or other conditions—have come into use or existence.

The reader will understand that wherever and whenever disease—whether of human, or of animal, or of fowl, or of vegetation—is referred to, *drugs have a specific and positive place in its prevention, treatment, or cure.* Drugs, therefore, come to be a most important, and—with the exception of food—*probably the most important item in the life of the State.*

Dating from 1900, progressive steps came rapidly in education, organization, legislation, diagnosis, and new drugs, as they relate to the human, to animals, to fowls, and to vegetation.

Educational facilities for training physicians, as judged by modern standards, were limited; while the facilities for training pharmacists were even more limited. In 1959 there are two handsomely equipped and well-staffed medical schools in Georgia. There are two schools of pharmacy in Georgia, neither of which is adequately equipped as to buildings, faculty, apparatus, or libraries; yet, despite this handicap they have justified their existence in training young men and women to serve the public in an ethical and professional capacity.

Some research is in progress in the medical schools; but very little research is in existence in the pharmacy schools in the study of the old drugs or in the creation of new ones. This lack of research in pharmacy in Georgia is not due to lack of interest on the part of the pharmaceutical researchers, or to a lack in their qualifications, but is due entirely to lack of financial support on the part of the State or of foundations. They are qualified, competent, and eager to begin a research program in a study of the old vegetable drugs, and/or in the creation of new drugs, if the facilities are provided.

The human, the animal, the fowl, and vegetation are all subject to diseases and may profit by such a research program.

There was only limited specialization in 1900 in medicine, and none in pharmacy. Today (1959) there is a high degree of specialization in medicine, and a beginning in pharmacy, all of which specialization (i.e., both in the field of medicine and in pharmacy) is definitely and positively in the interest of the public health and welfare.

There were very few hospitals in the State in 1900, and these were located in the larger cities. (Athens at that time was not large enough to justify a hospital). As judged by modern standards these hospitals were inadequately equipped and staffed. In 1959 there are 221 hospitals in Georgia, many of which are located in the small communities of the State, thus making hospitalization available to all the people of the State.

The "germ theory" of disease was just beginning to be generally accepted as a fact in 1900. The approach to asepsis was crude as compared to modern surgical asepsis. There was much dangerous floundering and fumbling in arriving at the present standard of efficiency in asepsis. Some of the disinfectants were frequently more dangerous to the patient than to the "germ." The "virus theory" of disease is a product of the present era. We are now in the midst of an intensive research program to determine, if possible, whether drugs will be effective in the prevention and cure of virus diseases, as has been true of diseases of germ origin.

As for anaesthetics, Dr. Crawford Long had used sulphuric ether as early as 1842. Chloroform and nitrous oxide were also

℞ DRUGS IN THE MODERN ERA   237

used, with ether, as the anaesthetics of choice, even though they were dangerous under some conditions, causing serious after-effects and even death. Today there is a long list of modern anaesthetics which are safer and more nearly devoid of dangerous after-effects. Anaesthetics and aseptic agents are the drugs which pharmaceutical industry has given to the world to make modern surgery possible.

The narcotic drugs, Opium, Laudanum, Morphine, Heroine, Cocaine, were prescribed by physicians and sold in drug stores in 1900 as indiscriminately as aspirin is prescribed and sold today. In 1907 the pharmacists of Georgia were successful in having enacted legislation which prohibited the sale of these products except on prescriptions. But for this legislation, and Federal legislation which came seven years later, addiction to narcotics might and could have been the most serious health problem in the State.

During this half-century, a large number of new drugs came into existence, many of which proved to be dangerous for purposes of self-medication. Again, recognizing their responsibility in safeguarding the people of Georgia so far as drugs are concerned, the pharmacists of the State sponsored the enactment of the so-called "Dangerous Drugs Act," which limits the use of these drugs to prescriptions. And, again, Georgia was among the first of the States to adopt legislation of this character.

A State Board of Health for Georgia was created by legislative enactment in 1875. But, failing to secure appropriations for maintaining its operation, the Board ceased functioning in 1877 and was not restored to activity until 1903, when an annual appropriation of $3,000 was provided.

The activities of the Board increased and expanded from year to year. Today the Georgia Department of Health ranks with the best in the United States and commands the respect and confidence of all the health professional groups in the State, as well as the people of Georgia. In the opinion of the author, the State receives in services from the Department of Health a large return on the tax dollar invested in its operation. The value of these services cannot be expressed in terms of dollars and cents.

But, as in all cases of sickness or disease, the efficiency and the efficacy of the activities of the Department of Health depend to a large degree upon drugs. The vast majority of drugs which had been in use were of vegetable origin. But the year 1900 marked the beginning of the application of the process of synthesis in the manufacture of drugs. It was about this time when such drugs as Acetanilid, Antipyrine, Phenacetin, and Salol were accepted by the medical profession as safe and efficient. But the number of synthetic drugs to come into existence and into extensive use has increased since that time from year to year. Today, there is scarcely a week that passes but that one or more new synthetic drugs are announced, many of them proving invaluable in the prevention as well as in the treatment and cure of many diseases.

Among the synthetic drugs now in use, none approximates in volume the amount of aspirin that is manufactured each year entirely by synthetic processes.

Prior to the discovery of the possibility of producing salicylic acid by synthesis from coal tar products, such vegetable products as methyl salicylate (in the form of Oil of Wintergreen or Oil of Gaultheria) were the sources of salicylic acid. Aspirin is the acetyl derivative of salicylic acid, and, if we depended on the vegetable source for salicylic acid, aspirin would be very limited in quantity, and would probably sell for 10 cents to 25 cents per tablet.

Since the annual production of synthetic aspirin is 20 million pounds (or 28 billion 5-grain tablets), the manufacturing cost of which is approximately 12 million dollars, if we had depended on the natural or vegetable source of salicylic acid for the production of this much aspirin, the cost would approximate 80 to 90 million dollars.

Arsphenamine for the treatment of syphilis is another one of the synthetic products on which we depend, and there is no natural product comparable in safety and efficiency.

The synthesis of vitamins, of antibiotics, of the sulfa drugs, and innumerable other products gives us medication of a high degree of efficiency, and in any quantity which might be necessary. Considering the vast amount of risk capital involved and the many obstacles to be overcome by researchers, the medicinal agent cannot be considered an item of merchandise, for the agent chosen by the prescriber represents his choice and his judgment as to which drug is necessary to correct the disease condition revealed by the diagnosis.

The period 1900-1959 is replete with evidence of progress in the determination of the causes of disease, the methods of diagnosis and treatment, or prevention.

Whereas there was no formal meeting of minds of the various professional groups which were responsible for the promotion of

℞ DRUGS IN THE MODERN ERA 239

the many evidences of progress, there was formal recognition of all available health knowledge, as supplied by the various members of the health groups, or from laboratories of basic research. This constitutes a *team* contribution; and team action must, of necessity, prevail in order to continue the program of progress.

As a result of cooperative action and effort on the part of pharmacists, physicians, and other health agencies, and the utilization of all available scientific knowledge, many of the diseases which were uncontrollable so far as treatment or prevention was concerned, prior to 1900, have, in this first half of the century, been eliminated as a menace to the health and life of the people of Georgia.

Looking at the record of this half-century, the author feels justified in reiterating the statement previously made that perhaps more progress in the diagnosis and treatment of disease has come in this half-century than through all previous centuries combined; and, further, that next to foods, drugs may be the most important item in our lives.

In reviewing the large number of diseases which had been generally fatal, but are now controllable by the use of modern drugs, it is hoped that the reader will experience the thrill that comes to those of us who have seen these evidences of progress come into existence—progress which we conceive to be an omen that still further strides toward conquering disease will be made.

For the convenience of the reader, we are considering grouping the human diseases according to the following system:
1. Those which have definitely proven to be controllable by drugs;
2. Those which show promise of being controllable by drugs;
3. Those which have not yet responded to present drug treatment methods.

HUMAN DISEASES WHICH HAVE BEEN CONTROLLED BY DRUGS AND ELIMINATED AS A MENACE DURING THIS HALF CENTURY, 1900-1959

Rabies

Rabies is of ancient origin, being described by various writers as early as the first century A.D. In 1885, Pasteur gave the first inoculation of antirabic vaccine.

Dr. Abercrombie, in his *History of Public Health in Georgia,* reports that Dr. B. W. Hunt, of Eatonton, Georgia, was the first human in the State to receive antirabic vaccine. In 1898 there was no antirabic vaccine in Georgia. Therefore Dr. Hunt went to the Pasteur Institute in Europe for treatment.

The State Department of Health began the preparation and distribution of antirabic vaccine in 1908, having taken over a proprietary vaccine business in Atlanta, for which a fee of $140 was being charged for treatment. From 1908 to 1913 there were 3,348 cases treated with this vaccine in the State.

There has been difficulty in getting through the Legislature any enforceable legislation requiring the vaccination of dogs and other animals for preventive purposes. The same applies to various other diseases involving vaccination.

Smallpox

Well into the 20th century, epidemics or sporadic outbreaks of smallpox were common in the State. Every community of any size had a building which was known as a "pest-house," where these unfortunates were incarcerated during the infectious period.

In 1911, smallpox was reported prevalent in practically all parts of the State, but did not reach epidemic proportions.

In the first ten years of its existence the Georgia Department of Health distributed 180,000 vaccine points without charge to the people. However, for lack of space and equipment, the State Department of Health did not manufacture the vaccine. In the 20th century, vaccine has, of course, become readily available, and smallpox as a health menace in Georgia has disappeared. But this has occurred as a result of less resistance to the practice of vaccination. There was no state-wide law compelling vaccination, but a law has been enacted which enables County Boards of Education to require all school children to be vaccinated for smallpox prior to their entrance into public school.

The reader will bear in mind that, prior to the appearance of Dr. Jenner's vaccine prepared from kine-pox, the practice of "inoculation" with smallpox virus was commonly practiced. This meant, of course, that the person so inoculated had the disease and, if he recovered, was immune to further attack. Smallpox vaccine today is, of course, administered by inoculation, but the kine-pox developed in the individual is without serious symptoms and is non-contagious, while giving complete protection against smallpox.

Pharmaceutical industry is now supplying the tools for the pre-

℞ DRUGS IN THE MODERN ERA

vention of this, one of the oldest and most deadly scourges which history records.

Diphtheria

Diphtheria was long considered a dangerous and frequently fatal affliction of children, but is now preventable and curable.

The Georgia Department of Health began the manufacture of Diphtheria Antitoxin in 1909 and distributed it to physicians and to local Boards of Health. Diphtheria Antitoxin was first admitted to the U.S. Pharmacopoeia in 1910, being the forerunner of all other antitoxins.

The antitoxin was primarily for curative purposes, but the Diphtheria Toxoid came somewhat later, to be used for preventive purposes. The toxoid was made Official in the U.S. Pharmacopoeia XIII (1940-1950).

Note: Hooper's Medical Dictionary (1841) does not mention diphtheria.

Pellagra

Prior to 1920 and the discovery of vitamins, the cause was not known and the incidence of pellagra in Georgia was high. The mortality rate approached one hundred per cent.

Dr. Henry R. Slack of LaGrange, a former Secretary of the Georgia Pharmaceutical Association and later engaged in the practice of medicine in Georgia, came very close (without realizing it) to the discovery of vitamins when he stated in a published article that the disease pellagra was fatal, but that the patient should be made more comfortable with a "well-balanced diet."

Tetanus

Tetanus is one of the long-known and recognized dangerous, infectious diseases. Prior to the manufacture of Tetanus Antitoxin and Toxoid, it was fatal in a high percentage of cases. Both the Antitoxin and the Toxoid are now recognized by the U.S. Pharmacopoeia. The Toxoid is used as a preventive, and the Antitoxin, as a curative agent.

Hooper's Medical Dictionary (1841-Volume I) says of the disease: "Attacks persons of all ages, sexes, temperaments, and complexions; but the male sex more often than the female, and those of a robust and vigorous constitution, than those of a weak habit."

Hookworm

This disease was first reported in Georgia by Dr. C. A. Smith in 1902. It was demonstrated at that time that the disease was widely distributed, particularly in the sandy-soil areas of the State, and among those who were known as "dirt-eaters" or whose habit was to go "barefooted."

Dr. Abercrombie reports that in one county, over a five-year period, 76,776 children and adults were treated for the disease. The treatment for the disease is safe and efficient. Preventive measures involve the abandonment of the surface toilet.

Typhoid Fever

For many years the cause was not known, the incidence was high, and there were epidemics in most communities almost annually. No person and no community (whether rural or urban) was safe from infection because there existed no known preventive measures.

In 1900, there were 17,000 reported cases. In 1900, the mortality rate in Georgia was high, 1,766 deaths being reported (with unreported or undiagnosed cases probably a multiple of this number). In 1924, the number of deaths reported in the State had decreased to 549. *In 1921, there were only 12 counties* in the State *that reported no deaths from typhoid fever.*

Treatment was entirely empirical since there was no known specific. The treatment, whatever it was, extended over weeks; recovery periods, if any, extended over months.

Today, pharmaceutical industry supplies as tools: Vaccine for preventive purposes, and Antibiotics for curative purposes.

The danger of typhoid fever is now a thing of the past, but most persons in the upper age bracket can recall with horror the anxieties of the years when typhoid fever was prevalent in most communities of the State.

Malaria

Unknown to the American Indian, the disease came into the Colony with the early settlers, very probably with the African slaves.

Although the cause of the disease was not known until approximately 1900, it is known that the disease spread rapidly in

℞ DRUGS IN THE MODERN ERA

the Colony and State and for many years was so prevalent in some areas that practically one hundred per cent of the inhabitants of the area were, in time, infected.

Quinine, or Cinchona Bark, helped to control the symptoms; but, until the malaria mosquito was eliminated in the 20th century by drainage of stagnant waters, little progress was made in preventing the disease.

The malarial unfortunate rarely died of the disease, but was "sick" and unable to work. The native usually used the term "puny" to describe his condition.

Those areas of the State which were shunned on account of malaria now are among the most prosperous.

Quinine, or Cinchona Bark, was for many years the only agent for the treatment of malaria, and quantities of it, supplied by the Department of Health of the State, were distributed to the public through free dispensaries located in the malarial sections. Atabrine and Plasmochin were synthetic products which made their appearance in 1933, as a substitute for, or adjunct to, Quinine.

The Engineering Division of the State Department of Health deserves the credit for the elimination of the malarial mosquito by its program of drainage and of oil treatments.

Syphilis

The ravages of the disease in the early years of the life of Georgia, in all strata of society, were alarming, and the incidence was increasing from year to year. Every conceivable drug of all the earlier periods, as well as of later periods, was called into use. The inorganic drugs of choice in the treatment were Mercury and Iodides, and the prescription files of the early drug stores will reveal hundreds of thousands of prescriptions for these items, with no assurance of a cure, or even mitigation of the disease, but with the extreme danger of chronic mercurial poisoning.

The most popular general treatment of earlier days was known as the "alterative treatment," an "alterative" being defined as an agent which "restores normal metabolic processes." The vegetable "alteratives" embraced a number of well-known drugs, including Sarsaparilla, Stillingia, Bloodroot, Poke Root, Colchicum, Prickly Ash, Yellow Dock, Red Clover, and Sassafras. This latter group of vegetable drugs constituted the basis for a number of proprietary, highly advertised "blood" and "syphilitic" remedies.

The syphilis organism was discovered in 1905. The Wassermann Reagent Test for the diagnosis of syphilis came in 1906, and Ehrlich's Salvarsan or "606" or "Arsphenamine" came in 1909. With the advent of this product, and antibiotics (which came later), progress is being made in the elimination of syphilis as a menace. Pharmaceutical industry supplies these tools.

Gonorrhoea

Gonorrhoea was an accompanying menace with syphilis to the people of the State. The treatment for many years consisted of injections of lead, zinc, or copper salts, which had no effect other than an astringent or styptic action, which frequently resulted in severe strictures.

The internal treatment involved the use of various vegetable diuretic drugs such as Balsam of Copaiba, Sandalwood, and others. But there was no cure for the disease until the appearance of the sulfa drugs in the 1920's, and the antibiotics in the 1940's. Pharmaceutical industry has supplied these tools.

Diabetes

Prior to 1922 this disease was considered one hundred per cent fatal. But under Insulin treatment, sufferers from the disease now are assured of a normal, active life including a normal life span. Insulin is the only known specific for this disease; and even though a monopoly exists in its manufacture, the price to the one-half to three-quarters of a million sufferers has been steadily reduced. Pharmaceutical industry, and pharmaceutical industry alone, supplies the tools for the treatment of diabetes.

If President Thomas Jefferson were alive, he would probably write Drs. Banting and Best to say to them what he wrote to Dr. Jenner (on the subject of smallpox vaccination): "You have erased from human afflictions one of its greatest; mankind will know that you have lived."

Pneumonia

Long known, and considered one of the most dangerous disease conditions, pneumonia was widely distributed in the State, common to all ages, races, and sexes, the incidence high, and, as late as 1900, recovery slow and extremely uncertain. This situation prevailed until the appearance of the sulfa drugs (1920) and the antibiotics (1940's), under which treatment recovery is

℞ DRUGS IN THE MODERN ERA

now considered almost certain and rapid. Pharmaceutical industry supplies the tools.

Tuberculosis

For many years tuberculosis was so prevalent in Georgia that this disease bore the title, "Public Health Menace Number One." It still occupies a place on the list of health problems.

While much progress is being made in its diagnosis and treatment (by the use of modern drugs), tuberculosis remains a serious health problem. Battey Hospital at Rome, as administered by the State Department of Health, is rendering a wonderful service to tuberculosis sufferers and their loved ones. The disease is arrested in many instances, and the patient is thereby enabled to assume a normal place in life, with a normal life expectancy.

Tularemia, Typhus, and Undulant Fever

All of these diseases appeared in the State in the period 1928-1933, but fortunately not in epidemic form. They seem to be yielding to modern drug treatment. Prevention of these diseases involves the use of rodenticides and parasiticides, since infection is carried to the human by parasites on various animals.

Amoebic Dysentery

This disease appeared in epidemic form in at least one area of Georgia as late as 1933. It would be interesting to determine whether there is any relationship between this disease and "The Fluxes" of Colonial days. "The Fluxes" were successfully treated with Ipecac; and Emetine, its active constituent, is generally accepted today as the remedy of choice in the amoebic dysentery of this era.

Poliomyelitis

Polio is the last of the dread diseases of past years to be apparently controlled by the administration of Salk's Vaccine. Again, pharmaceutical industry, not only at the risk of multimillions of dollars in capital and research investment, but also at the risk of its professional reputation, has provided this tool.

Other diseases which are now (1959) considered controllable by the use of modern drugs include the following:

Cholera	Endocarditis
Gas Gangrene	Mastoiditis

Certain Types of Meningitis
Plague
Whooping Cough (Pertussis)
Scarlet Fever
Yellow Fever
Tuberculosis

Some human diseases which have not yet yielded to control by drugs (1959), but all of which are being intensively studied, and, if progress in this second half century is comparable to that of the first half, will have their number materially reduced:

Encephalitis
Nephritis
Hepatitis
Colitis
Pancreatitis
Arthritis
Rheumatic Fever
Leukemia
Cancer
Arteriosclerosis
Coronary Diseases
Hypertension
Mental Diseases
The Common Cold
Influenza
Asthma
Pleurisy
Neuritis
Epilepsy
Heart Disease

ANIMAL DISEASES AND THEIR CONTROL BY DRUGS

The reader will understand that from the Colonial Era well into the 20th century, the diseases of domestic animals were frequently treated by the human medical practitioner, or by some individual without any formal professional training, who was known as a "horse doctor." Veterinary education, legislation, licensure, and practice in Georgia are products of the modern era.

There are at this time in the State approximately 300 licensed veterinary graduates who are registered in the Office of the Joint Secretary of Examining Boards and recognized—along with pharmacists, physicians, dentists, and nurses—as members of the health team.

Progress in the treatment, control, and prevention of animal diseases is shown in the charts below, the progress in drug treatment being listed in three categories.[1]

The asterisk preceding the name of the disease indicates that the disease may be transmitted to the human by one or more of the following domestic animals: dog, cat, hog, sheep, horse, cow.

---

[1] All data referring to animal diseases supplied by Dean Thomas J. Jones, School of Veterinary Medicine, University of Georgia.

ANIMAL DISEASES WHICH HAVE RESPONDED TO DRUG THERAPY

(Causative Agent: Bacteria, Parasitic Mites, Fungi, or Viruses)

- * Anthrax
- * Brucellosis
- * Glanders
- * Hemorrhagic Septicemia
- * Leptospirosis
- * Tuberculosis
- Paratuberculosis
- * Pseudotuberculosis
- * Salmonellosis
- * Swine Erysipelas
- * Listeriosis
- * Vibriosis
- * Tularemia
- Lamb Dysentery
- Ulcerative Lymphangiitis
- Hepatitis
- Pancreatitis
- Peritonitis
- Nephritis
- Enteritis
- Pneumonitis
- Blackleg
- Malignant Edema
- Bacillary Hemoglobinuria
- Black Disease
- Purpura Hemorrhagica
- Scours
- Navel Ill
- Paratyphoid Fever
- Strangles
- * Sancoptic Mange
- Dermodectic Mange
- * Actinomycosis
- Equine Influenza
- Swine Influenza
- * Encephalomyelitis
- * Cowpox
- Ornithosis
- * Encephalitis

*A Chart showing a more complete list of animal diseases which are transmitted from animals to man appears in the Appendix of this volume, p. 433.

ANIMAL DISEASES BROUGHT UNDER PARTIAL CONTROL BY PREVENTIVE VACCINATION

(Causative Agent: Virus, Bacteria, or Toxins)

- Hog Cholera
- Canine Distemper
- Feline Distemper
- * Rabies
- Infectious Canine Hepatitis
- Blackleg
- * Hemorrhagic Septicemia
- * Leptospirosis
- Tetanus
- Malignant Edema
- Pleuropneumonia
- Botulism
- Sheep Enterotoxemia
- Feline Pneumonitis

. . . . . .

ANIMAL DISEASES NOT YET UNDER CONTROL

Aujeszhy's Disease (Mad Itch)
Scrapie
* Foot and Mouth Disease (Aphtha Epizootica)
Malignant Catarrh of Sheep and Cattle
Bluetongue of Sheep and Cattle
* Calf Diphtheria
Leukemia
* Vesicular Stomatitis
Texas Tick Fever
Hemoglobinuria
Cat-Scratch Fever

POULTRY DISEASES CONTROLLABLE BY DRUGS[2]

Bacterial Diseases: Pullorum disease; Fowl cholera; Fowl typhoid; Paratyphoid infections; Infectious coryza; Erysipelas infection.

Parasitic Diseases: Coccidiosis; Blackhead.

POULTRY DISEASES BROUGHT UNDER PARTIAL CONTROL BY DRUGS

Bacterial Diseases: Chronic respiratory disease complex; Infectious Sinusitis; Arizona (paracolon) infections; Ulcerative enteritis; Infectious hepatitis.

Virus Diseases: Ornithosis and Psittacosis; Infectious synovitis; Bluecomb disease.

Parasitic Diseases: Hexamitiasis; Roundworms; Tapeworms; Lice; Mites; Ticks; Fleas.

POULTRY DISEASES UNCONTROLLABLE BY DRUGS

Fungus Diseases: Aspergillosis; Favus; Thrush.

Bacterial Diseases: Fowl tuberculosis; Botulism; Staphylococcic infections; Streptococcic infections; Moraxella Anatipestifer in Young Ducks; Colibacillosis.

Virus Diseases: Fowl pox; Infectious laryngotracheitis; Avain Leukosis complex; Newcastle disease; Infectious bronchitis; Avain encephalomyelitis; Equine encephalomyelitis; Virus hepatitis (ducks).

2. Data supplied by Dr. Samuel C. Schmittle, Director, Poultry Disease Research Center, University of Georgia, College of Agriculture.

℞ DRUGS IN THE MODERN ERA 249

Parasitic Diseases: Trichomoniasis (upper and lower digestive tract); Leucocytozoon infection; Flukes; Spirochetosis; Sarcosporidiosis; Malarial infections.

DISEASES OF PLANTS[3]

Those Diseases Controllable With Drugs

Apples: Scab; Bitter rot; Black rot; Blotch; Fire-blight.

Peaches: Brown rot; Scab; Leaf curl; Nematodes.

Cotton: Anthracnose boll and seedling; Angular Leaf spot; Rust-Deficiency-K or M.

Peanuts: Leaf spot.

Tobacco: Blue Mold; Angular Leaf spot; Black shank; Nematodes.

Cucurbits (Cantaloupes, Cucumbers, Watermelons, Squash): Downy Mildew; Anthracnose; Angular Leaf spot; Gummy Stem blight; Nematodes.

Tomatoes: Early blight; Gray mold; Late blight; Bacterial spot; Blossom-end rot; Nematodes.

Florist Plants: Soil Organisms, including Nematodes.

Wheat: Smut.

Oats: Smut; Helminthosporium blights.

Pine Seedling Nurseries: Fusiform rust.

DISEASES OF PLANTS

Those Diseases Which Need More Research With Drugs

Apples: Root rot complex.

Peaches: Root rot complex; Virus Diseases; Phony; Rosette.

Grapes (American type): Black rot; Virus complex.

Cotton: Seedling blight; Nematodes.

Peanuts: Southern blight; Nematodes.

Tobacco: Viruses.

Cucurbits (Cantaloupes, Cucumbers, Watermelons, Squash): Viruses.

Tomatoes: Mosaic; Bacterial wilt.

3. Data supplied by Dr. Julian H. Miller, Department of Plant Pathology and Plant Breeding, College of Agriculture, University of Georgia.

Insect-borne Diseases of Plants[4]

Fungus Diseases*

(*Carriers:* Beetles, Aphids, Maggots, Bees, Flies, Mites, Grasshoppers, Borers). Dutch elm disease; Chestnut blight; Blue stain (Norway pine); Brown rot (peach, plum, cherry); Perennial canker (apple); Downy mildew (Lima beans); Blackleg (cabbage); Bud rot (carnations); Ergot (rye, barley, wheat, many grasses); Fusarium wilt (cotton); Plum wilt; Potato scab.

Bacterial Diseases*

(*Carriers:* Beetles, Bees, Wasps, Flies, Aphids, Leaf-hoppers, Maggots, Plant Bugs).
Cucurbit wilt (cucumbers, melons); Bacterial wilt or Stewart's disease (corn); Fire blight (apple, pear, quince); Bacterial soft rot (cabbage, potato, other vegetables); Olive knot (olive); Bacterial rot (apple).

Virus Diseases*

(*Carriers:* Leaf-hoppers, Flea beetles, Aphids, Grasshoppers, Plant bugs, Potato beetles, Whiteflies, Thrips).
Curly top (sugar beet, ornamental and wild plants); Peach yellows; False blossom (cranberry); Aster yellows (asters and many other plants); Streak diseases of corn; Dwarf diseases of rice; Spindle tuber (potato); Leaf roll (potato); Sugarcane mosaic (sugarcane, corn, sorghum); Bean mosaic; Mosaic of crucifers (cauliflower, cabbage, turnip, mustard); Cucumber mosaic; Spotted wilt (tomato); Yellow spot (pineapple); Leaf curl (cotton); Yellow dwarf (onion).

The progress made in the elimination of many diseases as a menace to humans, animals, fowls, and plants as a result of the appearance of new drugs and new methods of diagnosis and treatment is most significant and impressive, even to those of us who have witnessed the progress come into existence step by step during this first half of the 20th century, and whose lives have been spent in close association with disease and drugs.

In the case of the human diseases which have come under control by drugs, many thousands of lives have been saved, and the

---

*(Note: Control measures—Insecticides in the form of dusts and sprays).

4. C. L. Metcalf and W. P. Flint (Rev. by R. L. Metcalf), *Destructive and Useful Insects.* (3rd Ed.), 1951.

℞ DRUGS IN THE MODERN ERA

average span of life has been raised some 20 years during this first half century.

In the case of the animal, fowl, and plant diseases which have come under control by drugs, the economic welfare of the people of the State has been improved by some multi-millions of dollars. Successful agriculture in all of its branches, animal husbandry, dairying, and the poultry industry, has been made possible and profitable through disease control by drugs.

These new drugs did not come into existence by accident or by chance, but as a result of the coordination of all scientific knowledge as it was revealed by basic research in the broad fields of chemistry and biology; and the adaptation of this knowledge to the creation of new drugs through some process of nature (as in the case of vaccines, antitoxic sera, toxoids, antibiotics, vitamins, et al.); or by the process of synthesis (as in the case of the sulfa drugs, atabrine, plasmochin, aspirin, and many others).

New methods of diagnosis, new knowledge of body functions both normal and abnormal, new theories of diseases, new techniques in treatment—all of these things accompanied the appearance of new drugs.

This new knowledge of new drugs, new diagnostic techniques and methods of treatment—all had to await the slow process of education as it evolved from the limited facilities for the training of pharmacists, physicians, and other scientific workers of the early years of the century, to the high standards of the present era.

We like to think of this advance in the treatment and prevention of disease as coming at the hands of what should be recognized as "Georgia's Health Team," composed of those educated specialists in the various specialized health services who are guided by team effort and team spirit. The nucleus of such a Health Team is suggested here:

A Proposed Health Team

Registered Professional Groups in Georgia—1958
- Pharmacists 2,262
- Physicians 3,800
- Dentists 900
- Nurses 11,500
- Veterinarians 300
- *Hospitals* 221

State Department of Health 1
City and County Departments of Health . . . 82
Professional Schools and Colleges
  Pharmacy 2
  Medicine 2
  Dentistry 1
  Veterinary 1
  *Hospitals (Past and Present) Offering
    Nurse Training 58
Pharmaceutical Industry—With Manufacturing Plants Located in Various Parts of the United States, 1100 retail drug stores and 9 wholesale companies in Georgia

The term "Pharmaceutical Industry," as used in this volume, is intended among other things to cover the following processes:

1. The identification of the crude drug as it is found in nature, whether of the vegetable, the animal, or the mineral kingdom.
2. The collection, curing, storing of drugs, or the products from which drugs are obtained.
3. The standardization of drugs by chemical, biological, or physical assay.
4. The determination of the active principle of drugs, vegetable and animal.
5. The manufacture and packaging of pharmaceutical products.
6. The determination of the pharmacological or therapeutic action of drugs.
7. The determination of the safe dosage of drugs.
8. The coordination of all basic research, whether chemical or biological, and of all available scientific knowledge having to do with drugs.
9. The synthetic manufacture of products which are similar to, or identical with, natural products; and/or the creation of entirely new products.
10. The distribution of drugs to the public via wholesale and retail drug stores of the State, the drug store an integral link in the system since it is the intermediary between the drug product, the physician, and the public.

With the existence of the high standards of education for the

---

*Note: A large percentage of the registered nurses of Georgia had their training in hospitals outside the State.

individual in each of the specialized fields; with a recognition on their part of their responsibilities to minister to the health needs of our people; with a sense of the values of "team effort" and coordination; with the recognition that personal aims and ambitions must be secondary to professional service; with this program of health care operating under our system of free enterprise unhampered by governmental regulation—the standard of health care for the people of Georgia would be second to none in the world, and we could reasonably expect that even more progress in health matters could be recorded in this last half of the century than has come in the first half.

On preceding pages, attention has been called to the large number of diseases of humans, animals, fowls, and plants which have not yet come under control by drugs but which await new drugs at the hands of pharmaceutical industry, so that they will be placed in that large group of "Controlled Diseases."

We all recognize that it is the function of pharmaceutical industry to provide the tools for the treatment of disease; but to discharge this responsibility, the industry is dependent upon the availability of properly trained men and women.

Most of the state universities, and many of the endowed institutions in America, include a school of pharmacy as one of the professional schools. It is in these pharmacy schools that the student acquires the "research spirit" which, under the guidance of the instructors, can stimulate him to research achievements.

But, unfortunately, educational administrators have not yet been made aware of the possibility of research achievement in the field of drugs, and therefore have not encouraged or demanded or provided equipment and personnel for a research program which might conceivably become a contribution of untold value and possibilities for the health of humans, animals, fowls, and plants. THERE IS NO GREATER POTENTIAL OF GENERAL SERVICE TO A PEOPLE.

Every school of pharmacy should be supported by State or Foundation appropriations to the end that research in the field of drugs is made not only possible but mandatory; for therein is determined the health of all forms of life—animal and vegetable.

The most obvious field of drug research in Georgia at the moment applies in the plant world; for, whereas there is no large pharmaceutical manufacturing establishment in the State, Mother Nature is manufacturing for us untold valuable drug products which may never have been viewed as to their potential drug values by modern research. But the American Indian and the settlers of the State for many generations found the locally growing plant products of value in the treatment and prevention of disease in the animal world. It must be further borne in mind that these and all other plants in the State are themselves subject to disease.

With the multiple thousands of plants growing wild, or growable, in the various soil and climate areas of the State, it is a shortsighted—and conceivably a dangerous—policy not to have in operation a continuing program of scientific research properly financed by State or Foundation appropriations. The schools of pharmacy offer the medium through which research in drugs should be conducted.

This second half of the 20th century will be known in history as the beginning of the Atomic Era. During all of the first half of the century, the atom was defined as "the limit of the divisibility of matter." The splitting of the atom, therefore, marks a historic era, but whether for good or evil is yet to be determined.

The revolution in our way of life—which has already begun and which will extend far into the future—resulting from the splitting of the atom, will involve disease and medication; and here again, provision must be made for research in new drugs for new diseases which will surely evolve.

A program to meet the health needs of the future whether of human, animal, fowl, or vegetation should be pointed toward these objectives:

1. A higher and still higher quality of training for specialists in the field of disease and drugs.
2. A continuing program of research in the field of disease and drugs.
3. The distribution of drugs through specialists who recognize the dangers as well as the values of drugs.

Supplement A

MEDICAL EDUCATION

Medical College of Georgia

DR. W. H. GOODRICH, a member of the faculty of the Medical Department of the University of Georgia, has recorded the first 100 years of its history, 1828-1928, from which recording much of the data given here is taken.

The Charter of the Medical Society of Augusta conveyed the right "to receive, hold, and enjoy real and personal property for its use and benefit," and allowed it to receive bequests or donations. Goodrich states that the language of the Charter is such that "it is inferable that the Society was to erect a Medical College at Augusta."

A Legislative Act was passed December 20, 1828: "To establish and incorporate the Medical Academy of Georgia," and the following doctors were named Trustees—Drs. William R. Waring, John Carter, Lewis D. Ford, Ignatius P. Garvin, Benjamin A. White, Samuel Boykin, William P. McConnell, Walter H. Weems, William Graham, Thomas P. Gorman, Alexander Jones, Milton Antony, John J. Boswell, Thomas Hoxey, J. P. Scriven, William C. Daniel, Richard Banks, Henry Hull, John Dent, Thomas Hamilton, Tomlinson Fort, Nathan Crawford, O. C. Fort, and John Walker.

The Trustees were to set up "such principles, rules and regulations" as they deemed necessary, and to provide a curriculum, with such professors and officers "as best calculated to perpetuate same and promote the improvement of the pupil in the several branches of the healing art."

The Trustees were authorized to confer the degree of Bachelor of Medicine on "such as in their judgment may be worthy of the same," the graduates to be allowed to practice medicine and surgery as fully as if licensed by the State Board of Physicians.

It was decided that three professors would be sufficient for the present. One should lecture on Anatomy and Surgery (Dr. Wm. R. Waring); one, on Materia Medica, Chemistry *and Pharmacy* (Dr. Lewis D. Ford); and one, on Institutes and Practice of Medicine, Midwifery and Diseases of Women and Children (Dr. Milton Antony).

(Author's note: Note that instruction in Pharmacy was provided not for the purpose of granting a degree in Pharmacy but for the benefit of the physician who would probably sell and dispense his own drugs.)

Dr. Ford, the Professor of Pharmacy, was later to become Dean of the Academy.

The first session of the Academy opened on October 1, 1829, with these gentlemen as students: E. A. Eve, R. B. Hibler, G. M. Newton, O. T. Hazzard, James Casslin, John Turner, and R. A. Ware.

Dr. Waring having resigned to move to Savannah, Dr. I. P. Garvin was named for the vacancy.

As an Academy, the institution could not be accredited because the M. D. degree was not conferred. Students having one term of lectures could not be given credit in other medical colleges.

To meet this condition, the name of the institution was changed by Legislative Act in December, 1829, to "The Medical Institute of the State of Georgia," and the Trustees were authorized to confer the M. D. degree on completion of two full courses of lectures of 4 months each, "the second term to be completed in this institution, and the first to be completed in this or some other reputable College of Medicine."

In May, 1830, the faculty was increased to six professors, "the lectures to be given in such hours as the Professors shall agree among themselves." Fees were set as follows: Matriculation—$5.00; Graduation—$10.00; Professor of Anatomy—$20.00; Professor of Chemistry—$20.00; Professor of Surgery—$15.00; Practices—$15.00; Materia Medica—$15.00; Midwifery—$15.00.

In 1832 the Legislature was asked for financial aid either by grant or by lottery in the amount of $10,000 to $25,000.

In April, 1833, the following students received the M. D. degree: Isaac Bowen (Thesis—"Blood" in Greek); E. A. Eve (Thesis—"Dyspepsia"); E. W. Grimes (Thesis—"Dysentery"); John Borden (Thesis—"Asthma"). During the summer, the faculty procured, at their own expense, apparatus for their courses of instruction.

In 1833 the Legislature was again asked for funds, and to change the name to the "Medical College of Georgia." The Legislature appropriated $10,000 and 50 lots on the City Commons.

$5,000 was given by the City of Augusta, the College agreeing to furnish medicines and medical service to the sick poor in the hospital and to prisoners in jail for a period of ten years.

In 1834 construction of the College building was begun. In the same year the faculty raised $6,000 and Dr. Dugas was sent to Europe to purchase an anatomical museum, chemical apparatus, etc. He returned in September "with an excellent collection and the nucleus for a medical library."

1836. In January, the faculty announced publication of *The Southern Medical Journal.* This was said to be the first medical journal published in the South.

1838. In conformity with the program of instruction in other medical schools of the country, the Trustees authorized the faculty to proceed with a program of instruction covering two terms of 4 months each for the Bachelor's degree and the same requirements for the M. D. degree. The faculty was never pleased with the 4 months' term, and in 1835 they addressed a communication to other schools and colleges of medicine over the country suggesting that a conference be held with the hope of getting all schools of medicine to agree to increase the length of the terms from four to six months. But none of the other colleges concurred in this movement. The faculty set up, on their own, a program calling for two terms of 6 months each, but the students promptly left the institution to enter other schools where the 4 months program prevailed. In 1838 the Medical College of Georgia reluctantly returned to the 4 months program. Of interest to pharmacists, it will be noted that Dr. Ford, Dean of the Medical College, who was also Professor of Pharmacy, was the person who proposed this increase in the requirements for the M. D. degree.

1859. In this year the Medical College at Augusta again appealed to the Legislature for financial aid. This aid in the amount of $10,000 was granted, under the condition that the Medical College of Georgia "shall annually from this time henceforth as long as they shall keep said sum, instruct, matriculate, lecture, and graduate 20 young men in Georgia who may be unable to pay their own expenses, to be selected by the Governor —two from each Congressional District and four from the State-at-large."

1861-1864. Now comes the Civil War, and with it the students in all of the colleges of Georgia—and the teachers—were called to arms. And, along with the other colleges in Georgia of every nature, the Medical College of Georgia closed its doors as a teaching institution but used the buildings as a hospital for the period of the War.

1865-1866. Following the Civil War the Medical College of Georgia was reopened on the first Monday of November, 1865. And in 1866 George W. Raines was made Professor of Chemistry and Pharmacy, along with a number of other changes from the original faculty which preceded the Civil War.

1872. The Trustees made overtures to the Trustees of the University of Georgia requesting that the Medical College of Georgia be made "The Medical Department of the University of Georgia," and the Minutes of the Board of Trustees of the University, September 30, 1872, record the following statement: "In regard to the proposed connection of the Medical College in Augusta and the University, this Committee (Laws and Discipline) recommend that the Board assent to the same and appoint a committee to arrange details."

The agreement between the Medical College of Georgia and the University of Georgia (July 5, 1873) set up the following specifications:

"Article 1—The Medical College of Georgia shall hereafter be styled 'The Medical College of Georgia being The Medical Department of the University of Georgia.'"

"Article 2—The control of its affairs shall be vested in the local Board of Trustees (of the Medical College), having full power to fill vacancies within their own body and their own faculty."

"Article 3—The local Board and the Faculty shall determine the granting of medical diplomas, and such diplomas shall be signed by the Chancellor and the Medical Faculty, sealed with the Seal of the University of Georgia, then delivered to the graduates in the City of Augusta."

"Article 4—The expenses of the Medical College shall be borne by the local Board who shall have the disposal of its receipts. No liability for the debts or expenses shall be incurred by the University of Georgia."

"Article 5—An ultimate power of control over the regulations and appointments of the Medical College shall be in the Board of Trustees of the University of Georgia to be exercised when they deem it necessary."

"Article 6—An Act of the Legislature may be applied for to sanction the change of name, its union with the University as above stated, and such other changes as may be necessary."

1892. The School raised its standards by requiring three terms of 6 months each, and the entrance requirements were raised to that required for second-grade teachers in the schools of Georgia.

1894. A Nurses Training School, one of the first in Georgia, was organized.

1900-1901. The standards were again raised, and all students were required to attend 4 terms of 6 months each before being permitted to appear before the Board for examination for the M.D. degree.

1911. The College still struggling for existence, Dean W. H. Doughty appeared before the General Assembly of Georgia and offered the entire plant to the University of Georgia. The Legislature accepted it, and thus the Medical College became in fact as well as in name an integral part of the State University.

The financial and academic problems of the College now seemed to be cared for, so far as the future was concerned, and from this point the school has expanded rapidly in financial support, in faculty personnel, and in facilities, especially insofar as hospital features are concerned. It now maintains a "Class A" rating by the accrediting agencies, and its research program has been outstanding, thus assuring its place as a service institution in the State of Georgia.

The Atlanta Medical College

The following statement of the history of the Atlanta Medical College has been recorded by Henry Morton Bullock in his book, *A History of Emory University*, 1936, Chapter 15.

In 1853 a small group of doctors, under the leadership of Dr. John G. Westmoreland, conceived the idea of forming a medical school in Atlanta. On February 14, 1854, the Legislature granted its charter under the title "The Atlanta Medical College," naming as trustees L. C. Simpson, J. I. Whitaker, John Collier, Hubbard Cozard, Daniel Hook, John L. Harris, William Herring, Green B. Haygood, and James L. Calhoun.

The original faculty of May, 1855, consisted of the following members: M. G. Slaughter, professor of anatomy; John W. Jones, professor of theory and practice of medicine; Jesse Boring, professor of obstetrics and diseases of women and children;

W. F. Westmoreland, professor of surgery; J. E. Dubose, professor of physiology; G. T. Wilburn, professor of surgical and pathological anatomy; J. J. Roberts, professor of chemistry, and J. G. Westmoreland, professor of materia medica and dean.

The founders chose a summer term running from May 1 to September 1, and 78 students enrolled in the first session of the College, 1855. There were five lectures daily, with some practical instruction provided. Candidates for the degree of Doctor of Medicine were supposed to be 21 years of age, of good moral character, and have attended two full courses of lectures, and submit a thesis on some medical subject.

Dr. J. G. Westmoreland, in addition to serving as dean, was also named treasurer and financial agent for building and equipping a College building. It was largely through his efforts that a building was completed by the opening of term in May, 1856.

In the opening year, 1855, the College launched the *Atlanta Medical and Surgical Journal*, a publication to which John P. Logan was named first editor.

In 1857 the Chair of obstetrics and diseases of women and children being vacated, Dr. J. S. Powell filled the position.

In 1858 a dispensary was established, with two professors in charge.

In 1860 financial difficulties plagued the College, and affairs at the College reached a very low point. Students were reduced and funds were badly needed.

Then the Civil War came to the South and to Atlanta. The Atlanta College closed, but the building was used as a hospital, somehow escaping the flames.

On August 16, 1865, the faculty met again for the first time since the War, in the office of Professor Powell, with Drs. Logan, Means, and the two Westmorelands also present. The need for doctors was urgent and the poverty-stricken students could not afford the time and money for two years' instruction. This emergency resulted in a winter course of lectures in addition to the summer course. This was evidently done to speed up graduation and licensing of doctors for practice.

In the years 1866-67-68, a disagreement came about in the faculty which finally resulted in the withdrawal of Dr. Powell from the faculty and the creation of a new medical college under the name of the Southern Medical College (1878-1898) with Dr. Powell as Dean.

1891. The School of Pharmacy was made an integral part of

the Atlanta Medical College, bearing the title, "The Atlanta College of Pharmacy." Dr. George F. Payne was named Dean.

The Southern Medical College

From facts set forth in Bullock's History comes the following account of the Southern Medical College.

1891. The enrollment for this year at Southern Medical College is given as 90 students and 35 graduates.

Dr. Powell had visions of an expanded educational institution, and one of the first developments in his scheme involved the creation of a dental department about 1889, and he *contemplated opening a pharmaceutical and a law department*. The dental department did open and had over 100 students enrolled, but the other departments either did not materialize or had a very brief existence.

1892. The Southern Medical College erected a new building on Butler Street opposite Grady Hospital, which was then in the process of construction. Later the building for the dental department was placed just north of the medical department. Bullock states: "These new buildings adjoined the buildings of the Atlanta Medical College and presented a sort of hand-to-hand business—because medical education was on a proprietary basis in those days."

That the Southern Medical College was lured to its new site was due to the fact that it was desirable to be near the Grady Hospital. For six years the two schools operated as next-door neighbors.

The Atlanta College of Physicians and Surgeons

Continuing with some of the facts in Bullock's history, come the following accounts:

1898. The deans of the two medical schools, Dr. W. S. Elkin of the Atlanta College, and W. S. Kendrick of the Southern College, worked out a plan by which the two rivals might be merged. The dental department of the Southern Medical College and the pharmaceutical department of the Atlanta Medical College bore the same relation to the new college as they had to their parent organizations. The new school was named "The Atlanta College of Physicians and Surgeons," and opened with an enrollment of 333 students, of which number 214 were studying medicine, 88 dentistry, and 31 pharmacy.

1900. At the commencement Dean Kendrick announced the decision of the faculty to require four courses of lectures for the degree, to be effective by 1901.

1905. Some differences of opinion in regard to administration of the College came about. Dean Kendrick and several other members of the faculty resigned and proceeded immediately to organize the Atlanta School of Medicine.

1907. Meanwhile, the salary for full professorships at the A. C. P. S. was $300 per year, which meant that all the professors were carrying on a regular medical practice. But attention is called to the fact that Dr. F. S. Harris, who came from the Jefferson Medical College to take the newly created Chair of Pathology and Bacteriology in 1901, was apparently the first actual full-time technical man employed in teaching medicine. His salary was $1200 per year.

1908. With much trepidation, the equivalent of a first-grade teacher's certificate was required for admission and this in turn was raised to 4 years of high school work in the fall of 1912.

1910. Throughout the life of the A. C. P. S., the Southern Dental College (under Dean Foster) and the Atlanta College of Pharmacy (under Dean George F. Payne) operated as practically independent enterprises. In 1910 the School of Pharmacy was abolished, "among other reasons to provide laboratory space for embryology, histology and neurology," Bullock states.

The Atlanta School of Medicine

In 1905 a group of practitioners and teachers of the Atlanta College of Physicians and Surgeons organized a new college under the name and title "The Atlanta School of Medicine" and arrangements were made (on a temporary basis) to share the building of the Atlanta Dental School.

Because of the prominence of the faculty members of both schools the A. C. P. S. and the new college, and the sharp rivalry that developed, the town was divided into factions. Four weeks after the organization meeting in 1905 the school was in actual operation, with 220 students drawn from eight Southern States. Of that number 21 were graduated at the end of the first course of lectures. Heartened by this success, which was far beyond the hopes of the founders, the faculty announced that the term would run for seven instead of the usual six months, and that four years of work would be required for the degree. The admission requirement was practically nil (but on a level with requirements of other schools of that period), though the faculty claimed a high quality of teaching.

The Atlanta School of Medicine was vigorous and at times militant in its publicity, boldly striking out at conditions in many medical schools where the students go all the way through without ever seeing a patient sick enough to be in bed. The reason for this emphasis on the bedside was that it was not then permitted in the hospitals of Atlanta and therefore was not available to students of the Atlanta College of Physicians and Surgeons. But the Atlanta School of Medicine had set up its own hospital, including an obstetrical ward.

The increasing cost of equipment and instruction made it difficult for both colleges to maintain themselves, and to meet the rising standards of the American Medical Association and the Association of American Medical Colleges. Seeing the handwriting on the wall, a motion was passed by the faculty in the spring of 1908 to have the Atlanta School of Medicine seek affiliation with the University of Georgia. But nothing came of this proposal. It did put the faculty in the frame of mind to listen to the proposal of the A. C. P. S. to consolidate the two institutions by 1913.

The Atlanta Medical College

The desire to secure the approval of medical accrediting agencies, as well as financial difficulties in which both were involved, was a prominent factor in bringing the two institutions together; that is, the A. C. P. S. and the Atlanta School of Medicine. Agreeing on the conditions of consolidation, both schools also agreed on the name of the new institution, which was to be chartered and incorporated under the name "The Atlanta Medical College."

1913-1915. To qualify for accreditation, admission requirements had to be raised. But these new admission requirements seriously affected the enrollment of freshman students. It became increasingly clear that without generous financial endowment the Atlanta Medical College could not survive.

Emory University School of Medicine

1915. The Atlanta Medical College merged with Emory University in this year, and the University on its part agreed to appropriate $250,000 to endow the School, and was to build a new hospital to enlarge the teaching facilities. There was evidently no argument among the trustees of the Atlanta Medical College about merging with Emory, for it is reported by Bullock that "they were most cordial to the proposal." On June 28, 1915, the Atlanta Medical College deeded their entire holdings to Emory University.

1917. Instruction continued, however, in the downtown location while the University was busily engaged in the erection of the buildings. But in the Fall of 1917, freshman and sophomore years of medical instruction were moved to Emory, and the facilities for upperclassmen were greatly improved by the opening of the new J. J. Gray Clinic Building on the downtown campus.

Higher entrance requirements, and the stiffening of the scholastic standards, resulted in a sharp drop in enrollment—from 490 students in 1915 to 238 students in 1916.

The entrance of the United States into World War I seriously and immediately affected the Emory School of Medicine, for part of the class of 1917 was graduated a month in advance at the request of the Navy Department. Many faculty members were drawn into the service or governmental activities connected with the War—totalling no fewer than 47 of the professors, who, along with practitioners of Atlanta, formed the Emory University Hospital Unit, under the command of Dr. E. C. Davis. At the end of the War there were said to be in the Unit 52 officers, 291 men, and 96 nurses. The hospital had under its care 2,237 patients.

The Savannah Medical College

According to the laws of Georgia, the Savannah Medical College was granted a Charter in 1838, but this College was not activated until 1853. One of the incorporators of the school was Dr. William R. Waring, who had been named as a faculty member of the Augusta Medical College in its beginning.

The Savannah Medical College was in active operation up to the beginning of the Civil War and closed during that period. The building, however, was used for hospital purposes during the War.

After the Civil War, the College was reopened. As late as 1870 the Savannah Medical College was operating on the basis of two terms of four months each. But it was a financial struggle to keep open, and in 1880 the College was forced to close for lack of financial support, even though the General Assembly of Georgia had appropriated $15,000 for its support in 1871.

OGLETHORPE MEDICAL COLLEGE

There seems to be evidence that in Savannah a sharp rivalry existed among certain groups of the medical profession, as indicated by the fact that, even though the Savannah Medical College had suffered for lack of financial support, another medical college was proposed and activated in 1856 under the name of Oglethorpe Medical College.

This College closed during the Civil War and did not reopen following the War. Both of these schools, however, provided in their faculties a professor of chemistry and pharmacy, which, as in the case of the Augusta Medical College, did not mean that a degree in pharmacy was contemplated or was ever granted.

In 1855 a proposition was submitted orally to the Trustees of Emory College whereby the Oglethorpe Medical College should be united and associated with Emory as one of Emory's departments. The proposal was "respectfully declined," however, by Emory's Trustees.

SOUTHERN BOTANICO MEDICAL COLLEGE—*1839*

During the early days of the development of a program of medical education in the State there were two schools of thought, one, the Allopathic group, being referred to as the "regular" school and the other being referred to as the Thomsonian, Botanic, or Eclectic school. Feeling between the two schools of thought was very bitter. So, following the incorporation of the college at Augusta and the school at Savannah which were specified as being "regular" colleges, in 1839 a medical college under the name "The Georgia College of Eclectic Medicine and Surgery" was chartered. During its early life, the College was located in Forsyth, Georgia. But in 1846 the school was moved to Macon, and its name was changed to the Southern Botanico Medical College. This school was said to have graduated several hundred doctors prior to the Civil War.[1]

Like other colleges in the State, it was closed during the period of the Civil War, but after the War the school reopened under the name "The Reform Medical College of Georgia."

---

1. Jones, *Education in Georgia*.

In 1881 the school moved to Atlanta. In 1884 it merged with a similar college under the new name of "The Georgia College of Eclectic Medicine and Surgery." As late as 1889 this medical school reported an enrollment of 300 students, but closed several years later, never to reopen.

In addition to the "regular" system of the practice of medicine and the Herbalist, Thomsonian or Botanic schools of thought, there came into the State, in 1852, the Homeopathic system, members of which group had been coming into Georgia probably for a number of years. But as a group they were recognized by law in 1852 "to practice physic on the Homeopathic system, and to charge and collect compensation for their services." The practice of Homeopathy was extensive enough in Georgia to make it necessary for the pharmacists of the State to carry homeopathic remedies, but the school of thought of Homeopathy was never popular enough for the development of a school or college for the training of homeopathic doctors in Georgia.

Dalton Medical College—1866

In the year 1866 the Dalton Medical College, Dalton, Georgia, was granted a charter by the Legislature. The following persons were incorporators: Jesse R. McAfee, Chas. P. Gordon, Baxter B. Brown, Samuel W. Fields, Moses Quinn, E. C. Cochran, L. P. Gudger, John K. Osborn, F. A. Rushenburg, Henry W. Renfrowe, and David Emerson. Section 3 of this Act gave the incorporators power to "select professors from their own body or from any of the medical colleges of the United States, to advance and promote the improvement of its pupils in the science of medicine, surgery, and medical jurisprudence."

There is no available evidence to indicate that this school was ever activated or ever functioned.

SUPPLEMENT B

PHARMACEUTICAL EDUCATION

SLOW as was the development of a program for the education of physicians in Georgia, the process extended over a period from 1733 to 1828 before even a beginning was attempted; and another 100 years was to elapse before there was a generally recognized demand for pharmaceutical education on the part of the profession itself or the public.

The preceptorship system of training for both medicine and pharmacy for the first hundred years of the life of the Colony and State had served a useful function and purpose. But as the time approached for the beginning of the separation of medicine and pharmacy into their specialized fields, the need for a different type of training in the field of medicine from the preceptorship type was recognized by most practitioners, and plans were initiated for the establishment of a medical college, even though it would, of necessity, be on a very simple and crude basis, judged by present-day standards. But it was a beginning.

The preceptorship system of training seemed more nearly adapted to pharmaceutical training than to medical, even though the preceptor might have been a physician-pharmacist.

The preceptorship system was so deeply entrenched in the training of pharmacists that as late as 1875, when the Georgia Pharmaceutical Association was organized, the Constitution of that Association set as one of its aims: "To regulate the system of apprenticeship and employment, so as to prevent, as far as possible, the evils flowing from deficient training in the responsible duties in the preparing, dispensing, and selling of medicines."

The framers of the Constitution of the Georgia Pharmaceutical Association might have, very properly, set up standards for the governing of the preceptor, as well as the appentice, for so far as the young apprentice was concerned, the choice of his preceptor could be the most important decision of his life. For then, as now, there were good and bad preceptors—as illustrated by the advertisement of the furniture dealer whose advertising slogan is "Good and bad furniture for sale."

The framers of the Constitution of the GPA were themselves products of preceptorship training of generations of preceptors, whose background of experience may have been as much medical as pharmaceutical. But, nonetheless, they were men of character and of high ethical principles. Having passed through the tragedies of the Civil War and the still more tragic era of the Reconstruction Period, they were men of mature mind and body and were aware of the need for an organized effort in the interest of the profession and of the public whom they were to serve, which resulted in the creation of the GPA.

Whereas up to that time (1875) there had been no organized program of education for pharmacists, there were evidently some persons in pharmacy who were recognized as being educated. For the Constitution refers to "the educated and reputable apothecaries and druggists" as being united toward certain objectives.

The apprentice-preceptorship system for the training of pharmacists was to continue under the Constitution. But there were certain qualifications the apprentice should present before beginning his period of training, among which was a certain amount of basic general education. One Georgia pharmacist of the vintage of 1880 specified that in his opinion the apprentice should present evidence of a basic education, including "a knowledge of Greek and Latin."

As a first major objective of the Association, the passage of laws seemed to constitute the most urgent need, with the result that a "Poison Law" was enacted the year following the organizational meeting, to be followed six years later (1881) by the passage of the first Pharmacy Act, with the creation of the first "Board of Pharmaceutic Examiners."

This Board of Examiners, and all succeeding Boards, was to become promptly aware of the educational background of the applicant who applied for license to practice pharmacy, many of whom, though perhaps well trained in the manual or technical phases, might be lacking in general educational training.

This first Board (1881) had no precedent to guide it and no authority under the existing law to introduce new standards of measurement differing to any marked degree from those which had been followed by the Medical Board of Examiners. But this Board, and all succeeding Boards, was to be charged with the responsibility of acquainting their fellow pharmacists with the increasing need for "reasonable" educational requirements, basic as well as technical, and comparable in quality to those required of persons applying for medical practice in the State.

Education of adults, particularly those steeped in tradition, is a slow, tedious, and discouraging process, and it was fifty years before real educational standards were established by law as a prerequisite for license, and this step came as a result of the insistence of the various Boards of Pharmacy as they were named from year to year.

Prior to, and subsequent to, this first Board, the period of apprenticeship seems to have been set at a minimum of three years, and there seems to have occurred a gradual breakdown in the preceptorship practice and responsibilities, for the speakers and the writers of that period began the use of the term "three years of *experience,*" and eventually changed this to read *"experience* clause," in referring to prerequisite requirements for licensure. And for fifty years after 1881 this was to be the only prerequisite for licensure.

With the gradual disappearance of the term "apprentice" and "preceptor" the "preceptor" was replaced by the "employer," and the "apprentice" by the term, "clerk." The loose term "three years of experience in a drug store" was meaningless, for "experience" might have been confined to work in a drug store as delivery boy, fountain employee, or as janitor. It was a sad day for pharmacy in Georgia when the preceptor was replaced by the employer, every one of whom could and should have been a "preceptor" in the highest interpretation of the word. It would be a happy day for the profession and for the public if every employer, whether pharmacist or businessman, would assume the full responsibilities of preceptorship with his employee.

During this fifty-year period (1881-1933) of continuation of the "experience clause" in determining the qualification of the applicant for license, one or more schools of pharmacy were opened with the endorsement of or at the insistence of the Boards of Pharmacy, schools with ample laboratory facilities and teaching personnel for the training of all the pharmacists needed for replacement, and for modest expansion in the number of new stores. But the old "experience clause" system was to continue to prevail for many years, even though the college curriculum extended over a period of two terms of only six months each, with no previous educational requirements for entrance to the school or college.

During all the years when the "experience clause" was in effect, there were some older men, as well as younger men, who, desiring a license to practice pharmacy, completed the requirements under the "experience clause," and who, for financial reasons, could not attend a school or college of pharmacy within or without the State.

Prior to the examination before the Board, many of these applicants sought the service of some pharmacist who had long experience and perhaps some educational advantage beyond the average, who would coach them in the subject matter of the examination.

For a time this coaching service proved of value to the individual and the profession. But when the service feature of the coaching was commercialized by others in the establishment of "Quiz Schools," the practice proved eventually to be a disservice to the individuals and to the profession alike, rather than a service. For these "Quiz Schools" soon expanded their appeal to students from a state level to a national level. Students were advised of the low educational requirements in Georgia, and the ease with which a license could be obtained, and hundreds of them came from every section of the United States, from Cuba, from Puerto Rico, Mexico, and South America, in the hope of receiving a Georgia license by which they might reciprocate back into their home state or country. But many of the Boards of Pharmacy in the other states refused to recognize the Georgia license, and numbers of those having received the Georgia license and not being able to reciprocate out of the State, remained in Georgia as competitors of Georgia pharmacists.

Thus it was that eventually Georgia's Boards of Pharmacy, humiliated under the stigma that Georgia had become, according to their own statements, "the dumping ground for the United States," introduced and pushed through to enactment legislation requiring graduation from a recognized school or college of pharmacy.

The first serious movement toward the establishment of a school of pharmacy in Georgia came in 1887 following the founding of the Georgia School of Technology, which was located in Atlanta. The School of Technology was to be operated as a branch of the University of Georgia under commissioners who were, in turn, under the direction of the Trustees of the University.

Individual members of the Georgia Pharmaceutical Association and the Georgia Board of Pharmacy thought they saw an opportunity to secure a state-supported school of pharmacy, rather than one operated on a proprietary basis, or as a unit in a Medical College, and promptly approached the Trustees of the University through Henry W. Grady as intermediary, who was himself a Trustee of the University. In due time Grady reported to the Association that the Trustees expressed interest in the matter of the establishment of a school of pharmacy, and would proceed toward its establishment. But in the meanwhile some disagreement arose in the Association as to the location of the school, some arguing that it should be at the Medical College at Augusta, others that it should be in Macon because of its central location, and still another group, for Savannah as a site. In addition to the problem of satisfying the different groups in the Association, one of the main buildings of the School of Technology was destroyed by fire. This, in addition to these arguments about the location of a school of pharmacy, resulted in the abandonment of the idea of the establishment of a school of pharmacy at the School of Technology in Atlanta.

The Atlanta Medical College, already offering instruction in pharmacy for the benefit of medical students, decided to open a College of Pharmacy as an integral part of The Atlanta Medical College, both of which schools were to be operated on a proprietary basis. This College of Pharmacy was opened for students September, 1891, under the deanship of Dr. George F. Payne, and under the name, The Atlanta College of Pharmacy. But in 1910 the Medical College abandoned the operation of the College of Pharmacy. The College of Pharmacy continued to operate, however, in new quarters, under the ownership of Dr. Payne until his death in 1923, when it was continued in operation by Messrs. Carl Owen and W. A. Medlock, until it was closed in 1927.

Even though there were still no educational requirements for license to practice pharmacy for a number of years thereafter, in 1903 there were three new schools of pharmacy to open their doors in September (in addition to The Atlanta College of Pharmacy). The new schools were Mercer University School of

Pharmacy in Macon, the Southern College of Pharmacy in Atlanta, and the University of Georgia School of Pharmacy in Athens. No one has been able to explain this sudden rush into pharmaceutical education, for there was no prospect of many students, nor was there any unusual demand for pharmacists coming into practice other than those coming under the "experience clause" or the preceptorship system. The Pharmaceutical Association and the Board of Pharmacy, out of their hope that college-trained pharmacists would elevate the professional status of the profession, may have influenced Mercer and the University of Georgia to enter the field in competition with The Atlanta College, already in operation, and the Southern College, which was to open that year. Little did these four schools realize that within a few years, and for a number of years thereafter, they would have one or more "Quiz Schools" as competitors, a type of competition they were ill-prepared to meet.

MERCER UNIVERSITY

The 1902-03 catalogue of Mercer University, a denominational school owned and operated at Macon by the Baptist Churches of Georgia, carried the following announcement: "The Mercer School of Pharmacy will begin its first session September 21, 1903. This conception and organization are the result of a long-felt need for a School of Pharmacy in Georgia directly connected with an institution of higher learning. Though the effort was made two years ago to connect such a school with Mercer University, at that time the laboratory equipment of the University was not adequate, and the school was not organized, but the erection of the new Science Hall before the opening of the next session, removes the difficulty, and the school will be thoroughly provided for."

"One new professor, M. A. Fort, was added to the teaching force, while the needs of the chemistry course were met by the Chemistry Department under Professor J. F. Sellers, who was made Dean of the new School, and the needs of biology were met by that department under Professor G. W. Macon. Three druggists of the City of Macon, T. A. Cheatham, Max Morris, and Mallory H. Taylor, served as lecturers in some related field."[1]

The following information is taken from Mercer's 1903-04 catalogue:

1. From a letter of Dr. Spright Dowell, President Emeritus, Mercer University.

℞ SUPPLEMENT B 273

SCHOOL OF PHARMACY

Faculty

P. D. POLLOCK, LL.D., PRESIDENT

J. F. SELLERS, M.A., DEAN,
Professor of Chemistry.

G. W. MACON, Ph.D.,
Professor of Biology.

M. A. FORT, A.B., Ph.C., M.D., SECRETARY,
Professor of Pharmacy.

(To be supplied)
Professor of Materia Medica.

T. A. CHEATHAM, Ph.G.,
Lecturer on Pharmacy.

MAX MORRIS, Ph.G.,
Lecturer on Materia Medica.

MALLORY H. TAYLOR, Ph.G.,
Lecturer on Pharmaceutical Chemistry.

The prescribed courses in the above catalogue are set out on page 89-100 inclusive. The student attendance for the first year was thirty-two and the maximum enrollment was forty-eight in 1905. There was a gradual decrease in enrollment and the school was discontinued in 1918. The average enrollment during the fifteen-year period was 23 and only six students were enrolled the last year. It was hoped that the income from student fees would provide the necessary income for maintenance, but the results were disappointing and this announcement was made in 1918: "The Pharmacy School has been suspended as a war measure. It may probably be restored next year."

[Author's Note: But the School did not reopen following the War.]

Following Dr. J. F. Sellers, as Dean, there came to Mercer Dean W. F. Gidley and, finally, Dean C. A. Struby.

During the 15 years of its existence, there must have been between 200 and 300 graduates of the Mercer School of Pharmacy. In the list of its graduates will be found the names of a number who have played an important part in building the profession of pharmacy in the State and Nation, and who have reflected great credit on their Alma Mater.

SOUTHERN COLLEGE OF PHARMACY[2]

The Southern College of Pharmacy was chartered in 1903 by Hansell W. Crenshaw, M.D., and Edgar A. Eberhart, Ph.D.

The institution opened October first, 1903, in quarters on the fifth floor of a building at the corner of Marietta and Broad Streets in Atlanta. The Ph.G. certificate was granted upon the completion of two terms of study, running from October to April and from April to October.

Like most other professional schools of that period, Southern was a proprietary institution, owned by Dr. Crenshaw and Dr. Eberhart, whose financial interest was sold to Dr. R. C. Hood, who in turn gave a one-fourth interest to an associate, W. B. Freeman. But this interest held by Freeman was later bought by Mrs. Hood.

The College occupied several different sites before being located in its present building in 1932. Eventually, the requirement for graduation changed from the two terms of six months each in 1922, to three terms of nine months each, and, finally, to the four-year course in 1935, on the completion of which the degree Bachelor of Science in Pharmacy was awarded.

In 1938 the College became a non-profit institution, and the deed to the institution was vested in a Board of Trustees, under a Charter.

The College was accredited by the Council on Pharmaceutical Education in 1942; elected to membership in the American Association of Schools and Colleges of Pharmacy; the Naylor Fund was established; Dean Hood retired as Dean in 1951, with Dr. Minnie M. Meyer as Acting Dean; a campaign to raise $400,000 in 1952 was undertaken; Dr. M. A. Chambers was employed as Dean in 1953, who resigned in 1957, to be followed by Dr. Oliver M. Littlejohn as Dean.

UNIVERSITY OF GEORGIA

In comparison to other state universities in so far as the number of students was concerned, the University of Georgia was, at the beginning of the century, a small institution composed of the College of Arts and Sciences and the Lumpkin Law School.

Walter B. Hill, the Chancellor of the University at that time,

---

2. The facts regarding Southern College were supplied by a member of the Southern College of Pharmacy Faculty. In 1959, Southern College of Pharmacy was merged with Mercer University.

envisioned the expansion of the functions and services of the University by incorporating a number of new schools into the system.

The 1958 catalogue of the University carries a list of the Schools that have been added over the years, and the order in which they came.

  The School of Pharmacy . . . . . . (1903)
  The College of Agriculture . . . . . . (1906)
  The School of Forestry . . . . (1908)
  The College of Education . . . . . . (1908)
  The College of Business Administration . . (1913)
  The School of Journalism . . . . . . (1921)
  The School of Home Economics . . . . (1933)
  The School of Veterinary Medicine . . . (1946)

It is a tribute to the pharmacists of the State of that time that the School of Pharmacy should be the first unit to be added in a plan for a major expansion of the first chartered State University, in accordance with Chancellor Hill's dream for the University.

It is of interest to note that the School of Pharmacy was the only one of the additional schools Chancellor Hill had envisioned that he lived to see come into existence, his death coming in December, 1905, following the opening of the School in September of that year. It was Chancellor D. C. Barrow who was to carry forward the program Chancellor Hill had planned.

It would be interesting to know what was in the mind of Chancellor Hill and the Trustees of the University that influenced them to select the School of Pharmacy as the first of the new schools to become an integral part of the State's largest educational institution. It could have been their recognition of the important part educated pharmacists might play in a public health program for the State that was then just in process of formation.

The School of Pharmacy was authorized by the Trustees at the June meeting of the Board, 1903, but there was some delay in the opening of the School, due to the absence of proper housing for the necessary classrooms and laboratories. Fate intervened, however, when fire destroyed Science Hall in 1904 and it was replaced by the present Terrell Hall, which was designated by the Trustees to house the Department of Chemistry and the School of Pharmacy.

The building was ready for occupancy in September, 1905,

and the first group of students, small in number, matriculated at that time, and the offices, classrooms, and laboratories were located in the basement of Terrell Hall, and due to the small number of students these quarters came to be the home of the School for 35 years.

Like other professional schools of the State at that time, the School of Pharmacy was to be self-sustaining from the tuition and laboratory fees paid by the students. But the number of students continued small, and the fees were totally inadequate to support even one full-time instructor.

Dr. Samuel C. Benedict, a practicing physician in Athens and University physician, was named Dean of the School and Professor of Materia Medica, on a part-time basis.

The curriculum was to extend over two terms of nine months each, on the completion of which the certificate Graduate in Pharmacy (Ph.G.) was to be granted. The two-year program of study, the degree offered, and the curriculum content paralleled those in the older Schools of Pharmacy in America.

Arthur J. Palmer, a practicing pharmacist, was elected Professor of Pharmacy, also on a part-time basis, but after one year he resigned. Mr. J. W. Galloway, also a practicing pharmacist in Athens, succeeded him, but also on a part-time basis. The number of students continued small, and none of them returned for the second year.

At the end of the school year June, 1907, consideration was given to closing the school in view of the small number of students and the competition of the three other schools in the State, but the decision was reached to put the School of Pharmacy on a definite permanent basis, with the following changes:

1. The charge for tuition and laboratory fees was discontinued.

2. A very modest budget was adopted, with an appropriation of $500 for equipment, $600 honorarium for the part-time Dean and Professor, and $1200 to employ a full-time Instructor in Pharmacy.

3. Robert C. Wilson, a practicing pharmacist in Athens was elected as Instructor in Pharmacy on a full-time basis.

On the opening of college in September, 1907, four students who had been registered the previous year returned for their second year, and these four students constituted the first graduating class in 1908: C. E. Brinson, A. Dwight Deas, William H. Hatcher, and J. A. Redfearn.

There being at that time no educational requirements for the licensure and practice of pharmacy, and no educational requirements for admission to the School of Pharmacy, it was agreed between Chancellor Barrow and the Faculty of the School that the School should set as its first objective the establishment of proper educational standards for the practice of pharmacy in the State, not only as a requirement for the issuance of a license, but also for the admission of students into the School of Pharmacy.

The first step was to require 4 units (or one year) of high school before admission to the School of Pharmacy of the University; the second step was to require two years (or 8 units), and, finally in 1912, graduation from high school or 12 units became the minimum for entrance.

The Chancellor and the Board of Trustees agreed with the Pharmacy Faculty that the objective of the School should be to graduate a few students of high quality rather than to lower educational standards and to graduate large numbers. The result of this decision was that for a number of years the enrollment continued small, and the number of graduates was still smaller. It should be pointed out, however, that for a number of years, it was still possible to secure a license in Georgia to practice pharmacy under the "experience clause" without any educational requirements.

Along with the other schools of pharmacy in the United States, the schools here in Georgia were operated on a two-year basis for graduation. But in 1926 the University of Georgia School of Pharmacy abandoned the two-year curriculum and installed a four-year program of study which led to the degree, Bachelor of Science in Pharmacy (B.S.Phar.).

A number of university and independent schools of pharmacy had been offering a four-year course *in addition to* the two-year course and continued to do so. It is believed that the University of Georgia was the first institution *to abandon all short courses* with the installation of the four-year course.

The four-year program has come to be the minimum requirement for all schools of pharmacy in the United States, and this will be increased to five years in 1960.

The Georgia Board of Pharmacy and the Georgia Pharmaceutical Association were zealous in their desire for proper educational prerequisites for license, but it was a slow process to secure proper legislation to raise the standard of education until finally, in 1933, legislation was enacted specifying graduation from a generally recognized school or college of pharmacy as the prerequisite for licensure.

Dr. Benedict continued as part-time Dean and Professor until his death in 1914. And, at that time, Robert C. Wilson was made Director of the School, and three years later was made Dean, in which capacity he served until his retirement in 1949, when Dr. Kenneth L. Waters succeeded him as Dean.

After being housed in the basement of Terrell Hall for 35 years, the School was moved into New College in 1939. The second and third floors of this, the second oldest building on the campus (1822), were remodeled to give, for the first time in the life of the School, ample office, classroom, and laboratory facilities for the enrollment of that time.

Following the World War II period there came such an influx of students that the ground floor and basement of the building were needed. Extensive remodeling provided ample space to house the Robert W. Woodruff Dispensing and Pharmacology Laboratories, the Dean's Office, two professors' offices, and a classroom. The basement provides the Manufacturing Laboratory and the Animal Room.

These facilities were deemed necessary to accommodate the maximum enrollment of 150 students. But, in 1958, 265 students are now crowded into this area.

The next and most urgent step should be the erection of a modern building, properly equipped to serve the undergraduate school and to provide space and facilities for an expanded research program in the health field of humans, animals, fowls, and plant life, thus to enable the profession of pharmacy in Georgia to assume its proper place and to function in all expanded public health programs that may come in the future.

Supplement C

LAWS GOVERNING THE PRACTICE OF MEDICINE AND PHARMACY, 1825-1958

THE reader will bear in mind that, for one hundred and fifty years following the establishment of the Colony, pharmacy and medicine were not distinguished one from the other by law or by practice, since, in most instances, the individual served in a dual capacity without formal educational requirements or professional background of training and experience other than that offered by the preceptorship system.

As early as 1804, there was formed in Savannah an organization under the name "The Georgia Medical Society." But it is not known whether this was to exclude apothecaries from the organization, or whether there were any individuals so designated for membership in the Society, or whether the physician members were also practicing pharmacy. Following this organization there came a similar organization in Augusta in 1822. But, whereas this was called a "Medical Society," the records show that many of the incorporators of the Society were actively engaged in pharmaceutical practice as well as medical practice. Both of these Societies set themselves up on a local level as examiners for those who were to practice medicine (and/or pharmacy).

It is therefore significant that we should agree that all legislation designated as medical legislation in 1825 also applied to and controlled pharmaceutical practice, and, for some fifty years or more, the laws applying to pharmacists were written by physicians, and all licensing of pharmacists until 1881 was done by the Medical Examining Board. The photostat which appears below in the illustration p. 280 documents the authority of the Board of Medical Examiners.

After 1881, the Georgia Pharmaceutical Association assumed

The Board of Physicians of the State of Georgia.

To all to whom these presents shall come.

Marshall A. Petal is hereby Licensed as Apothecary and Druggist in conformity with an Act of the Legislature of the STATE of GEORGIA, entitled, "An Act to regulate the Licensing of Physicians to Practice in this State." In testimony whereof, we have hereunto subscribed our names, and affixed the Seal of the Board, at Milledgeville this twenty first day of December 1866

Saml. G. White — President

Thos. H. Carey Secretary.

the responsibility of writing the laws to regulate the practice of pharmacy, and these pharmacy laws are tabulated chronologically from 1875 to 1959. Since physicians were writing the laws for the control of the practice of pharmacy, they granted themselves the right to be given a license to practice pharmacy without examination and without restriction, the license being automatically awarded upon showing of a diploma from a medical college, or a license to practice medicine.

As evidence of the above fact, the earliest law (1825) affecting the practice of pharmacy is quoted in full:[1]

"PHYSICIANS." "AN ACT TO REGULATE THE LICENSING OF PHYSICIANS TO PRACTICE IN THE STATE OF GEORGIA." [NOTE:—This Caption was amended in 1832 to include the practice of pharmacy—which see Laws 1832.]

Section 1. No physician is to commence the practice of medicine without a license.

Section 2. Penalty for violation is $500.00; and, if second offense, imprisonment may be imposed, but not exceeding two months; one-half fine to go to State Treasury and other half to the informer.

Section 5. The Board of Medical Examiners is established. A diploma from any medical college entitles person to license to practice medicine or pharmacy or both without examination.

Section 6. The first Board of Examiners was composed of the following physicians: "T. Fort, Antony, Scriven, West, Watkins, Harlow, Baber, White, Powell, Weems, Graham, Gerdine, Ridley, O. C. Fort, Hamilton, Daniel, Dent, Garemore, Jones, and Richardson."

Section 8. Persons practicing medicine (or pharmacy) at the time of the passage of this Act are exempt from examination.

Section 9. No apothecary within this State, *unless he is a licensed physician,* shall be permitted to vend or expose to sale any drugs or medicines without previously obtaining a license from the Board of Physicians created by this Act; and every apothecary so vending or selling drugs or medicines contrary to the provisions of this Act shall be liable to all the penalties imposed by this Act upon physicians and surgeons practicing without a license: provided, that nothing herein contained be construed to prevent shopkeepers from vending or exposing to sale medicines already prepared, and provided also, that the law does

---

1. *Laws of Georgia of Force, 1820-1829,* University of Georgia Library.

not apply to persons already engaged in this exclusive brand of merchandising (apothecary).

Section 10. The Board has power to examine all who apply for license to practice pharmacy, to pay the same fee as applied to physicians, that is, $5.00.

Section 11. To prevent delay and inconvenience, a single member of the Medical Board may grant a temporary license where a person makes application for such; but this provision may not apply to a person who has previously been denied or refused a license.

1828

"AN ACT TO ESTABLISH AND INCORPORATE THE 'MEDICAL ACADEMY OF GEORGIA' AT AUGUSTA, DECEMBER 20, 1828."[2]

This was the first professional school or college to be organized in Georgia. The curriculum provided for lectures in medicine, and in pharmacy as an aid to physicians who were to dispense medicines.

1829

By an Act of the Legislature the name of "The Medical Academy of Georgia" was changed to "The Medical Institute of the State of Georgia." The name of this institution was to be changed several times in later years. It is now (1959) "The Medical College of Georgia."

1831

"AN ACT TO ALTER AND AMEND THE ACT OF 1825."[3]

This original Act of 1825 had been re-enacted. The amendments and alterations included the following:

Section 1. A provision against fraud in applying for license: "Wherever the Board of Physicians have any doubts as to the qualifications of any applicant for license, they may proceed to examine him, even though he may present a diploma from a medical college, and either grant or refuse license."

Section 2. "The Board has the authority and the duty to prescribe such course in reading as in their opinion may be necessary and proper to those who intend to pursue the practice of medicine

---

2. *Laws of Georgia of Force 1820-1829*, University of Georgia Law Library.
3. *Laws of Georgia, 1831*, p. 152.

under private instructors, which course in reading shall be published in at least two of the Gazettes of the State, and shall be obligatory of all who may apply to the Board for license after expiration of two years from time of publication."

Section 3. "It shall not be lawful for the Board of Physicians to license any person who does not present satisfactory testimonial of good moral character."

1832

An Act was passed to amend the original law of 1825, to read as follows:

"AN ACT TO REGULATE THE LICENSING OF PHYSICIANS IN THIS STATE, TO PREVENT APOTHECARIES VENDING AND EXPOSING TO SALE WITHIN THIS STATE DRUGS AND MEDICINES WITHOUT A LICENSE FROM THE BOARD OF PHYSICIANS, AND TO PREVENT MERCHANTS, SHOPKEEPERS, AND ALL OTHER PERSONS FROM COMPOUNDING AND PREPARING DRUGS AND MEDICINES, OR EITHER."[4]

1835

"AN ACT TO PROHIBIT THE EMPLOYMENT OF SLAVES AND FREE PERSONS OF COLOR FROM COMPOUNDING OR DISPENSING MEDICINES IN DRUGGISTS' AND APOTHECARIES' STORES, AND TO COMPEL DRUGGISTS AND APOTHECARIES TO KEEP ARSENIC AND OTHER DANGEROUS POISONS UNDER LOCK AND KEY."[5]

Section 1. "That from and after the first day of January next, any person or persons having in his or her or their employment any slave or free person of color in any apothecary shop or druggist's store in this State, in the apothecary branch of the business, in putting up, compounding, or dispensing, purchasing, or vending any drug or drugs, medicines of any description, kind or sort whatsoever, shall be guilty of a high misdemeanor; and on conviction thereof shall be fined the sum of $100 for the first offense, and $500 for the second offense, one-half of the fine going to the informer and the other half to the State."

Section 2. "Every druggist or apothecary, or any other person, vending any medicines of a poisonous quality shall not vend the same to any person or persons of color under the penalty aforesaid."

4. *Laws of Georgia, 1832,* p. 131.
5. *Ibid.,* 1835, p. 268.

Section 3. "Permission is granted to employ a Negro or free person of color in that branch of their business not having to do with dealing with poisons."

1836

"AN ACT TO REVISE AN ACT TO INCORPORATE THE GEORGIA MEDICAL SOCIETY PASSED THE 12TH OF DECEMBER, 1804."[6]

1838

"AN ACT TO ESTABLISH AND INCORPORATE A MEDICAL COLLEGE IN THE CITY OF SAVANNAH UNDER THE TITLE 'THE SAVANNAH MEDICAL COLLEGE.'"[7]

Section 1. The incorporators were the following: W. R. Waring, Wm. C. Daniel, John M. Berrien, Robt. M. Charlton, Wm. T. Williams, Jos. W. Jackson, Wm. Law, and the Reverend Edward Neusville.

1839

An Act was passed establishing the Southern Botanico Medical College.[8] The school was to be located at Forsyth, Georgia. The Board of Incorporators were the following: Jesse George, James Dowdle, Jesse Sinclair, Alfred Brooks, Reddick Pierce, Josiah E. Nunnally, Steven G. Cotten, Joseph Bankston, Wm. H. Fonerden.

1845

"AN ACT TO AMEND THE CHARTER OF THE MEDICAL COLLEGE OF GEORGIA, AND TO EXEMPT THE FACULTY AND STUDENTS FROM JURY DUTY DURING THE COLLEGIATE TERM."[9]

"AN ACT TO AMEND AN ACT AUTHORIZING THE ESTABLISHMENT OF THE SOUTHERN BOTANICO MEDICAL COLLEGE OF GEORGIA, SO AS TO AUTHORIZE THE BOARD OF TRUSTEES OF SAID COLLEGE TO MOVE TO THE CITY OF MACON WHENEVER IN THEIR JUDGMENT IT SHALL APPEAR TO SAID BOARD EXPEDIENT OR CONDUCIVE TO THE INTEREST OF SAID INSTITUTION."[10]

6. *Laws of Georgia,* 1836.
7. *Ibid.,* 1838, p. 156.
8. *Ibid.,* 1839.
9. *Ibid.,* 1845, p. 153.
10. *Ibid.,* 1845, p. 153. Act approved Dec. 27, 1845.

1847

"AN ACT TO ESTABLISH A BOTANICO MEDICAL BOARD OF PHYSICIANS IN THIS STATE AND FOR THE BETTER REGULATION OF THE BOTANIC OR THOMSONIAN PRACTICE OF MEDICINE" (and Botanic or Thomsonian Pharmacy).[11]

Section 1. "No person or persons except graduates of the Southern Botanico Medical College shall be allowed to practice physic or surgery on the Botanic or Thomsonian system of medicine, *or any of the branches thereof (pharmacy),* or in any case to prescribe for the cure of disease for fee or reward unless he or they shall have been licensed to do so in the manner hereinafter prescribed."

Section 2. "And be it further enacted; that all bonds, notes, promises and assumptions made to any person or persons except to said graduates not licensed in the manner hereinafter mentioned, the consideration of which shall be services rendered or medicines prescribed or furnished as a Botanic or Thomsonian physician or surgeon in the treatment or management of disease, shall be and they are, hereby declared utterly void and of no effect."

Section 3. The creation of a Board of Physicians and Surgeons to be known as the Botanico Medico Board of Georgia, to examine all applicants for license to practice under this system.

Section 5. "*No Botanic or Thomsonian pharmacist* within this State, unless he be a graduate as aforesaid, or a licensed Botanic or Thomsonian physician, shall be permitted to vend or expose for sale Botanic or Thomsonian medicines without previously obtaining a license from the Board created by this Act; and every person so vending or exposing to sale such medicines shall be subject to the disabilities imposed by this Act, on Botanic or Thomsonian physicians practicing without license: Provided that nothing herein contained be so construed as to prevent merchants or shopkeepers from vending or exposing to sale Botanic or Thomsonian medicines already prepared."

Section 6. "The (Botanico) Board of Physicians created by this Act shall have the power to examine any apothecary who may apply to it for a license touching their knowledge of drugs and pharmacy, and on finding such persons qualified, shall grant such license and receive therefor the same fees as provided in this Act for license to practice medicine or surgery ($5.00)."

11. *Ibid.,* 1847, p. 234.

Section 7. "To avoid delay and inconvenience, a single member of the Board of Physicians may grant temporary license to last no longer than the next meeting of the Board; but no temporary license may be given if the person has previously been refused license by the Board."

Section 8. "The Board may examine a person who presents a diploma wherever there are doubts of the qualification of the applicant."

Section 9. Authority is given to prescribe a course of reading for applicants.

Section 10. The Board may grant temporary or perpetual license.

Section 11. Good moral character is demanded of applicants.

Section 15. The names of the Board: "Wm. Fisher, James Buys, L. C. Quinn, John Coxe, M. S. Bellenger, J. Sinclair, L. Bankston, James T. Ellis, and J. Bryan."

"AN ACT TO REVIVE AND KEEP IN FORCE AN ACT ENTITLED 'AN ACT TO REGULATE THE LICENSING OF PHYSICIANS TO PRACTICE IN THIS STATE' ASSENTED TO THE 24TH DAY OF DECEMBER, 1825."[12]

Section 1. The above is hereby enacted.

Section 2. The names of the Board (Regular): "L. D. Ford, J. P. Garvin, G. M. Newton, H. M. Moore, J. Branham, B. F. Keene, E. A. Broddus, H. T. Shaw, R. Banks, G. D. Phillips, J. Persons, W. J. Johnson, M. A. Franklin, J. M. Greene, T. Fort, B. A. White, C. G. Paine, T. F. Green, George D. Case, H. K. Burroughs: Provided that the graduates of the Botanical Medical College and the licentiates of a legally constituted Medical Board of Botanic Physicians be fully exempted from the operation of the said Act, as revised."

1849-1850

"AN ACT TO COMPENSATE PHYSICIANS AND SURGEONS WHO SHALL BE SUMMONED BY THE SHERIFF OR CORONER OF COUNTY TO MAKE POST-MORTEM EXAMINATION FOR THE INFORMATION OF JURIES OF INQUEST."[13]

Here is recorded (what appears to be) the first instance where individuals are granted license to practice medicine and to charge for services either under the Botanic system or the Regular sys-

12. *Ibid.,* 1847, p. 237.
13. *Laws of Georgia,* 1849-50, p. 335.

tem *by Act of the Legislature.* A number of instances will occur where action similar to this prevails, with the result that eventually there was a large number of individuals practicing medicine and/or pharmacy in the State whose licenses were granted by the Legislature without the person having taken an examination.

"AN ACT TO AUTHORIZE JEPTHA B. STEPHENS TO PRACTICE MEDICINE UNDER THE BOTANIC SYSTEM AND TO CHARGE FOR HIS SERVICES."[14]

"AN ACT TO AUTHORIZE DANIEL SIKES OF THE COUNTY OF TATNALL TO PRACTICE MEDICINE IN SAID COUNTY, CHARGING COMPENSATION THEREFOR WITHOUT A LICENSE, AS NOW BY LAW PROHIBITED."[15]

1852

"AN ACT TO ENDOW THE SOUTHERN BOTANICO MEDICAL COLLEGE AT MACON, GEORGIA."[16] APPROVED JANUARY 21, 1852. THE SUM APPROVED WAS $5,000.

"AN ACT TO AUTHORIZE GEORGIA BIRD OF THE COUNTY OF TALIAFERRO; FREDERICK SHAFFER OF MUSCOGEE COUNTY; L. D. WYATT OF GORDON COUNTY; T. BATTLE AND HENRY L. BATTLE OF HANCOCK COUNTY; WILLIAM P. RICHARDS OF LUMPKIN COUNTY; WILLIAM C. DABBS OF FLOYD COUNTY; B. A. C. BONNER OF THE COUNTY OF CASS; H. H. LUMPKIN AND DANIEL B. HEAD OF THE COUNTY OF CARROLL; FREDERICK FREEMAN OF CLARKE COUNTY, AND LEANDER B. BATTLE TO PRACTICE PHYSIC ON THE HOMEOPATHIC SYSTEM, AND TO CHARGE AND COLLECT COMPENSATION FOR THEIR SERVICES."[17]

1854

"AN ACT TO AUTHORIZE WARREN FREEMAN OF THE COUNTY OF BIBB TO PRACTICE PHYSIC ON THE HOMEOPATHIC SYSTEM, AND TO CHARGE AND COLLECT COMPENSATION FOR HIS SERVICES."[18]

In various Acts of 1854 the following individuals were authorized by the Legislature to practice medicine and charge and collect

---

14. *Ibid.,* p. 336.
15. *Ibid.,* p. 336.
16. *Laws of Georgia,* 1852, p. 300.
17. *Ibid.,* p. 352.
18. *Ibid.,* 1854, p. 504.

compensation for the same: Drs. William D. Quinn and James H. Lane of Wilkes County; Madison Greenwood of Rabun County; James R. Fulsom of Lowndes County; H. W. Wootten of Carroll County; James J. Garrison of the County of McIntosh; Ransom Rogers, Senior, of the County of Screven; Claiborne H. Jones of the County of Upson; Azariah Burnett of Dade County; James O. Hunt of the County of Harris; Asa Houston Langston of Hart County; Tomlin F. Brewster, a minor, of Cherokee County; Charles H. Andas of Hancock County; O. Profitt of Jasper County; Joel Turner of Elbert County.

"AN ACT TO AUTHORIZE ALL PHYSICIANS WITHIN THE STATE OF GEORGIA HAVING RECEIVED A DIPLOMA FROM ANY MEDICAL COLLEGE WITHIN THE UNITED STATES TO PRACTICE PHYSIC IN THIS STATE AND TO CHARGE FOR THE SAME WITHOUT LICENSE."[19]

Section 1. "All persons having received a diploma from any medical college in the United States be, and they are, hereby authorized to practice physic within the limits of this State and to charge and collect for the same without license."

Section 2. Notes, mortgages, or other evidences of debt for services to people without a license are void.

"AN ACT TO INCORPORATE THE ATLANTA MEDICAL COLLEGE AND FOR OTHER PURPOSES THEREIN MENTIONED."[20]

The Trustees named were the following: L. C. Simpson, Jared A. Whitaker, John Collier, Hubbard Cozart, Daniel Hook, John L. Harris, William Herring, Green B. Haygood, and James M. Calhoun, and "their successors" in office.

1856

"AN ACT TO AUTHORIZE DRS. J. J. M. GOSS OF JACKSON COUNTY, BAILY WHITE OF HANCOCK COUNTY, MANFORD J. JONES OF MARION COUNTY, ISAAC H. HALL OF TROUP COUNTY, F. N. HARDMAN OF FULTON COUNTY, B. H. C. BEEMAN OF GORDON COUNTY; BE AND THEY ARE HEREBY AUTHORIZED TO PRACTICE MEDICINE UPON THE ECLECTIC SYSTEM AS TAUGHT AT CINCINNATI, OHIO, AND TO COLLECT AND CHARGE THE USUAL FEES."[21]

19. *Ibid.,* 1854.
20. *Ibid.,* 1854, p. 501.
21. *Ibid.,* 1856, p. 500.

1860

"AN ACT TO REGULATE THE PRACTICE OF PHYSIC IN THE COUNTY OF ELBERT, AND FOR OTHER PURPOSES."[22]

Section 1. "That all laws authorizing any person to practice physic and collect for the same who is not a graduate of some properly recognized medical college, and has not a diploma for the same, are hereby repealed so far as they relate to the *County of Elbert.*"

1861

"AN ACT TO CONSTITUTE AN ECLECTIC BOARD OF PHYSICIANS TO EXAMINE AND LICENSE YOUNG MEN TO PRACTICE MEDICINE UPON THE ECLECTIC SYSTEM, AND TO LOCATE THE SAME IN THE TOWN OF ATHENS, GEORGIA."[23]

Section 1. "Be it enacted by the General Assembly of the State of Georgia that I. J. Goss, of Jackson County; M. P. Alexander, of Hall County; J. D. Beecham, of Franklin County; Travis Latner, of White County; H. S. Brady, of Madison County; and their successors in office, be and they are hereby constituted an *Eclectic Board of Physicians,* to examine and license young men to practice medicine upon the Eclectic or Progressive System, and the said Board shall conform to the same rules and regulations as are provided for the government of the Allopathic Board of Physicians located at Milledgeville, Georgia.

Section 2. That the said Board shall hold its sessions annually in the Town of Athens, Georgia, on the first day of April, and shall continue in session as long as may be necessary to transact the business of said Board.
Assented to December 19, 1861.

Code of Georgia, Chapter 4:[24]

Section 1338. "Any white person who has received a diploma from any medical school or medical college of the Confederate States without regard to the school is authorized to practice medicine to the extent of the powers given in said diploma subject to the provisions hereinafter set forth."

22. *Ibid.*, 1860, p. 212.
23. *Ibid.*, 1861, p. 116.
24. *Code of Georgia, 1861,* Chap. 4, p. 260.

Section 1339. "ALLOPATHIC BOARD OF PHYSICIANS ESTABLISHED." Authority and duties set forth.

Section 1340. Duties of the Allopathic Board of Physicians are set forth. Among the duties is to grant licenses to physicians; also *to grant licenses to apothecaries* upon their standing a satisfactory examination as to their knowledge of drugs and pharmacy.

Section 1341. Provision is made for temporary license, similar to the one already noted.[25]

Section 1344. There is also established a Board of Physicians of the Reform Practice of Medicine, who are to have the same authority and perform the same duties "herein before set forth."

Section 1346. Penalties are set up for any person practicing medicine for a fee who does not hold a license. The penalty is $500 for the first offense, and for the second, imprisonment of not more than two months, one-half of fine to inure to the informer, the other half to the educational fund of the County.

Section 1348. Neither Board can license persons to practice in a School of medicine different from their own. Physicians belonging to a School of medicine not represented by a Board of Physicians may practice under their diplomas alone, and if they have none, are liable as if they had no license and were required to have them.

Section 1349. The fee for license is set up at $5.00.

Section 1350. Physicians who were in practice prior to the 24th of December, 1847 are exempted from all the provisions of this Chapter.[26]

Section 1351. "No person in this State, except a licensed physician, shall vend or expose to sale any drugs or medicines without first obtaining a license therefor from one of said Boards.

Section 1353. "Druggists are exempted from obtaining said license who were engaged in such business prior to the 24th of December, 1847, and who continue so at the adoption of the Code, and merchants or shopkeepers may deal in medicines already prepared if patented, or, if not patented, legally warranted by a licensed druggist."

1863

"AN ACT TO AUTHORIZE AUSTIN W. BERRY OF HANCOCK COUNTY TO PREPARE AND VEND DRUGS AND MEDICINES, AND TO DO ALL

---

25. *Code of Georgia, 1861,* Chapter 4, pp. 260-262.
26. *Code of Georgia, 1861,* Chapt. 4, p. 262.

OTHER MATTERS AND THINGS PERTAINING TO SAID BRANCH OF BUSINESS AS A REGULAR LICENSED DRUGGIST."[27]

Section 1. This Bill is assented to because of the petition of a very large proportion of the citizens of Hancock County for its passage, including the physicians of the County.

1866

"AN ACT TO INCORPORATE THE DALTON MEDICAL COLLEGE, DALTON, GEORGIA."[28]

The following are named as the incorporators: Drs. Jesse R. McAfee, Charles P. Gordon, Baxter B. Brown, Samuel W. Fields, Moses Quinn, E. C. Cochran, L. P. Gudger, John K. Osborn, F. A. Rushenburg, Henry W. Renfrowe, and David Emerson.

Section 3. The incorporators are authorized to select professors from their own body or from any of the medical colleges of the United States, to advance and promote the improvement of its pupils in the science of medicine, surgery, and medical jurisprudence.

1867

Code of Georgia, 1867, Paragraph 806.[29]

Practitioners of law, physic and dentistry shall pay an annual tax of $5.00 each, (and register their license in the Office of the Clerk of the Inferior Court).

Code of Georgia.

Sections 53-54.[30] Concerns adulterated drugs or adulterated liquor. In case damage accrues to purchaser, the seller thereof shall be liable for damages in the injury done.

Section 54. If a vendor of drugs and medicines, by himself or his agent, either knowingly or negligently furnishes the wrong article of medicine, and damage accrues from the use of the drug or medicine, the vendor is liable for damages.

---

27. *Laws of Georgia,* 1863, p. 226.
28. *Laws of Georgia,* 1866, p. 200.
29. *Code of Georgia, 1867,* Paragraph 806, page 161.
30. *Ibid.,* Paragraph 29.

1871

Physicians are exempted from jury duty provided they are in the active practice of their profession.[31]

"AN ACT TO EXTEND THE USEFULNESS OF THE SAVANNAH MEDICAL COLLEGE BY APPROPRIATING $15,000."[32]

This is an amendment to the original Act, and entitles the Board of Trustees to increase its membership to twenty-five (25). It is specified that the State does not own any lien on the property.

1872

"AN ACT TO REGULATE THE PRACTICE OF DENTISTRY AND TO PROTECT THE PEOPLE AGAINST EMPIRICISM IN RELATION THERETO IN THE STATE OF GEORGIA."[33]

Section 1. Prohibits anyone from practicing dentistry who is not a graduate of a dental college or who has not received a license from a Board of Dentists.

Section 10. Provision that dentists who have been in practice prior to the passage of this Act are exempt from all the provisions of same.

1873

Code of Georgia, 1873.[34]

Section 1408. Prescribes punishment for keeping a drug or apothecary store without first acquiring a license as required by law.

Laws of Georgia.
An Act was passed repealing certain phases of the Medical Law specifying the setting up of means by which a license may be revoked for cause.[35]
All regularly practicing apothecaries are exempt from jury duty.[36]

1875

Provision for garnishment of daily or weekly wages only for Board of Physicians is extended to include, when consideration

---

31. *Laws of Georgia, 1871.*
32. *Ibid.*
33. *Laws of Georgia, 1872,* p. 27.
34. *Code of Georgia, 1873.*
35. *Laws of Georgia, 1873,* p. 23.
36. *Ibid.,* p. 31.

for the debt is "medicine furnished by any physician, surgeon, druggist or apothecary to said employee or his family."[37]

PHARMACY LAWS OF GEORGIA, 1875-1958

The Georgia Pharmaceutical Association was organized and began its distinctive and valuable functions on October 20, 1875, and the time seemed appropriate that pharmacists themselves should, out of their experience, begin to dictate the laws governing the practice of their profession.

1876

In cooperation with the State Board of Health, composed at that time of physicians only, the Pharmaceutical Association was active in drafting a "Poison Law" to govern the sale and distribution of poisons, and to aid in its legislative enactment.

"AN ACT TO REGULATE THE SALE OF POISONS IN THIS STATE."[38]

Schedule A. The poisons are listed.
Schedule B. Names of the individual poisons are given, with specifications how they shall be labelled and packaged, and setting up the specification that the druggist must carry a poison book and register in such book the name of the person, the name of the poison sold, and for what purpose to be used, and the quantity of poisons and the date; that the book shall be open to inspection by law officers or others.
The "Poison Law" was enacted during the Legislative Session of 1876, thus becoming the first pharmaceutically sponsored law. This law, like those to follow, was specifically in the interest of the public health, safety and welfare.

1881

"AN ACT TO ESTABLISH A BOARD OF PHARMACEUTIC EXAMINERS, AND TO PRESCRIBE THE POWERS AND DUTIES OF SAID BOARD, AND TO REGULATE THE COMPOUNDING AND VENDING OF MEDICINES, DRUGS, AND POISONS IN THE STATE OF GEORGIA, AND TO PROVIDE A PENALTY FOR THE INFRINGEMENT OF THE PROVISIONS OF THIS ACT."[39]*

37. *Laws of Georgia, 1875,* p. 22.
38. *Laws of Georgia, 1876,* p. 24.
39. *Laws of Georgia, 1881,* p. 184.
*This is the basic law that was to govern the practice of pharmacy for many years. It has been amended many times.

Preamble:
Whereas in all civilized countries it has been found necessary to restrict the traffic in medicines and poisons, and to provide by law for the regulation of the delicate and responsible business of compounding and dispensing the powerful agents used in medicine; and, Whereas the safety and welfare of the public are endangered by the sale of poisons by unqualified or ignorant persons; and,
Whereas the power of physicians to overcome disease depends greatly upon their ability to obtain good and unadulterated drugs and skillfully prepared medicines, and the sophistication and adulteration of drugs and medicines is a species of fraud which should be prevented and suitably punished; therefore

Section 1. The General Assembly of the State of Georgia do enact that within sixty days after the passage of this Act, the Governor of the State shall appoint five experienced druggists or practical pharmacists who shall have been actually engaged in the drug business for the past three years immediately preceding their appointment, and these five druggists shall constitute the Board of Pharmaceutic Examiners, who shall hold their office for the term of three years or until their successors shall have been legally appointed and qualified; that three members of said Board at any regular, called, or adjourned meeting shall constitute a quorum for the transaction of business; that any vacancy which may occur on said Board shall be filled by the Governor for the unexpired term.*

Section 2. Members of the Board shall take the Oath prescribed by the Constitution of the State of Georgia for state offices, and shall file same in the Office of the Secretary of State, who upon receiving the said Oaths of Office shall issue to each of the said Examiners a certificate of appointment.

Section 3. After appointment and qualification, the Board of Examiners shall meet and organize, elect a chairman. The Board may adopt such rules, regulations, and by-laws as they shall deem necessary to carry into execution the provisions of this Act.

Section 4. Said Board shall meet at least once every twelve months at such place as the majority of the Board may determine, and may hold such special meetings as frequently and at such places as the proper discharge of its duties shall require; the same to be convened by order of the Chairman, and the rules or by-laws shall provide for the giving of the proper notice of the

---

*Names of this first Board of Examiners are given in the Appendix.

℞ SUPPLEMENT C 295

time and place of such meetings to members of the Board and the public.

Section 5. It shall be the duty of said Board to grant license; first, to pharmacists who, after three years' experience in a drug store kept by a licensed apothecary or pharmacist, have graduated from a college of pharmacy acknowledged by the American Pharmaceutical Association, and who shall exhibit to the said Board a diploma of the same; second, to pharmacists who have obtained a diploma from an authorized foreign college or institution or examining Board, and who shall exhibit the same to the Board of Pharmaceutic Examiners; third, to physicians who are graduates of a *regular* medical college and who shall exhibit their diplomas to said Board; also to druggists who shall produce to said Board satisfactory evidence of having been engaged in the drug business for a period of ten years next preceding the time of application; also to druggists who have attended a college of pharmacy acknowledged by the American Pharmaceutical Association for at least one term or session and who have been engaged in the drug business for at least nine years previous to the time of applying for the said license; fourth, to druggists who after three years' experience in a drug store kept by a licensed apothecary or pharmacist shall have passed a satisfactory examination before said Board of Pharmaceutic Examiners. All licenses granted shall be signed by a majority of the whole Board and shall specify the grounds upon which such license is granted and shall be in such form as the Board shall prescribe.

Section 6. All persons applying for examination and license shall pay to the Board of Pharmaceutic Examiners the sum of $15.00, and, if passing the examination, shall be furnished with a license as hereinbefore provided, for which no further fee shall be required or paid. Should the applicant fail to stand a satisfactory examination, no fee shall be required for a subsequent examination, such subsequent examination not to be granted within six months after the first. It shall be the duty of the Board to keep a record of its transactions in a book to be kept for that purpose by one of the members, said book to be turned over to their successors in office.

Section 7. This section provides for the registration of license in the Office of the Ordinary of the County where the licentiate resides or intends to conduct drug business. For each registration the Ordinary shall receive fifty cents to be paid by the party so registering, and a certificate of such registration stating the terms of the same shall be given him by said Ordinary.

Section 8. States that no person "shall engage in the compounding or vending of drugs, medicines or poisons within this State without a full compliance with this Act; except, first, such druggists as are exempted from the operation of the present law by the statutes of the State of Georgia and such druggists as have heretofore obtained license and are legally authorized by existing laws to vend drugs and compound poisons and chemicals; second, physicians putting up their own prescriptions and dispensing medicines from their own office; third, merchants selling family remedies not poison, as prescribed and allowed by Section 1409 of the Code of Georgia of 1873; fourth, assistants in drug stores where the manager of said drug store has complied with the requirements of this Act."

Section 9. Any person who shall violate the provisions of either of the two preceding sections of this Act, or shall register fraudulently, shall be guilty of a misdemeanor and upon conviction shall be punished by fine not to exceed $100 and imprisonment not to exceed three months, either or both at the discretion of the Court. In all cases of prosecution under this Act, the burden shall be upon the defendant to show his authority. "Be it further enacted that all fees for examination and license, and one-half of the fines collected from convictions under this Act shall be paid to the Board of Pharmaceutic Examiners to defray the expenses of the same and as compensation for their services."

Section 11. "Be it further enacted that this Act shall take effect from and after the date of its passage."

Section 12. "Be it further enacted that all laws and parts of laws militating against the provisions of this Act are hereby repealed." Approved September 29, 1881.[40]

Unlicensed Drug or Apothecary Store.

"AN ACT TO AMEND SECTION 1408 OF THE CODE OF 1873 WHICH PRESCRIBES THE PUNISHMENT FOR KEEPING A DRUG OR APOTHECARY STORE WITHOUT FIRST PROCURING A LICENSE AS REQUIRED BY LAW."[41]

Section 1. Provides that Section 1408 of the Code of Georgia of 1873 be amended as follows:
"Any person violating the preceding Section is liable to indict-

---

40. *Laws of Georgia,* 1881, p. 184.
41. *Laws of Georgia,* 1881, p. 67.

ment, and on conviction shall be punished as prescribed in Section 4310 of the Code of Georgia of 1873. The onus of proof is upon the defendant to show his authority."
This Act approved September, 1881.

1882

An Amendment to the Act Creating the Board of Pharmaceutic Examiners.[42]

Section 1. Provides for the original Act to be amended as follows:
"In the fifth Section of said Act, after the words 'to physicians who are graduates of a *regular medical college* and who shall exhibit their diplomas to said Board,' the following words should be added, to wit: 'and to physicians who were practicing medicine prior to the first of January, 1847, who shall produce satisfactory evidence that they were so practicing,' so that said clause shall read as follows: 'to physicians who are graduates of a *regular* medical college and who shall exhibit their diplomas to said Board, and to physicians who were practicing medicine prior to the first of January, 1847, who shall produce satisfactory evidence that they were so practicing.'"

1884-1885

Regulating the Sale of Morphine.

"AN ACT TO PRESCRIBE THE MANNER OF SELLING THE SULPHATE AND OTHER PREPARATIONS OF MORPHINE IN THIS STATE, AND FOR OTHER PURPOSES."[43]

This Act provides for a scarlet paper wrapping for any container of any Sulphate or other preparation of Morphine, as well as for a scarlet label lettered in white letters, plainly naming the contents. Violators are guilty of misdemeanor, and subject to fine of $10 to $50.

1889

Amending the Act Establishing the Board of Pharmaceutic Examiners.[44]

Section 1. Amends the original Act by changing the name

---

42. *Laws of Georgia,* 1882, p. 146.
43. *Laws of Georgia,* 1884-85, p. 134.
44. *Laws of Georgia,* 1889, p. 89.

"Board of Pharmaceutic Examiners" to the "Georgia State Board of Pharmacy." It also directs the Governor of the State to appoint five experienced druggists or practical pharmacists from the list of names of ten persons submitted by the Georgia Pharmaceutical Association who shall have been actually engaged in the drug business within this State for the three years immediately preceding their appointment. That these five experienced druggists or practical pharmacists so appointed shall constitute the Georgia State Board of Pharmacy; one of whom shall hold his office for one year, one for two, one for three, one for four, and one for five years, or until his or their successors shall have been legally appointed and qualified; and that at each and every annual meeting thereafter the Georgia Pharmaceutical Association shall submit to the Governor the names of five persons with the qualifications herein before mentioned, and the Governor shall appoint from said names so submitted one member of said Board who shall hold his office for five years or until his successor is duly appointed and qualified. This Act shall not affect the term of the present Board.

Section 3. Provides for the election of a chairman and a secretary from the membership of the Board.

Section 4. Provides for reciprocation of license with other state Boards.

Section 5. Provides for an examination and license fee of $5.00 and an annual renewal fee of $2.00 to be paid to the Board of Pharmacy. "All monies received for renewals in excess of $600 shall be paid into the Treasury of the Georgia Pharmaceutical Association, and said Board shall make an annual report to the Georgia Pharmaceutical Association."

Section 6. Inserts in original Act a clause concerning adulteration of drugs, to be inserted after Section 8 of the original Act, as follows: "No person shall within this State manufacture for sale or offer for sale or sell any drug, medicine, chemical or pharmaceutical preparation which is adulterated."

Section 10. Gives the State Board of Pharmacy authority to demand samples of any drug, medicine, chemical or pharmaceutical preparation for analysis of such drug.

Section 11. Empowers the Board of Pharmacy to "employ an expert chemist or analyst to examine into the so-claimed adulteration and report upon the result of his investigation, and if said report justifies such action, the Board shall cause the prosecution of the offender."

1890-1891

AN ACT AMENDING SECTION 5 OF ORIGINAL PHARMACY LAW OF 1881, AS AMENDED IN 1889.[45]

"That Section 5 of the original Act creating the Board of Pharmaceutical Examiners be so altered and amended that it shall hereafter read as follows:

Section 5. It shall be the duty of the Georgia State Board of Pharmacy to grant license; first, to druggists who, after three years' experience in a drug store managed by a licensed apothecary or pharmacist, shall have passed a satisfactory examination before the said Board of Pharmacy; second, *to such physicians,* * graduates of a regular medical college, and to such graduates of schools of pharmacy as shall have passed satisfactory examination before said Board of Pharmacy; third, to pharmacists who have obtained license from such other State Boards of Pharmacy as may be recognized by said Georgia State Board of Pharmacy. All licenses granted shall be signed by a majority of the whole Board, shall specify the grounds upon which such license is granted, shall be in such form as the Board shall prescribe, and shall be posted in a conspicuous place in the place of business of such licentiate; provided that this Act shall not apply to physicians who are graduates of medical colleges in good standing and who have been practicing medicine for five years at the time of the passage of this Act."

1893

Permanent Licenses by State Board of Pharmacy.

"AN ACT TO AMEND AN ACT APPROVED 1881, AND AMENDED IN 1889, AS CONTAINED IN THE CODE OF GEORGIA, PAGE 1482, 83, 84, AND FOR OTHER PURPOSES."[46]

This amendment provides for a *permanent* license to be granted at the time of examination, upon payment to the Board the sum of $15.00.

Approved December 1, 1893.

---

45. *Laws of Georgia*, 1890-91, Vol. I, p. 234.
46. *Laws of Georgia*, 1893, p. 107.

*Prior to this time physicians were not required to stand examination for license to practice pharmacy.

1904

"AN ACT TO AMEND SECTION 1492, VOLUME I, OF THE CODE OF GEORGIA, PROVIDING FOR THE APPOINTMENT AND QUALIFICATION OF MEMBERS OF THE GEORGIA STATE BOARD OF PHARMACY, SO AS TO PROVIDE THAT ONLY RETAIL DRUGGISTS WHO ARE NOT CONNECTED WITH ANY COLLEGE OR SCHOOL OF PHARMACY SHALL BE QUALIFIED TO APPOINTMENT ON SAID BOARD OF PHARMACY; TO PROVIDE FOR THE FILLING OF VACANCIES ON SAID BOARD, AND FOR OTHER PURPOSES."[47]

Section 1. Provides an amendment which requires that, to be qualified as members of the Board of Pharmacy, appointees shall be "registered druggists who shall have been actually engaged in the retail drug business within this State for three years immediately preceding the submitting of their names, *and who are not connected with any college or school of pharmacy.*"
This amendment was approved August 15, 1904.

Georgia State Board of Pharmacy, Meetings.

"AN ACT TO AMEND SECTION 1495, VOLUME I, OF THE CODE OF GEORGIA, PROVIDING FOR MEETING OF THE STATE BOARD OF PHARMACY, AND FOR OTHER PURPOSES."[48]

This Act provides that the Board shall meet at least twice every 12 months, and may also hold special meetings as they require, to be convened by the chairman, after proper notice of meeting is given to members of Board and to the public.
Approved August 12, 1904.

Georgia State Board of Pharmacy, Licenses By.
"AN ACT TO AMEND SECTION 1497, VOLUME I, OF THE CODE OF GEORGIA, PRESCRIBING THE MANNER OF GRANTING LICENSES BY THE GEORGIA STATE BOARD OF PHARMACY, AND FOR OTHER PURPOSES; SO THAT AFTER AMENDMENT THE SECTION SHALL READ:

'All persons applying for examination and license shall pay to the Board of Pharmacy the sum of $15.00, and if passing the examination, shall be furnished with a license as herein before provided. Should the applicant fail to stand a satisfactory examination, no fee shall be required for a subsequent examination or subsequent examinations. It shall be the duty of the Board to

---

47. *Laws of Georgia*, 1904.
48. *Laws of Georgia*, 1904, p. 60.

keep a record of its transactions in a book to be kept for that purpose by the Secretary of said Board to be turned over to his successor in office. The salary of the Secretary of the said Board shall be ten percent of the gross receipts annually. All necessary expenses of the Board to be paid out of receipts, and the remainder to be equally divided between the members of the Board. Said Board shall make an annual report to the Georgia Pharmaceutical Association.' "[49]

1907

Narcotic Drugs, Sale of, Regulated.
"AN ACT TO PROVIDE AGAINST THE EVILS RESULTING FROM THE TRAFFIC IN CERTAIN NARCOTIC DRUGS, AND TO REGULATE THE SALE THEREOF."[50]

This Act makes it unlawful to furnish persons with any of the following drugs, or any salt or compound thereof, or any preparation containing the following, except upon the original written orders or prescription of a lawfully authorized physician or practitioner of medicine, dentistry or veterinary medicine, which order shall be dated and signed, and shall contain the name of the person for whom prescribed, or the kind of animal for which ordered: Cocaine, Alpha or Beta Eucaine, Opium, Morphine, Heroine, Chloral Hydrate.

Section 2. Forbids physicians from prescribing any of the above drugs to habitual users, with the exception of persons under their professional care whose treatment necessitates the use of such drugs.

Section 3. Provides penalties for violations of this Act.
This Act was approved August 22, 1907.

1908

Inspection of Foods and Drugs.[51]
Section 1. Creates the position of Chief Food Inspector.
Section 2. Creates the position of Chief Drug Inspector, to serve under the Commissioner of Agriculture who shall make the appointment of the Chief Drug Inspector on the recommendation

---

49. *Laws of Georgia*, 1904, p. 61.
50. *Laws of Georgia*, 1907, p. 121.
    Georgia was the first or among the first of the states to pass narcotic legislation, which preceded the Harrison Act by seven years.
51. *Laws of Georgia*, 1908, p. 80.

of the Georgia State Board of Pharmacy, and whose salary shall be $1500 per year.

Section 3. Provides that in case of violations of this Law it becomes the duty of the Commissioner of Agriculture to prosecute the offenders.

1911

Drug Inspector, Chief, Appointment of, etc.
"AN ACT AMENDATORY OF AND TO MORE THOROUGHLY CARRY INTO EFFECT THE PROVISIONS OF AN ACT ENTITLED 'AN ACT TO PREVENT THE ADULTERATION, MISBRANDING, AND IMITATION OF FOOD FOR MAN AND BEAST, OR BEVERAGES, CANDIES, AND CONDIMENTS OR MEDICINES, DRUGS, LIQUORS, OR THE MANUFACTURE AND SALE THEREOF IN THE STATE OF GEORGIA, PRESCRIBING A PENALTY FOR THE VIOLATION THEREOF AND FOR OTHER PURPOSES, APPROVED AUGUST 17, 1908.' "[52]

Section 1. Raises the salary of the Chief Drug Inspector from $1500 to $2500 per annum. The duties of the Chief Drug Inspector are more clearly defined.

Code of Georgia, Paragraph 2099, Article 2.[53]
Specifies that the State Chemist shall examine all samples of drugs submitted by the Drug Inspector, and on examination of those products he shall report to the Commissioner of Agriculture, and suits for violations are to be filed in the name of the Commissioner of Agriculture.

"The term 'drug' as used in this Act shall include all medicines and preparations recognized in the U.S.P. and N.F. for internal or external use, and any substance or mixture of substances intended to be used for the cure, mitigation, or prevention of disease of either man or other animal."

1913

Food and Drugs Act Amended.[54]
This amendment defines specific use and meaning of term "misbranded" as it applies to drugs and articles of food. The Act states: "That for the purposes of this Act an article shall be deemed to be misbranded in case of drugs; first, if it be an imi-

---

52. *Laws of Georgia*, 1911, p. 170.
53. *Code of Georgia* (1911), Paragraph 2099, Article 2, p. 547.
54. *Laws of Georgia*, 1913.

tation of, or offered for sale under the name of, another article; second, if the contents of the package as originally put up shall have been removed in whole or in part, and other contents shall have been placed in such package, or if the package fail to bear statement on the label in as conspicuous letters as is, or may be, prescribed by the United States law or rules and regulations the quantity or proportion of any Alcohol, Morphine, Opium, Cocaine, Heroine, Alpha or Beta Eucaine, Chloroform, Cannabis Indica, Chloral Hydrate or Acetanilid, or any derivative, or any preparation of such drugs."

Section 2. Provides a new wording, as follows: "If in package form, the quantity of the contents must be plainly and conspicuously marked on the outside of the package in terms of weight, measure, or numerical count."

1918

"AN ACT AMENDING THE PHARMACY LAW HAVING TO DO WITH THE SALE OF POISONS FOR INSECTS."[55]

Paris Green, Arsenate of Copper, Arsenate of Lead, or any preparation containing any of these articles used for killing Lincoln Bugs, Cabbage Worms, Caterpillars, or similar insects, may be sold by merchants provided the labels, cartons and packages containing such preparations have the word "poison" printed across the face of each in red ink in type *not less than one-half inch in size:* all labels, cartons and packages containing such articles to show the kind and quantity of poison as the package contains, give specific directions for use, and antidote for such poisons as the package contains in letters of *not less than 3/8 inch in size.*

1919

Salary of Chief Drug Inspector. Amending the Laws of 1908 and 1911.[56] "The salary of the Chief Drug Inspector shall not exceed the sum of $3000 per year."

The first law had provided a salary of $1500, and the second law, $2500.

55. *Laws of Georgia,* 1918, p. 113.
56. *Laws of Georgia,* 1919, p. 281.

Alcohol, Regulation of Sale, Shipment, etc.[57]

This is an Act of the Georgia Legislature to comply with the Uniform State Law on the subject of Alcohol, and to provide for the allowance of purchase of duty-free Alcohol for certain scientific purposes.

1927

Georgia Board of Pharmacy Established.

"AN ACT TO PROVIDE FOR THE ESTABLISHMENT OF THE 'GEORGIA BOARD OF PHARMACY' REPLACING THE FORMER 'GEORGIA STATE BOARD OF PHARMACY.'"[58]

Section 1. Provides for the repeal of Sections 1722 through 1731, inclusive, of the Code of Georgia.

Section 2. Provides that the five members of the then-existing Georgia State Board of Pharmacy become the members of the Georgia Board of Pharmacy.

Section 4. Provides that no person shall be eligible for appointment to membership on said Board who is not a licentiate of the Board of Pharmacy of the State of Georgia, and who has not been actually engaged for a period of five years or more in the retail drug business. Section 4 also makes the following stipulation: "nor shall any person be eligible to appointment on said Board who has any official connection with any school or college of pharmacy." And, also, "that no member of the Board who has served one full term shall be eligible for re-appointment until there has intervened a period of one full term of five years from the date of expiration of his membership to the date of his re-appointment."

Section 5. Provides the annual election by the Georgia Pharmaceutical Association of a member to serve on the Board of Pharmacy in the vacancy created by the expiration of the term of office of one member. The Governor is required by law to make the appointment of this person chosen by the Georgia Pharmaceutical Association.

Section 6. Provides means for filling an unexpired term for a member of the Board. He shall be chosen from the next highest number of votes at the last annual convention of the Georgia Pharmaceutical Association.

57. *Ibid.*, p. 123.
58. *Laws of Georgia*, 1927, p. 291.

SUPPLEMENT C 305

Section 8. Provides that compensation of Board members shall be $15.00 per day while in actual performance of their duties, and, in addition, they shall receive their actual travel expense while in performance of their duties, such compensation to be paid out of the funds received by the Board under the provisions of this Act.*

Section 12. Provides that it shall be unlawful for any proprietor, owner, or manager of a drug store or pharmacy to allow any person in his employ, except a registered pharmacist, to compound or mix any drugs, medicines, or poisons, except an employee under the immediate supervision of a registered pharmacist.

Section 13. Provides that applicants for license to practice pharmacy must be not less than 21 years of age, and *shall have at least a high school education, with a minimum of 16 units* as are designated by the Association of Accredited Schools, and not less than 36 months experience in a drug store or place where drugs and poisons are dispensed by a licensed vendor, registered under the laws of his state Board, or, in lieu of the foregoing, be a graduate of a recognized school of pharmacy, provided this Act shall not be construed to affect a person who has had three years' practical experience under the direct supervision of a registered pharmacist at the time of the passage of this Act.**

Section 17. Provides for refusal to issue license for cause.

Section 18. Specifies who may compound or sell drugs. "No person shall engage in the compounding or vending of medicines, drugs or poisons within this State without full compliance with this Act, except: 1, such druggists as are exempted from the operation of the present law by the statutes of the State of Georgia, and such druggists as have heretofore obtained a license and are legally authorized by existing laws to compound and vend drugs, poisons, and chemicals; and, 2, physicians putting up their own prescriptions and dispensing medicines from their own office; and, 3, this item shall be construed in the interests of the public health and shall not be construed to prohibit the sale by merchants of home remedies not poison, or the sale by merchants of preparations commonly known as patent or proprietary medicines, when sold only in the original and unbroken packages: Paris Green, Arsenate of Copper, Arsenate of Lead, or prepara-

---
*This repeals and replaces the fee system of remuneration for Board members.
**This provision is the first step toward educational requirements.

tions containing any of these articles used for killing Lincoln Bugs, Cabbage Worms, Caterpillars, and all similar insects, provided the labels, cartons, and packages containing such preparations have the word 'poison' printed across the face and conform to the U.S. Pure Food and Drug Act, and general merchants other than druggists shall not be required to register under the provisions of this Act."

Section 19. "It shall be the duty of the Board to examine all applicants for license under the provisions of this Act, submitted in proper form, and to grant certificates of license to such persons as may be entitled to the same. It shall further be the duty of said Board to cause the prosecution of all persons violating the provisions of this Act, and in all such prosecutions the burden shall be upon the defendant to show his authority."

Section 21. Provides that the term "drug store," "pharmacy," or "apothecary," wherever used in this Act, shall be construed to mean a place where drugs, medicines or poisons are dispensed, compounded, or sold at retail under the direction and direct supervision of a person who is duly licensed and registered by the Georgia Board of Pharmacy to practice pharmacy in Georgia.

Section 22. Makes it unlawful for any person to take, use, or exhibit the title "drug store," "pharmacy," "apothecary," or any combination of such titles, or any title of like import, or any synonym or other term designated to take the place of such title, unless such place of business is in fact and in truth a drug store or pharmacy as defined in this Act.

Section 23. Provides for annual registration in office of Secretary of Board of Pharmacy.

Section 24. Provides that the Georgia Board of Pharmacy shall have the power and authority to make rules and regulations governing the action of the Board, and to make such other rules and regulations as they deem necessary to carry out the intent and provisions of this Act.

1931

State Government Reorganization. Executive Branches.[59]
"The Secretary of State is authorized to appoint a *Joint Secretary of Examining Boards* for all Boards having special Examiners: Veterinary, Public Accountants, Pharmacy, Osteopathy, Nurses,

---

59. *Laws of Georgia*, 1931, pp. 35-36.

Optometrists, Embalmers, Medical, Chiropractic, Dental, Barbers, Architects, Bar, Engineers, Firemen, Georgia Real Estate Commission. The office of Secretary of each of these Boards is abolished. Duties of the Joint Secretary are set up. Salary of the Joint Secretary is specified. His salary can never exceed the fees which he collects. All fees paid by applicants for examination for license are to be paid into the Treasury of the Secretary of State."*

1933

Pharmacy Board Act Amended.[60]

"AN ACT TO AMEND SECTION 13 OF THE PHARMACY BOARD ACT OF 1927, AND TO SET UP THE FOLLOWING NEW SECTION:"

Section 13. "That from and after January first after the passage of this Act, each applicant for registration as a pharmacist shall not be less than 21 years of age, and shall be a graduate of a generally recognized school or college of pharmacy, and, in addition, shall have had 12 months of practical experience in a drug store or place where physicians' prescriptions are dispensed by a licensed pharmacist registered under the laws of the state of his abode. Provided however that this Act shall not apply to those persons bona fide citizens of Georgia who, at the time of the passage of this Act, are actually employed in a place of business which is operated by a licensed pharmacist who is engaged in the compounding and filling of physicians' prescriptions, and who, within six months after the passage of this Act, file with the State Drug Inspector notice of their intention to apply for examination under this exemption, and who, within three years, present themselves for examination, and who file with the Board of Pharmacy evidence of graduation from an accredited high school and of having had at least three years' practical experience. Provided further that this Act shall not apply to those persons bona fide citizens of Georgia who, prior to the time of the passage of this Act, have had five or more years of experience in a retail drug store under the direct supervision of a licensed pharmacist, and who present themselves for examination before the Board of Pharmacy prior to January first, 1934."

*Up to 1959, there have been only two "Joint Secretaries," both of whom have been retail pharmacists.
60. *Laws of Georgia*, 1933, p. 210.

1935

Narcotic Drug Act (Known as the *"Uniform State Narcotic Act"*).[61]

The object of this legislation was to implement the Federal Harrison Anti-Narcotic Act by making it possible to prosecute violations in the State Courts as well as in Federal Courts.

"AN ACT TO REGULATE THE MANUFACTURE, SALE, POSSESSION, CONTROL, PRESCRIBING, ADMINISTERING, DISPENSING, COMPOUNDING, MIXING, CULTIVATION, AND GROWTH OF NARCOTIC DRUGS IN THE STATE OF GEORGIA."

Section 1. Gives definition for terms used in the Act.

Section 2. Limits ownership of Narcotics to authorized persons.

Section 3. No person shall manufacture, compound, mix, cultivate, grow, or by any other process produce or prepare Narcotic Drugs, and no person as a wholesaler shall supply the same, without first having obtained a license so to do from the State Board of Pharmacy.

Section 4. Specifies the qualifications for license to handle Narcotics.

Section 5. States the persons to whom sales may be made or who may dispense Narcotic Drugs on written orders; and defines lawful possession.

Section 6 A. Specifies the conditions under which pharmacists may dispense Narcotics.

Section 6 C. Specifies conditions under which a pharmacist may sell Narcotics to physicians, dentists, or veterinarians.

Section 7. A physician or a dentist in good faith, and in the course of his professional practice only, may prescribe, administer, and dispense Narcotic Drugs, or he may cause the same to be administered by a nurse or intern under his direction and supervision.

A veterinarian in good faith, and in the course of his professional practice only, and not for use by a human being, may prescribe, administer and dispense Narcotic Drugs, and he may cause them to be administered by an assistant or orderly under his direction and supervision.

Section 9. Requires every dentist, veterinarian, and physician or other person who purchases, or has in his possession, Narcotic

---

61. *Laws of Georgia*, 1935, p. 418.

℞ SUPPLEMENT C 309

Drugs to keep a record of all Narcotics he has received and all he has dispensed, but he need not record single doses. Manufacturers, wholesalers, apothecaries, hospitals, and all other persons or institutions who purchase Narcotics for resale or for dispensing, shall keep a complete record of drugs received and dispensed or sold.

Section 10. Provision is made for forfeiture of drugs taken up by a law enforcement official.[62]

Section 15. Provides that a record of conviction of a physician, apothecary, or dentist, be sent to the licensing Board or other officer, for disciplinary action, such as suspension of license, registration, reinstatement, et cetera.[63]

Alcoholic Beverages.[64]

Section 28. Provides that "nothing in this Act shall be construed to prevent registered licensed pharmacists or manufacturers of medicines, drugs, or those using grain alcohol for industrial or mechanical purposes, from receiving such grain and ethyl alcohol for legitimate use in those counties allowing permits to be issued; and in those counties who have voted against allowing permits to be issued, the pharmacists, chemists and manufacturers or others who may obtain grain and ethyl alcohol under existing laws shall be entitled to obtain same by applying to the Ordinary in such county refusing permits, and obtaining a permit therefrom, a copy of such permit to be retained by the Ordinary, one by the purchaser, and one sent to the distributor or manufacturer. A fee of one dollar shall be paid by the applicant to the Ordinary for such permit."

1937

Pharmacists Registration Fee.[65]

Section 84.1319 of Code of Georgia Amended; i. e. Code of 1933. "Every person who shall be duly licensed under the provision of this Chapter shall annually, before engaging in any business under license, register in the office of the Joint Secretary of State Examining Boards, and pay a fee of two dollars ($2.00) to the Secretary thereof."

62. *Ibid.*, p. 433.
63. *Ibid.*, pp. 435-436.
64. *Laws of Georgia*, 1935, p. 342.
65. *Laws of Georgia*, 1937.

1939

"AN ACT TO REGULATE THE SALE, POSSESSION, PRESCRIBING, AND DISPENSING OF CERTAIN DANGEROUS DRUGS, PROVIDING CERTAIN EXEMPTIONS, PROVIDING FOR ENFORCEMENT AND PENALTIES FOR VIOLATION THEREOF."[66]

Section 1. It shall be unlawful for any person, firm, corporation, or association to sell, give away, barter, exchange, distribute, or possess in the State of Georgia, Amytal, Luminal, Veronal, Barbital, Acid Di-Ethyl-Barbiturate, Sulfanilamide, Prontylin, Neo-Prontosil, or any salts, derivatives, or compounds of the foregoing substances, of their salts, derivatives, compounds, or any trademarked, or copyrighted preparation or compound registered in the U.S. Patent Office containing more than 4 grains to the avoirdupois or fluid ounce of the above substances, except on a prescription of a duly licensed physician as defined by this Act, and such prescription shall be compounded only by a registered pharmacist in accordance with the law of this State. The provisions of this Act shall not apply to the sale at wholesale by recognized drug jobbers or wholesalers and drug manufacturers, to pharmacists or drug stores, or to physicians qualified to practice their profession according to the law, or to the sale by pharmacists in drug stores to one another.

Section 3. Provides that "whenever a pharmacist dispenses a dangerous drug, as defined in this Act, he shall in each case place upon the container the following: name of the patient, name of the physician prescribing such drug, name and address of the drug store or pharmacy from which such drug was dispensed, together with the date of the prescription."

Section 4. Provides that "any physician, as defined in this Act, when prescribing dangerous drugs as set forth in Section 1 of this Act, shall in each case give the name and address of the patient, together with complete directions for administration." Physicians are required to comply with the provisions of Section 3 of this Act.

Section 5. Defines and limits possession and control of dangerous drugs.

---

66. *Laws of Georgia*, 1939, p. 288. (Known as "Dangerous Drugs Act"). This law was promoted by the pharmacists of Georgia, and Georgia was one of the very first states to adopt such legislation as being in the interest of the health and welfare of its citizens.

℞ SUPPLEMENT C 311

Section 6. It shall be the duty of all law enforcement officers to enforce all provisions of this Act.

Section 7. Any person violating any provision of this Act shall be deemed guilty of a misdemeanor, and upon conviction shall be punished as for a misdemeanor.

State Board of Pharmacy.

"AN ACT TO AMEND SECTION 42-102 OF THE CODE OF GEORGIA OF 1933 RELATING TO THE APPOINTMENT, DUTIES, AND SALARY OF THE CHIEF DRUG INSPECTOR, SO AS TO PROVIDE FOR THE APPOINTMENT OF SAID INSPECTOR BY THE GEORGIA BOARD OF PHARMACY, AND TO PROVIDE THAT HIS DUTIES SHALL BE PERFORMED UNDER THE SUPERVISION, DIRECTION, AND CONTROL OF SAID BOARD; TO AMEND SECTION 42-103 OF THE CODE RELATING TO HEARINGS AND PROSECUTIONS OF VIOLATIONS OF THE DRUG LAWS OF THIS STATE, SO AS TO VEST THE AUTHORITY TO HOLD SUCH HEARINGS AND DIRECT PROSECUTIONS IN THE GEORGIA STATE BOARD OF PHARMACY AND ATTORNEY-GENERAL; TO AMEND CODE SECTION 42-113 OF THE CODE OF 1933 RELATING TO THE EXAMINATION OF SPECIMENS OF FOODS AND DRUGS SO AS TO INVEST IN THE GEORGIA STATE BOARD OF PHARMACY JURISDICTION AND AUTHORITY OVER ALL MATTERS RELATING TO THE MISBRANDING OR ADULTERATION OF DRUGS, AND HEARINGS WITH REFERENCE THERETO; TO PROVIDE AN EFFECTIVE DATE FOR THIS ACT, AND FOR OTHER PURPOSES."[67]

Section 1. Places the responsibility for the Chief Drug Inspector's work on the Georgia State Board of Pharmacy instead of on the Commissioner of Agriculture.

Section 4. "That the purpose and intent of this Act is to divest the Commissioner of Agriculture of the authority to appoint the Chief Drug Inspector or to supervise, direct, or control his duties, and to vest the power of appointing the Chief Drug Inspector in the Georgia State Board of Pharmacy, and to provide that all of his duties shall be performed subject to the supervision, direction, and control of said Board; to consolidate all other powers and functions of the Chief Drug Inspector under the control, supervision, and direction of the Georgia State Board of Pharmacy in the interest of efficiency and of the public health, safety, and welfare."

Section 4 A. Provides that the General Assembly shall transfer funds now appropriated to the Department of Agriculture

---

67. *Laws of Georgia,* 1939, p. 228.

for the support of the Drug Department to the State Board of Pharmacy to carry out the provisions of this Act.

Section 4 B. This Act becomes effective January first, 1941. Approved March 24, 1939.

Foreign Medical Practitioners and Pharmacists.[68]

"AN ACT TO PROHIBIT THE STATE BOARD OF MEDICAL EXAMINERS AND THE STATE BOARD OF PHARMACY EXAMINERS FROM ISSUING A LICENSE TO PRACTICE PHARMACY OR MEDICINE IN THIS STATE TO ANY PERSON WHO WAS NOT BORN OR NATURALIZED IN THE UNITED STATES, OR WHO IS NOT A CITIZEN OF THE UNITED STATES; TO PROVIDE PENALTIES FOR THE VIOLATION OF THIS ACT; AND TO REPEAL ALL LAWS OR PARTS OF LAWS IN CONFLICT WITH THIS ACT."

Section 2. Provides certain exceptions.

Section 3. Provides for revocation or cancellation of license in medicine or pharmacy for cause.

1941

An Amendment to the Code of 1933, Section 42-102.[69]
This law is amended to authorize the State Board of Pharmacy to set the salary of the Chief Drug Inspector.

An Amendment to Uniform Narcotic Act, Code Number 42-028.[70]
An Amendment to add Isonipecaine (Demerol) to list of Narcotic Drugs.

1947

Dangerous Drugs Act Amended—Amending Title 42, Chapter 42-1.[71]

Code Number 42-102, 42-110, 42-701 are the items amended in this Act.

An Act to amend the Dangerous Drugs Act, of the Code of 1933, as amended, by adding wholesaling establishments and retailing establishments to the types of establishments which the Chief Drug Inspector is directed to visit and inspect.

68. *Laws of Georgia*, 1939, p. 319.
69. *Laws of Georgia*, 1941, p. 421.
70. *Ibid.*, p. 437.
71. *Laws of Georgia*, 1947, pp. 1463 ff.

R SUPPLEMENT C 313

Medicines, Drugs and Poisons—Board of Pharmacy. Chapter 84 Amended.[72]

"AN ACT TO AMEND THE FOLLOWING SECTIONS OF THE CODE OF GEORGIA, AS AMENDED, SECTION 84-1309, BY AUTHORIZING THE STATE BOARD OF PHARMACY TO ADOPT RULES AND REGULATIONS: SECTION 84-1312, BY REMOVING THE LIMITATION OF THE NUMBER OR PURPOSES OF THE MEETINGS OF SAID BOARD; SECTION 84-1316, BY SPECIFYING THE GROUNDS AND ESTABLISHING A PROCEDURE FOR REVOCATION, REFUSAL OR SUSPENSION OF LICENSE BY SAID BOARD, AND BY CREATING THE RIGHT OF APPEAL FROM ITS DECISIONS; SECTION 84-1317 OF THE CODE OF 1933, RELATING TO WHO MAY COMPOUND OR SELL DRUGS BY PROVIDING THAT THE SAID SECTION SHALL NOT APPLY TO PHYSICIANS, DENTISTS, AND VETERINARIANS PRESCRIBING OR PUTTING UP THEIR OWN PRESCRIPTIONS AND DISPENSING MEDICINES, NOR TO MERCHANTS SELLING PATENT OR PROPRIETARY PREPARATIONS, WHEN SOLD ONLY IN THE ORIGINAL AND UNBROKEN PACKAGES; AND TO PROVIDE THAT THIS ACT SHALL NOT APPLY TO MANUFACTURERS, DISTRIBUTORS, OR DEALERS SELLING, COMPOUNDING, OR MIXING POISONS, SPRAYS, OR DUSTS USED FOR AGRICULTURAL PURPOSES, OR TO BIOLOGICS OR REMEDIES USED BY FARMERS OR VETERINARIANS OR OTHERS FOR DISEASES IN POULTRY OR LIVESTOCK, OR TO REMEDIES OR POWDERS USED FOR DESTRUCTION OF RATS, BUGS, OR INSECTS OR PESTS, OR TO OTHER PREPARATIONS NOT INTENDED FOR HUMAN CONSUMPTION, NOR USE ON HUMAN BEINGS; SECTION 84-1318, BY PRESCRIBING CONDITIONS FOR THE COMPOUNDING OF DRUGS, MEDICINES OR POISONS; SECTION 84-1319, BY REQUIRING CERTAIN INFORMATION FROM, AND PAYMENTS OF, AN ANNUAL FEE BY REGISTERED PHARMACISTS, AND BY PROVIDING A PENALTY FOR VIOLATION OF SAID SECTION; AND TO AMEND SECTION 84-9920 OF THE GEORGIA CODE, BY PROVIDING A PENALTY FOR VIOLATION OF ANY PROVISION OF CHAPTER 84-13 AS AMENDED, RELATING TO THE COMPOUNDING OR VENDING OF MEDICINES, DRUGS, OR POISONS, AND TO AMEND SECTION 3 OF THE ACT ENTITLED 'AN ACT TO PROHIBIT THE STATE BOARD OF MEDICAL EXAMINERS AND THE STATE BOARD OF PHARMACY EXAMINERS FROM ISSUING A LICENSE TO PRACTICE MEDICINE OR PHARMACY IN THIS STATE TO ANY PERSON WHO WAS NOT BORN OR NATURALIZED IN THE UNITED STATES, OR WHO IS NOT A CITIZEN OF THE UNITED STATES, APPROVED MARCH 23, 1939,' BY

72. *Laws of Georgia*, 1947, p. 1471.

RESTRICTING THE APPLICABILITY OF THE PROCEDURE FOR REVOCATION OR CANCELLATION OF LICENSES TO WHICH REFERENCE IS MADE IN SAID ACT, TO LICENSES ISSUED BY THE STATE BOARD OF MEDICAL EXAMINERS, AND TO PROVIDE A PROCEDURE FOR REVOCATION OR CANCELLATION OF LICENSES ISSUED BY THE STATE BOARD OF PHARMACY; AND TO REPEAL ALL LAWS AND PARTS OF LAWS IN CONFLICT WITH THIS ACT, AND FOR OTHER PURPOSES."

Section 3. Amends Section 84-1316 of the Code of Georgia of 1933 so that it shall read as follows: "The State Board of Pharmacy may refuse to grant a license to any person found guilty of a felony or gross immorality, or who is addicted to the use of alcoholic liquors or narcotics, or other habit-forming drugs, to such extent as to render him unfit for the practice of pharmacy, and may, after due hearing, revoke or suspend a license for such cause, or for fraud in its procurement, or for any violation of any of the provisions of this Chapter, or for any violation of any rule or regulation of the Georgia Board of Pharmacy made pursuant to Section 84-1309 of the Code of Georgia of 1933."

Section 4. Provides that Section 84-1317 of the Code of Georgia of 1933, relating to who may compound and sell drugs, as amended, be further amended to allow an exception for "physicians, dentists, and veterinarians prescribing and putting up their own prescriptions and dispensing medicines."

Section 6. Provides that Section 84-1318 of the Code of Georgia of 1933 relating to the registration of pharmacists and druggists be amended to read as follows: "It shall be unlawful for any proprietor, owner, or manager of any drug store or pharmacy to allow any person in his employ except a registered pharmacist to compound or mix any drugs, medicines, or poisons for sale, except an employee under the immediate supervision of a registered pharmacist. No registered pharmacist shall have more than one drug store or pharmacy under his supervision. The proprietor, owner, or manager of any drug store or pharmacy shall have a registered pharmacist present and available in such drug store at all times during which drugs, medicines, or poisons are compounded or mixed."

Section 7. Provides for annual registration of pharmacists who are duly licensed under the provisions of this Chapter, and the payment upon registration with the Office of the Joint Secretary of State Examining Boards, of an annual fee of two dollars.

SUPPLEMENT C   315

Section 8. Provides that Section 3 of the Act prohibiting the foreign-born or un-naturalized pharmacist or physician from being issued license, be amended.

Section 9. Provides that Section 84-9920 of the Code of Georgia of 1933 relating to the granting of licenses to and the registration of pharmacists, be amended, so that it shall read as follows: "Any violation of any provision of Chapter 84-13 relating to the granting of licenses to and the registration of pharmacists, and to the compounding and vending of medicines, drugs, or poisons, shall be a misdemeanor."

Section 9 A. Provides that nothing in this Act shall require mixers of, manufacturers of, dealers in, or dispensers of, any agricultural poison, dust, spray, insecticide, fungicide, or rodenticide normally used for agricultural purposes, or not intended for human consumption, to conform to the provisions of this Act. Approved March 28, 1947.

Sulfanilamide Sales for Livestock and Poultry Diseases.[73]
This Act provides for the sale, purchase, and use of drugs of the Sulfanilamide or Sulfonamide group, manufactured for use in control of livestock and poultry diseases, to be bought and sold by persons other than licensed pharmacists and without the necessity of prescriptions.

Section 2. Specifies that all packages containing these sulfa drugs intended for use by animals shall have stamped on their label *"not for human use."*

Drugs Purchased by Poultry Dealers.[74]
This is a similar Act to the above, providing for purchase and use of Sulfaguanadine and Sulfathiazol in the treatment of poultry diseases, in powdered form and in original packages, with label marked *"for poultry only."*

1952

Condemnation of Vehicles Transporting Narcotics.[75]
AN ACT TO DECLARE AS CONTRABAND AND SUBJECT TO CONFISCATION AND CONDEMNATION ALL VEHICLES AND CONVEYANCES OF EVERY KIND, ALL BOATS AND VESSELS, AND VEHICLES FOR AIR TRANSPORTATION, USED IN TRANSPORTING, CONVEYING, REMOVING, OR STORING, ANY NARCOTIC DRUGS.

73. *Laws of Georgia*, 1947, p. 734.
74. *Laws of Georgia*, 1946, Adjourned Session, p. 135.
75. *Laws of Georgia*, 1952, p. 201.

1953

Chief Drug Inspectors' Assistants.[76]
"AN ACT TO AMEND SECTION 42-102 OF THE CODE OF 1933, AS AMENDED, TO PROVIDE FOR MORE THAN 2 ASSISTANT DRUG INSPECTORS, BUT NOT TO EXCEED 5."

1956

Sale of Drugs in Vending Machines.[77]
Code Number 84-1317 Amended.

"AN ACT TO AMEND CODE NUMBER 84-1317 OF THE 1947 CODE RELATING TO WHO MAY COMPOUND OR SELL DRUGS, SO AS TO PROVIDE THAT 'NO DRUG SHALL BE SOLD OR DISPENSED BY VENDING MACHINES'; TO PROVIDE A PENALTY FOR VIOLATION; TO REPEAL CONFLICTING LAWS; AND FOR OTHER PURPOSES."

Uniform Narcotic Drug Act Amended.[78]
This amendment provides for oral prescriptions for certain narcotic drugs, compounds thereof and derivatives thereof, under certain conditions; provides for the procedure connected therewith, and repeals conflicting laws.

Veterinary Use of Sulfanilamide and Sulfonamide Drugs.[79]
"AN ACT TO AMEND AN ACT RELATING TO THE SALE, PURCHASE, AND USE OF DRUGS OF THE SULFANILAMIDE OR SULFONAMIDE GROUP MANUFACTURED FOR USE IN THE CONTROL OF LIVESTOCK AND POULTRY DISEASES, OF THE CODE OF 1947, SO AS TO PERMIT THE USE OF SUCH DRUGS IN MIXED FEEDS, TO REPEAL CONFLICTING LAWS, AND FOR OTHER PURPOSES."

Section 2, as amended: Permits poultry and livestock owners in this State to buy and use such drugs for control of livestock and poultry diseases, with certain specifications.

[Author's Note: The enforcement of all the Pharmacy Laws is the responsibility of the Georgia State Board of Pharmacy.]

---

76. *Laws of Georgia*, 1953, p. 395.
77. *Laws of Georgia*, 1956, p. 724.
78. *Ibid.*, p. 19.
79. *Laws of Georgia*, 1956, p. 345.

Supplement D

THE GEORGIA PHARMACEUTICAL ASSOCIATION AND THE WOMEN'S AUXILIARY

IN VIEW of the importance of drugs in the prevention and treatment of diseases, of which there were many during the early years of the Colony and State, it is not generally understood why the profession of pharmacy did not sooner emerge as a distinctive and independent health unit in the State of Georgia. A brief review of conditions as they existed in the Colony and the State, beginning in 1733, may give the answer.

1. (1733-1750) The number of apothecaries who came into the Colony in proportion to the population was excessive, thus forcing them into other activities.

2. The number of physicians to the population was also out of proportion, and they were forced into additional activities for maintenance, one of which was the supplying of drugs.

3. The period during which self-diagnosis and self-treatment of disease became a necessity in most of the areas of the State and Colony, and was aided and abetted by the physicians in the publication of books on the subject for distribution to the public.

4. The period when the newspapers (first of Savannah and Augusta and then of other towns) carried the glowing advertisements of so-called "cures" for most diseases.

5. The absence of any facilities for professional education except the occasional opportunity for apprenticeship under a busy, and, many times, an ill-prepared physician-preceptor.

6. The complete lack of licensure requirements for either medicine or pharmacy until the passage of the first State Law in 1825, setting up a Board of Physicians to examine applicants for license to practice medicine or pharmacy, by providing that li-

cense to practice pharmacy was automatically granted to physicians without examination.

7. The first Medical College in the State came in 1828. Following the prevailing custom in such colleges in other states, the curriculum included lectures in the subject of pharmacy, not for the training of pharmacists, but for the instruction of the medical practitioner who would dispense the drugs he prescribed.

8. Under such conditions when all knowledge of, and dealings with drugs was vested in one individual, there was no incentive or opportunity to specialize in any phase of medical knowledge or practice, with the result that, for these many years, such conditions prevailed: there was very limited progress in the science of drugs and the diagnosis and treatment of disease. Real progress had to await the development of a high degree of specialization in medicine and in pharmacy.

Pharmacy in the more densely populated areas of the Eastern States advanced more rapidly as a professional entity than could be true in the case of Georgia, and this fact eventually resulted in the birth of the American Pharmaceutical Association in 1852. One of its objectives was to stimulate the creation of state pharmaceutical associations in the various states, and thus to unite all pharmacists of America in a program to promote the practice of pharmacy as a professional entity to serve in the interest of the health and welfare of the public.

The first Georgia pharmacist to become a member of A.Ph.A. appears to be Dr. Robert Battey of Rome, Georgia, who served as Third Vice-President of the Association in 1856, and was likewise the first Georgia pharmacist to serve as an official of A.Ph.A. He reported at this third Annual Meeting that "Pharmacy in Georgia is in a sad state; that in Rome and Floyd County there were 21 places selling drugs, only two of which were serviced by licensed pharmacists; that 'quackery' in Western Georgia was on the increase; that in the cities in the State physicians were gradually discontinuing the practice of dispensing drugs; and that there were 127 drug stores in the State." How this figure was determined he does not state, and this seems to be the only instance where the number of drug stores is referred to during this period.

Following his graduation in pharmacy from P.C.P., he graduated in medicine from Jefferson Medical College, and came to be a surgeon of national and international fame, though he continued his interest in pharmacy until his death in 1895.

Dr. Battey was joined in membership in A.Ph.A. in 1857 by Dr. John S. Pemberton of Columbus, Georgia, and Mr. John M. Clarke of Milledgeville. Dr. Pemberton made a name for himself as the creator of the formula of Coca-Cola, and Mr. Clarke came to be the first President of the Georgia Pharmaceutical Association, the first pharmacist to serve on the Medical Board for the examination of applicants to practice pharmacy, and to be a prominent figure in Milledgeville, the Capital of the State for a number of years.

In 1858 Messrs. Battey, Clarke and Pemberton were joined in membership in A.Ph.A. by Messrs. A. A. Solomons and W. W. Solomons of Savannah, who were the forebears of the present generations of Solomons now operating a wholesale drug business in Savannah. In 1859 the membership in A.Ph.A. was increased by the following members from Georgia: W. H. Warner of Rome, J. D. W. Nowlin of Rome, Fleming Grieve of Milledgeville, J. A. Taylor of Atlanta, W. A. Lansdale of Atlanta, Robert A. Massey of Atlanta, D. M. Smith of Atlanta, J. Henry Zeilin of Macon, and R. H. Land of Augusta.

In the year 1860 Mr. Theodore Schumann of Atlanta was the only individual from the State to join the A.Ph.A. Then came the great tragedy of America, the Civil War, with its horrible aftermath, with the result that no additional memberships in A.Ph.A. from Georgia were possible from the year 1861 to 1868.

But in the year 1869 William A. Cotting of Milledgeville was added to the membership, and in 1870 J. B. Huddart of Macon, and in 1878 the name of John B. Daniel of Atlanta, founder of the wholesale business now bearing his name, was added. Also, that of Frederick F. Peacock of Atlanta, and of Leonard W. Hunt of Macon, and of Frederick S. Mason of Rome. In 1873 the name of Foster S. Chapman was added, and in 1875 Hommer S. Tarrant of Augusta. In 1876 followed the names of Walter A. Taylor of Atlanta and John Ingalls of Macon.

Well into the 1870's in Georgia, physicians were still controlling the issuance of licenses to pharmacists, and they were also, under the law, claiming the right and privilege to be given a license to practice pharmacy on the presentation of a medical diploma, and without examination. No pharmacists were on the Board of Examiners prior to the naming of Mr. Clarke in 1872 though some effort had been made to place one or more pharmacists on this Board. But in 1875, the State Board of Health was concerning itself about the sale of poisons, and was proposing to introduce into the Legislature a "Poison Law" which of course would apply to and affect the druggists of the State.

The druggists of Atlanta and Macon, including all the A.Ph.A. members in the State, being aware of this intent of the State Board of Health, were very insistent that if a "Poison Law" was to be written, it should not be written by physicians or by the State Board of Health (which was composed of physicians), but that pharmacists should participate in drafting the legislation. This was a factor which resulted in a "Call" to the pharmacists of the State to get together to form an "Association."

So, in the summer of 1875, there was sent out from Atlanta a notice to the druggists of the State, this notice signed by Fred King of Atlanta and L. W. Hunt of Macon, published in the *Atlanta Herald* and in the *Macon Telegraph,* as well as in two or three journals, to the effect that the druggists of the State were to assemble in Macon on October 20th "to consider the organization of a pharmaceutical association, binding each other closer with ties of friendship, and to promote interest in the 'junior members' of the fraternity, and exciting the spirit of emulation and ambition; the interchange and dissemination of scientific researches; the framing of laws to be enacted that will result not only in the protection of the profession but to the public in general." (Excerpt from these newspaper notices.)

As a result of this notice, the Meeting was held in Macon in Freeman's Hall, at 8 o'clock on the evening of the 20th of October, 1875.

There appears to be no list of those who attended this first Meeting at Macon, but it was later reported that 20 or more druggists of the State responded to the "Call." No Minutes of this first Meeting seem to have been kept.

From a later Proceedings (1877) it develops that Mr. John M. Clarke of Milledgeville was called to the Chair, and that Dr. Fred King of Atlanta was requested to act as Secretary at this first Meeting.

Mr. Clarke, on taking the Chair, explained in a precise but graceful manner the object of the Meeting. A committee of three, consisting of Theodore Schumann of Atlanta, John Ingalls of Macon, and J. R. Jaynes of Dalton, was appointed to draft a Constitution and By-Laws for the governing of the Association, and this queer note is inserted. "The Committee returned after an absence of a few minutes with a copy of the Constitution and

By-Laws of the Tennessee Association, slightly altered, which was adopted as the Constitution and By-Laws of the Georgia Pharmaceutical Association. A number of copies were ordered to be printed, and the Secretary was ordered to distribute them among the members and to those druggists throughout the State who might apply for them." A copy of this Constitution and By-Laws appears herewith:

CONSTITUTION AND BY-LAWS OF THE GEORGIA PHARMACEUTICAL ASSOCIATION AS ADOPTED AT THE ORGANIZATIONAL MEETING OF THE ASSOCIATION—OCTOBER 20, 1875.

Article 1. Organization.

This Association shall be called the Georgia Pharmaceutical Association. Its aim shall be to unite the educated and reputable pharmacists and druggists of the State in the following objects: First, to establish the relations between druggists, apothecaries, physicians, and the people at large, upon just principles which shall promote the public welfare, and tend to mutual strength and advantage. Second, to improve the science and art of pharmacy by diffusing scientific knowledge among apothecaries and druggists, fostering pharmaceutical literature, developing talent, stimulating discovery and inventions, and encouraging home production and manufacture in the several departments of the drug business. Third, to regulate the system of apprenticeship and employment, so as to prevent as far as possible the evils flowing from deficient training in the responsible duties of preparing, dispensing, and selling medicines. Fourth, to secure the enactment of such laws as will be of mutual advantage to the profession and the public, suppressing empiricism, and, as much as possible, to restrict the dispensing and sale of medicines to competent druggists and apothecaries.

Article 2. Members.

Section 1. Every druggist and apothecary of good moral and professional standing, whether in business, retired from business, or employed by another, and those teachers of pharmacy, chemistry, materia medica, and botany, who may be professors in the colleges of pharmacy, (provided these colleges of pharmacy are acknowledged by the American Pharmaceutical Association), who, after duly considering the objects of the Association, and the obligations of its Constitution, are willing to subscribe to them, are eligible to membership.

Section 2. No person should be considered a member of the Association until he shall have signed the Constitution, and paid into the Treasury the sum of two dollars ($2.00) as the annual contribution for the current year. Any member may be expelled for improper conduct by a vote of two-thirds of the members present at an Annual Meeting.

Section 3. Every member shall pay in advance into the hands of the Treasurer the sum of two dollars ($2.00) as his yearly contribution, and is liable to lose his right of membership for neglecting to pay such contribution for two successive years.

Section 4. Members shall be entitled, on the payment of five dollars ($5.00), to receive a certificate of membership, signed by the President, one Vice-President, Secretary, and Treasurer, at the same time covenanting to return the same to the Secretary on relinquishing their connection with the Association.

Section 5. Resignation of members shall be made in writing to the Secretary. But no resignation shall be accepted from any one who is in arrears to the Treasurer. All resignations shall be acknowledged in writing by the officer who receives them, and shall be reported at the next Annual Meeting.

Section 6. Pharmacists, chemists, and other scientific men, who may be thought worthy of the distinction, may be elected honorary members. They shall not, however, be required to contribute to the Treasury; nor shall they be eligible to hold office, or vote at the Meetings.

Article 3. Officers.

Section 1. The officers shall be a President, three Vice-Presidents (who shall be elected annually), a Secretary, and a Treasurer, who shall be elected for a term of five years, and hold their offices until an election of successors.

Section 2. The President shall preside at the Meetings, and administer the Rules of Order usual in deliberative assemblies. He shall nominate all committees, except a majority of the members present direct a resort to a ballot, or other means. He shall present, at each Annual Meeting, a report of the operations of the Association during the year, with such information pertaining to its condition, prospects, and objects it has in view, together with such suggestions for its future management as may to him seem proper.

Section 3. In case of the absence or inability of the President, his duties shall devolve upon a Vice-President.

Section 4. The Secretary shall keep correct Minutes of the Proceedings, and carefully file all reports, essays, and papers received by the Association, and shall be charged with the editing, publishing and distributing of the Proceedings of the Association. He shall furnish the Chairman of every special committee with a list of its members, and a copy of the Minutes of its appointments. He shall have charge of all the correspondence, and shall notify each member of the time and place of every Meeting.

Section 5. The Treasurer shall collect and take charge of the funds of the Association. He shall pay out no monies, unless upon an order signed by the President, or a Vice-President, and attested by the Secretary. He shall present a statement of his accounts at each Annual Meeting, that they may be audited. He shall report to each Annual Meeting the names of such members as have failed to pay their annual contribution for the year.

Article 4. Meetings.

Section 1. The Meetings shall be held annually, or as the officers may from time to time determine: provided, That, in case of failure for any cause, the duty for calling the Association together shall devolve upon the President or a Vice-President.

Section 2. At the opening of each Meeting, the President—or in his absence a Vice-President—shall call the Meeting to order and preside. In case the President and Vice-Presidents are absent, the Association shall call the Meeting to order upon the order of any member acting as President-Pro-Tem. In the absence of the Secretary, the President shall appoint a Secretary-Pro-Tem.

Section 3. Seven (7) members shall constitute a quorum for the transaction of any business.

Section 4. The Order of Business at the first session shall be: 1—The roll of those in attendance shall be called by the Secretary. 2—The election of new members. 3—A committee to nominate officers for the ensuing year shall be appointed, to consist of five members, and to report at the opening of the second session.

Section 5. The order of business at the second session shall be: 1—The election of members. 2—Election of officers. 3—Reports of standing and special committees. The order of business at subsequent sessions shall be determined by the Business Committee, with the consent of the Association.

Section 6. In the discussion of all questions, and the transaction of all business, the ordinary rules of parliamentary bodies shall be enforced by the presiding officer, from whose decision, however, any member may appeal, and a majority of the Meeting shall thereupon decide. On the call of any member, "yeas" and "nays" shall be ordered, and the names and the manner of voting shall be entered on the Minutes.

Article 5. Committees.

Section 1. There shall be elected annually three standing committees—a committee on Papers and Queries, a Business Committee, and a committee on Legislation—each consisting of three members.

Section 2. A committee on Papers and Queries shall secure answers to such questions that would be of practical interest, and in other ways encourage a diffusion of practical information.

Section 3. The Business committee shall be charged with the transaction of all unfinished business from one Meeting to another, and with collecting, arranging, and expediting the business during the sessions of the Meeting.

Section 4. The Committee on Legislation shall examine into, all laws and regulations affecting the sale of medicines, and shall confer with the Legislature on all legal matters pertaining to the same.

Article 6. Amendments.

This Constitution may be altered or amended by a vote of three-fourths of the members present at any Annual Meeting—notice to so alter or amend having been given at least one session before a vote thereupon.

[Authors Note: Through the years the original Constitution has been rewritten, revised, and amended, from time to time. And particularly is this true of the By-Laws of the Constitution of the Georgia Pharmaceutical Association.]

A committee of five, appointed to bring in nominations for officers for the Association, was composed of the following: J. J. Pinckard of Macon; John Ingalls of Macon; Dr. Fred King of Atlanta; M. B. White of Forsyth; and P. R. Holt of Barnesville. This committee brought in the following recommendations for officers: President, John M. Clarke of Milledgeville; First Vice-President, John Ingalls of Macon; Second Vice-President, Theodore Schumann of Atlanta; Third Vice-President, J. R.

℞ SUPPLEMENT D   325

Jaynes of Dalton; Secretary, Dr. Fred King of Atlanta; and Treasurer, L. W. Hunt of Macon.

Following the election of officers, Dr. C. D. Nottingham of Macon, who was a member of the State Board of Health, appeared before the body and made the following statement:

As a member of the State Board of Health, I come before the Association to ask its cooperation in securing the enactment of such laws as will restrict the sale of poisons to competent druggists, so as to secure the public against the indiscriminate sale of such drugs by incompetent dealers. (Note: This law was passed in 1876.)

Furthermore, he congratulated the Association and prophesied a vast field of benefits for the profession of medicine in its broadest sense by such a move.

[Author's Note: It was approximately 60 years following this that pharmacists were placed on the State Board of Health as full-fledged members.]

After the withdrawal of Dr. Nottingham, a committee of three physicians of the Macon Medical Society appeared, and through its chairman (whose name is not mentioned in the reports) expressed a desire *to cooperate with the Association in the accomplishment of any work for the procurement of any laws that would redound to the future benefit of medicine and pharmacy.*

In addition to the names already mentioned at this first Meeting, the following names of people who were present are given who participated in the activities of this first Meeting: Mr. Schumann of Atlanta and Mr. R. B. Hall of Macon.

Prior to adjournment at half past eleven o'clock in the evening, some discussion arose as to where the First Annual Meeting of the Association was to be held. Finally, after much discussion, Macon was chosen over Atlanta as the place for the First Annual Meeting, to be held on the second Tuesday in April, 1876.

[Note: At half past eleven o'clock, the meeting adjourned after a most harmonious session, to meet in Macon on the day and date above mentioned.]

Apparently, there is no printed record of this First Annual Meeting except for the brief mention made of these two meetings (1875 and 1876) in the printed *Proceedings* of the Second Annual Meeting of 1877.

The following note appears in the *Proceedings* of the Second

Annual Meeting of 1877: "Proceedings of the First Annual Meeting of the Georgia Pharmaceutical Association in 1876: Pursuant to adjournment, the First Annual Meeting of the Georgia Pharmaceutical Association met in the City Hall of Macon at ten o'clock in the morning of Tuesday, April 11, 1876."

"In the absence of the President, Mr. John M. Clarke, the First Vice-President, Mr. John Ingalls, presided."

"On motion, the regular order of business was dispensed with, and the Proceedings of the called Meeting (1875) were read and adopted."

It appears that this first Annual Meeting, called for ten o'clock in the morning, was adjourned until three o'clock that afternoon, so that information could be obtained from the President, Mr. John M. Clarke, who lived at Milledgeville, as to why he was not present for the meeting. It developed that Mr. Clarke was confined to his place of business due to the fact that his assistant was either ill or out of Milledgeville.

There is a record that a committee of two was appointed to consider applications for membership. This committee was composed of L. W. Hunt, of Macon, and Theodore Schumann of Atlanta. They reported on the applications of the following gentlemen, who were duly elected:

Osceola Butler, Savannah	John G. Westmoreland, Atlanta
W. M. Mills, Savannah	
E. R. Beckwith, Macon	J. H. Logan, Atlanta
T. A. Cheatham, Macon	James Sharp, Jr., Atlanta

[Note: Whether this John G. Westmoreland, just mentioned, was Doctor John Westmoreland, who was connected with the Atlanta Medical College, is not known. But it is probable that this is one and the same person.]

The following standing committees were appointed for the ensuing year. Committee on Papers and Queries: Theodore Schumann, Chairman; J. M. Clarke, T. A. Cheatham. Committee on Legislation: John B. Daniel, Chairman; John Ingalls, John G. Westmoreland. Committee on Business: Roland B. Hall, Chairman; Osceola Butler, J. J. Pinckard.

Delegates to the American Pharmaceutical Association were John Ingalls, John M. Clarke, and Dr. Fred King.

There is included on pages 403-411 of this volume a complete list of all the officers of the Association, from 1875 to 1958.

℞ SUPPLEMENT D 327

Fortunately, we have a copy of the *Proceedings* of the Second Annual Meeting of the Georgia Pharmaceutical Association, which copy came to us from one of the libraries in an Eastern state. This is most fortunate in view of the fact that not one single copy of the Proceedings was available here in Georgia. This copy is now available in the General Library of the University of Georgia in Athens, and will be carefully protected and safeguarded through all time.

2nd Annual Meeting—1877

The Second Annual Meeting of the Georgia Pharmaceutical Association met in Atlanta on the second Tuesday in April, 1877. Since a copy of the Proceedings has been published and is available, a rather full account of what transpired at this Meeting will be given.

In his presidential address, President L. W. Hunt stated the following: "Georgia has over 300 druggists and apothecaries, and out of this number 112 were licensed October, 1874, with the license fee being $25.00."

It seems that a rapid increase in the membership in the Association was taking place. This is an alphabetical list of the members of the Association in 1877, and the towns from which they came:—

J. H. Alexander, Augusta
F. A. Beall, Augusta
E. R. Beckwith, Macon
E. M. Berry, Atlanta
A. H. Birdsong, Sparta
W. D. Boozer, Hogansville
R. M. Boyd, Atlanta
J. Bradfield, Atlanta
H. S. Bradley, Gainesville
— Brown, Dalton
T. F. Burbank, Cedartown
O. Butler, Savannah
A. G. Candler, Atlanta
T. A. Cheatham, Macon
J. M. Clarke, Milledgeville
J. W. Collier, Atlanta
J. J. Crawford, West Point
J. W. Crum, Conyers
W. H. Culpepper, Camilla
J. B. Daniel, Atlanta
J. T. Dozier, Cave Spring
N. B. Drewry, Griffin
E. J. Eldridge, Americus
W. L. E. Ellis, Hawkinsville
R. R. Evans, Atlanta
J. Faile, Hawkinsville
Amos Fox, Atlanta
R. B. Hall, Macon
E. R. Hirt, Atlanta
P. R. Holt, Atlanta
M. D. Hood, Columbus
G. J. Howard, Atlanta
L. W. Hunt, Macon
E. W. H. Hunter, Louisville
John Ingalls, Macon
J. R. Jaynes, Dawson
J. W. Jaynes, Rome
Fred King, Atlanta

J. O. King, Atlanta
R. H. Land, Augusta
L. A. Lee, Conyers
— Leilly, Fort Valley
— LeSewer, Fort Valley
J. H. Logan, Atlanta
J. M. Madden, Brunswick
A. A. Menard, Macon
C. R. Mann, Perry
T. L. Massenburg, Macon
— Mathews, Fort Valley
J. P. Miller, West Point
W. E. Miller, Atlanta
W. M. Mills, Savannah
Y. H. Morgan, Cochran
J. Patillo, West Point
George Payne, Macon
F. K. Peacock, Macon
A. G. Pease, Newnan
J. S. Pemberton, Atlanta
J. J. Pinckard, Macon
J. A. Polhill, Savannah
P. S. Powell, Cuthbert

J. W. Rankin, Atlanta
— Reese, Fort Valley
E. K. Root, Marietta
J. W. Sanders, Columbus
Theo Schumann, Atlanta
Harry Sharp, Forsyth
James Sharpe, Jr., Atlanta
A. W. Smith, Americus
J. A. Taylor, Atlanta
W. A. Taylor, Atlanta
R. Thomas, Valdosta
J. A. Thompson, Hawkinsville
E. G. Tidwell, Washington
J. Waterman, Talbotton
L. E. Welch, Albany
J. G. Westmoreland, Atlanta
M. B. White, Forsyth
W. H. Wimberly, Atlanta
— Wooten, Dalton
— Wright, Dalton
T. F. Young, Flowery Branch

This list comprises 81 members. This was a distinguished group of Georgia pharmacists. The names of many of them are intimately and definitely associated with the steps that were taken at that time tending toward modern pharmacy, as we know it today, particularly as regards the laws having to do with the practice of pharmacy. A number of individuals in this group were responsible for a beginning in the matter of legislation, setting up pharmacy as a distinct profession separated from the control of the medical profession as it had previously been. Most of those, perhaps all of them, who were physically fit, had passed through the tragic era of the Civil War and the Reconstruction days which followed. They were mature in years, in thinking, in experience, and had had some contact with the outside world beyond the State of Georgia, so far as pharmaceutical matters were concerned. No doubt, their contacts through the American Pharmaceutical Association, and perhaps their experiences during the Civil War, gave them some incentive and some background to begin to build an Association in Georgia. We owe them a debt of gratitude, and the names as recorded here are passed on into perpetuity in recognition of their service to the profession in the State.

Several of those pharmacists named in this list went on to be recognized nationally. In 1884, John Ingalls, of Macon, was President of the American Pharmaceutical Association, the first Georgian to be so honored. In 1902, Dr. George F. Payne, of Macon and Atlanta, was President of the American Pharmaceutical Association. Prior to Dr. Payne's election as President of A.Ph.A., he served as First Vice-President, in 1896 and 1898, and as Second Vice-President in 1901.

Other Georgia pharmacists in later years came to occupy positions of honor in the American Pharmaceutical Association, as well as in the National Association of Retail Druggists, the story of which will be recorded later in this volume.

It was customary at this time (1877) that on all important occasions of this kind, someone was selected to be known as the "Orator of the Day." The Pharmaceutical Association was following this practice in the choice of Mr. T. A. Cheatham, as the Orator of the Day on this occasion.

One of Mr. Cheatham's main arguments was for higher educational standards for the practice of pharmacy. He also condemned the practice, evidently extensive at that time, of the use of so-called "nostrums" and self-diagnosis and treatment of disease. He argued that the apprenticeship system which had prevailed had proved of value in the training of pharmacists. But he argued further that the requirements for apprenticeship should be watched very carefully, and as a preliminary to apprenticeship he believed that the student should have a good general or basic education, preferably offering evidence of his knowledge of Greek and Latin.

At this Atlanta Meeting in 1877, there were reported 45 members who answered to the roll call.

4th Annual Meeting—1879

Whereas there is no printed record of the *Minutes* of the 4th Annual Meeting of the Georgia Pharmaceutical Association, there is in existence a newspaper account of this 4th Annual Meeting, held in Savannah, Georgia, in 1879, at which time Osceola Butler of Savannah was serving as President.

The following members of the Association were present on this occasion:

J. H. Alexander, Augusta	W. M. Mills, Savannah
A. H. Birdsong, Sparta	Y. H. Morgan, Cochran
Osceola Butler, Savannah	J. W. Rankin, Atlanta
N. B. Drewry, Griffin	W. F. Reid, Savannah
W. L. E. Ellis, Hawkinsville	W. E. Miller, Savannah
W. L. Harrison, Savannah	J. F. Reilly, Savannah
G. M. Heidt, Savannah	Theo Schumann, Atlanta
W. F. Holloman, Waynesboro	Harry Sharp, Forsyth
	J. W. Solomons, Savannah
L. W. Hunt, Macon	L. C. Strong, Savannah
E. W. H. Hunter, Louisville	E. J. Tarpley, Dublin
John Ingalls, Macon	W. A. Taylor, Atlanta
E. J. Kieffer, Savannah	E. G. Tidwell, Savannah
J. Leddy, Savannah	C. B. Turner, Savannah
G. F. Symons, Brunswick	J. Weichselbaum, Savannah
J. M. Madden, Brunswick	E. S. Zittrouer, Savannah

A committee was named to select new members from current applications, and gave a favorable report on the following names:

F. Joerger, Brunswick	M. A. Barie, Savannah
W. A. Harrison, Savannah	J. T. Shuptrine, Savannah
H. Gallagher, Athens	E. A. Abbott, Savannah
G. T. Schaffer, Savannah	C. M. Hillsman, Savannah
Lewis Cass, Savannah	Lawrence Lippman, Savannah
H. W. Ellwood, Macon	
A. J. McCoy, Savannah	J. B. Abrams, Savannah
H. Burford, Savannah	St. J. R. Yonge, Savannah

The President announced that the following committee was to select officers for the ensuing year: G. M. Heidt, N. B. Drewry, J. M. Madden, E. J. Kieffer, and A. H. Birdsong.

According to the newspaper account, a financial report giving the status of the Association is given. This is the first recorded mention of finances, in which John Ingalls as Treasurer showed a balance on hand of $274.22, and asked that a committee be appointed to examine his books and vouchers; but, there being nothing in the Constitution or By-Laws providing for such a committee, someone moved that the report of the Treasurer be received without reference to a committee.

The person chosen to be the Orator of the Day, Mr. I. Zacharias, was unable to attend this reunion, but he sent his regrets at his inability to be present and chose Mr. Jacob Weichselbaum to read the oration for him. In the address Mr. Weichselbaum, Orator-by-Proxy, called attention to the value of the Association in elevating the profession of pharmacy.

The Committee on Applications returned a further favorable report upon the following applications for membership:

W. W. Lincoln, Savannah   W. E. Davies, Thomasville
R. E. Coster, Columbus   R. H. Tatum, Savannah
S. R. Pyles, Thomasville   T. S. Hawkeson, Augusta
J. A. Davenport, Americus

The following resignations were read and accepted:

V. L. Smith, Atlanta
R. Thomas, Valdosta
A. C. Pease, Newnan

An interesting paper was received from Mr. Zachariah replying to the query referred to him at the last Meeting, to wit: "Has the Experiment Been Tried to Cultivate Papaver Somniferum (Opium), And To Make Opium In the United States And With What Result?" The paper was read by the Secretary, and on motion was ordered to be filed. Unfortunately, it was not printed.

[Author's Note: This account of the 4th Annual Meeting was taken from a Savannah newspaper of 1879. It appeared in a scrapbook of the Kieffer family. The book was loaned by a member of this family to the author.]

At this 4th Annual Meeting of the GPA, Mr. Schumann of Atlanta, who was Chairman of the Committee on Legislation, made a statement with reference to the proposed Pharmacy Law, and submitted a draft of the Law to be presented at the next assemblage of the Legislature. This, so far as the records go, (except for the "Poison Law") is the first mention of any legislation sponsored by the Georgia Pharmaceutical Association. Of course, the original law passed in 1825, which set up the Medical Board of Examiners, did include legislation having to do with pharmacy, requiring those who were applicants for license to practice pharmacy to take an examination before the Board of

Medical Examiners. According to the *Proceedings* of the American Pharmaceutical Association, as stated there, this law of 1825 is the first law in the United States requiring a license for pharmacists. Whether this is authentic or not we cannot say.

Even though there is no published record of the Annual Meetings of the Association for 1878, 1879, 1880, and 1881, it must be recorded that the first Association-sponsored legislation, giving us our first basic Pharmacy Law, was enacted in 1881, (see Pharmacy Laws in Supplement C), and the first meetings of the "Board of Pharmaceutic Examiners" were held in 1881.

The first meeting of the Pharmaceutical Board was in Atlanta on November 9, 1881, at which time the Board organized with officers, and adopted some rules and regulations for governing the Board.

The first meeting of the Board for the purpose of examining applicants was held in Atlanta on December 17, 1881. The *Minutes* of the meeting shows a list of the names of the following who presented themselves for examination:

T. D. Dodson, Columbus
M. G. Little and T. C. Jones, Albany
C. O. Tyner, Atlanta
P. P. Reed, Savannah
R. P. Johnson, Smithville
B. E. Roughton, Sandersville
J. E. Jones, Fort Valley
J. H. Harper, Covington

Some of these applicants are reported as having failed, but they were awarded a "temporary license," good until the next meeting of the Board.

At this same meeting of the Board of Pharmaceutic Examiners, "honorary licenses" were issued to the following "gentlemen": Messrs. W. A. Taylor, Atlanta; W. W. Lincoln, Savannah; A. A. Solomons, Savannah; and Wm. Rook, Marietta.

In 1884, Dr. Henry Slack of LaGrange, who was Secretary of the Georgia Pharmaceutical Association for several years, secured copies of the Proceedings of the GPA for several years. During the time he was Secretary, of course, he preserved copies of the Proceedings, and fortunately had them bound. Just a few years prior to his death he gave them to the University of Georgia Library. Those copies are the only ones in existence today, so far as can be determined. They cover a period of from 1884-1889, the date of the 14th Annual Meeting.

℞ SUPPLEMENT D 333

9th Annual Meeting—1884

The 9th Annual Meeting of the GPA was held in Macon, Georgia, on the second Tuesday in April, 1884, at which time Mr. J. W. Rankin, President at that time, pointed out some important matters:

"*Our pharmacy law (of 1881), as far as I know, or have heard, is operating very well. It is a good law as far as it goes, and it probably is as desirable as any we could hope to obtain. I think it has protected the public in a large degree from incompetent or careless compounding of prescriptions, and has to some extent limited the sale of poisons to the legitimate pharmacists.* We hope soon to see the day when we shall have full protection in this matter. The general public do not (it would seem) yet feel sufficient interest in this business which is so important to them to assist us in having such laws passed as will protect them from danger. *Strange to say, the greatest and most determined opposition to a better law came from a quarter which was least expected, namely, the medical profession. This must have been from a total misapprehension of the interest and purposes of such a law, for I cannot conceive how or why there should be any clash of interests between physicians and pharmacists. It would seem to be the manifest interest of each to work together in all things pertaining to both professions.* Under all circumstances I would recommend that the matter be let alone for the present. *I feel sure that sooner or later, and in my opinion in the near future, the people will become educated to the necessity of a more stringent law to regulate pharmacy, and laws to prevent the adulteration of drugs, (particulary in the cities) and that we will then have a statute which will not only protect the public, but will elevate and dignify pharmacy.* I desire in this connection to call your attention to a movement to obtain the passage of a national Pharmacy Act. It is well worth your consideration."

Mr. Rankin makes this statement:

"*Pursuant to a resolution passed at the 8th Annual Meeting of the Georgia Pharmaceutical Association at Athens, in 1883, I had prepared and sent out to committees in each county, petitions to be signed requesting Congress to give tax-free alcohol for the manufacture of medicines, and for pharmaceutical preparations. In response to about 100 petitions sent out, we had 27 returned executed.* This is not as many as should have been perfected; but I think probably 20 or more were signed and sent direct to our members of Congress. *We have forwarded the 27 petitions to the Honorable Thomas Hardeman, Member-of-Congress-at-Large from our State, asking his attention, and have written also the Honorable N. J. Hammond, Member of Congress, and to Senators Brown and Colcourt, requesting their assistance."*

"It may not be out of place here to mention that this action, taken by this Association at Athens in 1883, *may be the beginning of the end of this Revenue business.*"

[Author's Note: Personified optimism is indicated in this last sentence of Mr. Rankin's.]

Mr. Rankin called attention to the fact that he sent a copy of the action taken here in Georgia to many of the other state associations and to many of the trade centers throughout the country, and when he told the National Wholesale Druggists Association in New York in October of the action taken by the Georgia Association, the same resolution was introduced before that body, and that the President of that splendid body of men vacated his seat and amended the motion by asking that "the whole Revenue system be repealed" and supported it with a ringing speech. The preamble recited that "the whole Revenue system is oppressive to the poor, unjust to the druggist, and not necessary to the support of the Government."

Mr. Rankin continued:

"I believe that the great mass of the people desire the total repeal of all the system of Internal Revenue taxation. I believe the whole country is ripe for it, and that an earnest word from you today, representing as you do one of the most honorable professions in the world and one which is free from selfish ends, an earnest word, I say, from this Association, sent by telegraph if you desire, cannot be overlooked or passed by at Washington. It is a war measure, imposed now on a country at peace with all the world, it is a system of oppression not in any way contemplated by our form of government, it is a grinding tax on the poor of the country; it places every pharmacist whether wholesale or retail on the footing of a rum seller. The revenue from it is not needed by the Government. It will surely seem that these were good and sufficient reasons for the repeal of this taxation. I grant that some will say that free whiskey would increase drunkenness. But that is hardly justified by the facts; make your liquor license high, and you do more to make a rum shop respectable than if whiskey was taxed $5.00 per gallon. But in my opinion this is

℞ SUPPLEMENT D

the time to strike, and I do hope this Association will speak its mind today."

Another item which Mr. Rankin discusses is the cutting of drug prices, which he condemns because he says it is unprofessional, and it is "unbusinesslike," he says, "because it deprives the seller of his legitimate profit and demoralizes the prices of the goods so cut, to the injury not only of all dealers and purchasers but even to the seller himself." He refers to the cutting of prices as "scalping," about which he says, "I believe the 'scalping' business will be short-lived."

[Author's Note: Mr. Rankin proved to be a poor prophet in this connection!]

Mr. N. I. Brunner, of Macon, discussing the question as to "Pharmacists versus Manufacturers," states:

"It has always been a mystery to the writer why it is that the retail druggists do not make more of their preparations than they do. There are a great number of very simple compounds that are bought from the wholesaler that the true apothecary could make himself. The only reasons that I can see why they prefer to *buy* rather than to *make* are laziness and ignorance."

Mr. Brunner bemoans the fact that he realizes he is leading a forlorn hope to stir up any interest in this subject.

He concludes with this statement:

"In conclusion, I beg of you gentlemen, one and all, to emancipate yourselves from this ready-made goods business, enlighten your physicians and customers of the true state of affairs, and a hearty reaction will soon set in that will redound to the credit of all pharmacists."

Dr. H. K. Main, of Dalton, read a paper in which he discussed the question as to whether the Quinine that was imported into this country in bulk was equal in quality to that of our own manufacture. He reported that he was now convinced that the imported product was equal in all respects to the home product.

Mr. R. H. Land, of Augusta, wrote a letter to be read at the Association on the subject: "Are We On the Retrograde?" He said: "Do not misunderstand me. I do not mean to say that our young men are less competent or less thoroughly prepared, but simply this: we are drifting silently and imperceptibly into mere merchants by urging our physicians in the use of the many 'elegant' preparations put up away from home, and sold to us at a high price, instead of preparing them ourselves."

The Secretary was ordered to call the roll of members at this 9th Annual Meeting, and the following answered to the roll-call:

N. I. Brunner	T. L. Massenburg
O. Butler	William Mills
G. D. Case	W. H. Morgan
S. J. Cassells	W. A. Pigman
J. S. Dozier	J. A. Polhill
S. C. Durban	J. H. Polhill
Dr. T. B. Gibbs	E. S. Parks
R. B. Hall	J. W. Rankin
R. C. Hall	S. G. Riley
L. W. Hunt	Theo Schumann
J. Ingalls	W. E. Shelverton
H. J. Lamar	G. D. Speight
H. J. Lamar, Jr.	J. W. Stanford
W. A. Loyless	E. J. Tarpley
C. B. Loyd	M. H. Taylor
T. W. McKeown	J. P. Turner
D. E. McMaster	G. S. Vardeman
H. K. Main	I. Zacharias

An interesting ballot is taken here on a question raised by George D. Case. The Secretary was requested to call the names of every person present, and as each name was read out, the member called should state whether he used the Old or the New Pharmacopoeia in the matter of the different preparations. The vote stood: "21 in favor of the Old, and 12 in favor of the New Pharmacopoeia."

An interesting age-old item, discussing the question of the cutting of prices, came up, the conclusion arrived at being "that it is only in the province of the manufacturer to uphold prices by refusing to sell to any druggist who cut stated prices."

Mr. Rankin offered a motion to instruct the Secretary "to have the Proceedings of the Association published *provided that sufficient advertisements could be obtained to cover the cost of same.*" This statement probably explains why there is in the history of the Association a frequent lapse of years when there is no publication of the Proceedings. This same motion was made in succeeding years, and sometimes it happened that advertisements were not available and, hence, no copies of Proceedings were printed.

℞ SUPPLEMENT D

10th Annual Meeting—1885

The 10th Annual Meeting of the GPA was held in Atlanta. There were about 60 people present at that Meeting when the roll was called, including quite a number of new members, but of course, mostly a number of the old faithful crowd. This has been true on down through the years.

Dr. S. C. Durban, President for that year, in his presidential address, urges higher professional standards on the part of the practitioners of pharmacy. He appeals particularly to the young men to study especially the subjects of chemistry and botany, in addition to the practical phases of pharmacy. He also includes mineralogy as one of the sciences that a pharmacist should be familiar with, and says: "The shop of the apothecary is oftentimes the school where the mind is trained to observation, taste development, and original investigations pursued, which results in giving to science a name to be enrolled among her worthy votaries,—results which often outlive the name of the discoverer."

Mr. W. A. Loyless discussed at some length this topic, "Has the Contract System or Rebate Plan Been, Or Is It Likely To Be, Of Advantage to the Retail Druggist?" He proves to his own satisfaction that the "rebate plan" then in vogue was of primary importance to the retail druggist, particularly in the purchase of proprietary products.

George D. Case, discussing the topic, "What Can Be Done To Encourage Young Men To Become Better Pharmacists," argues that the people want medicine, like miscellaneous goods, cheap. He says that "there are two principal causes of discouragement that keep old or young men from becoming better pharmacists."

His statement follows: "Chemistry is the keystone of the pharmacal arch. A young man can never become a proficient pharmacist until he becomes first at least tolerably well acquainted with this science. First, then, before receiving encouragement, every man should cross the threshhold of our profession with at least a decent knowledge of chemistry as his credential. Without this, his progress will be halting, unsatisfactory and unsafe."

As a result of a prize essay, R. H. Land, M.D., of Augusta, presented a paper on the subject, "What Plants Indigenous to Our State Can Be Gathered or Cultivated Profitably?" He mentions a number of products familiar to most of us in which he says: "In our gardens the Mints all grow luxuriantly, as do Hops, Belladonna, Hyoscyamus, Digitalis, Chamomile, Ricinus, and a thousand other useful plants which it would take too much time to enumerate." He says that there is not an acre of land in the State of Georgia which does not produce some plant of medicinal value. He calls attention to the fact that in the mountains of North Georgia we have the Seneka, Gaultheria, Kalmia, Guaiac, Sanguinaria, Asarum, Sassafras, Wild Cherry, Salix, Cornus, Ulmus, Styrax; and in the lower or sandy portion of the State, perhaps the most important official plants are: Stillingia, Spigelia, and Gelsemium. Phytolacca, Podophyllum, Chenopodium, and various other plants are mentioned.

Mr. Osceola Butler discusses the meaning of the words "disinfectant" and "antiseptic." The reader will bear in mind that the "germ theory" of disease was new at this time (1885). He illustrates by saying that "disinfection" means "any process by which the contagium of any given disease may be destroyed or be rendered inert," and he cautions against confounding "disinfectants" with the term "deodorant," "which merely cover or destroy offensive odors without affecting the contagia." He also compares disinfectants with antiseptics, which he says are "fatal to the growth and multiplication of 'microzymes.'" He makes this statement: "The best method of dealing with infected air is to replace it by ventilation, of open fireplaces." He suggests for the disinfection of excreta a solution of bichloride of mercury, 1/1000; solution of carbolic acid, 5%; solution Labarraque, 1 ounce to one quart water; permanganate of potash, 10 grains to one quart water; sulphate of iron, one pound to one gallon water; solution chloride of lime, which is both cheap and very efficient, he states. He calls attention to the fact that solution chloride of lime is commonly called "chlorinated lime."

Mr. John Ingalls, addressing the Association as delegate to the A.Ph.A., calls attention of the group to the fact that he has been elected President of the Association, the first native Georgian to hold this office. His report is also interesting in this respect: He was also delegate to the National Retail Druggists Association, which body was meeting in Milwaukee on August 25th and 26th, whereas the A.Ph.A was meeting on August 26-29, an occurrence which today would be considered most unusual.

Mr. Schumann, addressing the 10th Annual Meeting, argues for the manufacture in the drug store of many of our important chemical products, claiming that they can be manufactured of just as high degree of purity and strength as the manufacturer makes them, and at a considerable saving; as witnessed by the fact that he claims to make Biniodide of Mercury for $1.47, but the price of the manufacturer is $4.82 for this product. And he makes White Precipitate for $.47 for 9 ounces, whereas the list price is $.54 for 9 ounces. He also mentions a number of other items in this connection.

On the second day of the 10th Annual Meeting, Dr. J. S. Pemberton of Atlanta discussed a paper which had been read by Mr. Schumann the day before. In a masterly manner, he referred to the profession of pharmacy and the high standard we should strive to achieve. He took the position that the day was not far distant when the profession would be honored and looked up to, and it would be the duty of every young man to qualify himself "for the important station he will undoubtedly occupy, sooner or later."

Mr. W. A. Loyless read a paper on the subject of price-cutting. He stated, "The price-cutter is a wrecker who is both unwilling to make a fair, legitimate profit himself and determined no one else shall." He stated further that, "When you once start cutting, you set in motion an avalanche which sweeps down with irresistible force and momentum, carrying with it not only yourself but others, with fearful rapidity, down the steep incline, and buries yourself and them in one common grave."

At this Meeting a committee on legislation was instructed to cooperate with the National Wholesale Druggists Association in an effort to repeal an Internal Revenue Tax on alcohol for the use of druggists.

Various members of the Association, including Dr. Pemberton, Mr. Hunt and Mr. Schumann, discussed the question of the sale of drugs by general merchants, and offered this resolution:— "Resolved, that the Board of Pharmaceutical Examiners be requested to ask the Ordinaries of the State to give information with the names of such merchants as may be compounding and selling such medicines contrary to law, and that said Board proceed at once to prosecute all violators."

[Author's Note: So far as can be determined, this is the first recorded instance where the responsibility of the Board of Pharmacy for the prosecution of violators of the Pharmacy Law is called to the attention of the Association.]

Mr. Rankin again discusses the matter of the tax on alcohol. He says:

"The price of alcohol at the present time is $2.30 per gallon, and the tax on it is $1.70, which leaves $.60 per gallon as the actual cost of the alcohol delivered in your store."

He argues further that the general public, particularly the poor, suffers because the price of all medicines containing alcohol is largely increased because of the tax, which he pronounces unjust, especially in view of the fact that the Government receives a small net revenue, a large portion of it being consumed in collecting it.

Dr. Henry R. Slack of LaGrange, who holds both the M.D. degree and the Ph.G. degree, and has acted as Secretary of the Association for several years, reads an essay on the subject of "Chemistry." The paper reviews the theories in regard to chemistry at that particular time, considered then to be very advanced theories.

Mr. R. H. Land, of Augusta, reads an essay on Pharmacy. His opening sentence reads as follows: "Pharmacy embraces much that is good, much that is true, and much that is beautiful. In its everyday relations to the community in which we live, it brings us in contact with human nature in every phase; in its scientific relations it unfolds the wonders of botany, chemistry and mineralogy, and the kindred sciences, as well as the laws of physics. As an art or practice, either in preparing, compounding or preserving substances for the purposes of medicine, it brings to light the simple arrangements and the grand results that arise from the union and disunion of nature's own trades and treasures." He draws a beautiful picture of the basic sciences: of chemistry, botany, physics, and related sciences, as they merge into the one great group of the phases of pharmacy. In the course of his remarks, however, Mr. Land introduces a somewhat sour note when he says that when any young man considers entering the profession of pharmacy, he must be told that he is making a serious mistake unless he goes into it *with the expectation of leaving hope behind,* so far as the "pleasures of the world are concerned." He says, "If, after being fully informed of all this, he is willing to undertake the study of pharmacy, we may hope to make a useful member of the profession out of him, and will not hesitate at undertaking his instruction."

11th Annual Meeting—1886

The 11th Annual Meeting of the GPA convened in Savannah in April, 1886. The printed list of active members for that year is composed of only 54 names, approximately one-half as many active members as were reported the year before. Only 39 of the active members were reported as being present at the first session.

President H. G. Hutchinson of Atlanta, in the opening paragraph of his address, states: "Like all other Associations ours has had to contend with trials and difficulties. But nothing has so militated against its growth and prosperity as the indifference and apathy of so many of our brethren."

And he continues: "As a result of this lack of concert of action, we are today oppressed by laws that were put upon us without our approval, and are kept upon us to our detriment and injury." He illustrates what he means by this by citing the tax on alcohol and the retail liquor dealers' tax of $25.00, which he says could never have been passed if the retail druggists of the country had been organized and had fought it.

President Hutchinson also recites the fact that at last session of the Legislature a bill was passed which required that a red label would have to be placed on any quantity of Morphine that was sold over the counter. He complains not so much about the passage of this law, but about the fact that the Pharmaceutical Association was not consulted about the matter.

The President also complains about the "seduction of the average physician, who is induced to prescribe ready-made prescriptions."

Secretary H. R. Slack reported on the query that had been proposed: "Is A Mixture Of Nitric And Carbolic Acid Explosive?" "If so, what proportions so result?" Mr. Slack commented: "Mixing strong nitric and carbolic acid does produce an eruption of sufficient violence to be denominated an 'explosion.' It is equal to or exceeds that caused by iodine to turpentine."

Dr. J. S. Pemberton, who was later to evolve a formula for Coca-Cola, delivered an essay entitled, "An Essay On Guarana, Caffeine, and Coca." He discussed Guarana and other sources of Caffeine, and gave the constitutional action of Caffeine and the conditions under which it is advised. He claimed that Caffeine obtained from the Kola Nut was superior to that from any other source. He concluded his discussion of Caffeine with this statement: "What a grand fact it is that the good things of life are cumulative, and the bad, eliminative. Hence, Caffeine supersedes Guarana." In discussing Coca, Dr. Pemberton said: "Never in the history of the medical world has a remedial agent, within so short a space of time, risen from the comparative obscurity to such practical as well as real importance to the medical profession as Coca and its alkaloids."

The Legislative Committee urged the Association to contact their Senators and members of the national House of Representatives to induce them to vote for the repeal of all Internal taxes. Following are the reasons:

"1. Such taxes have always been unpopular.
2. They are inquisitorial in character.
3. They are special in their nature.
4. They are taxes upon goods produced in our own country.
5. They interfere with freedom of trade among the states.
6. They violate the unwritten law of the land which is to draw the revenue from the Customs and not from the Excise.
7. The Internal Revenue Taxes are war measures and always have been.
8. They were enacted to raise money to meet the wants of the Government in the late Civil War, and for no other purpose, with the understanding that these taxes were to be abolished when the exigencies of the Government no longer demanded them."

The Legislative Committee also called attention to the various rates per gallon on Distilled Spirits, as follows:

"Commencing with 20 cents per gallon in 1862, it rose to 60 cents per gallon in 1864, and to $1.50 in June of 1864, and to $2.00 by December, 1864. Then it dropped to 50 cents in 1868, to be followed by an advance to 70 cents in 1872, and to 90 cents per gallon in 1875."

The Committee quotes the Hon. D. D. Pratt, Commissioner of Internal Revenue, who in his annual report of 1875 refers to the fact that a "reasonable rate of 50 cents per gallon tax produced a more satisfactory revenue than when the tax exceeded $2.00 per gallon."

Mr. P. C. Magnus offered a prize of $20.00 for the best line of chemicals and fluid extracts made by a clerk in any retail store in the State. [Author's Note: Mr. P. C. Magnus came to be one of the largest importers of volatile oils and perfume products in the United States. His firm, under the name of Magnus, Mabee, and Renard, is still in existence at the present time (1959).] In 1886 Mr. Magnus was a retail pharmacist in Rome, Georgia.

12th Annual Meeting—1887

The 12th Annual Meeting of the GPA was held on Cumberland Island off the Georgia Coast, April 12, 1887.

President Stanford, in his presidential address, stated that he "viewed with pride the improvements and progress made in our profession in the last eleven years since its organization." "But," he said, "I regret to say that the laws of our State have been and are now such as to hinder rather than encourage our noble profession." "The doctors manage to get elected to the Legislature and have passed from time to time such laws as are beneficial to their profession, while we pharmacists like my friend Colonel Lamar, and some others I might name, decline to accept these honors (if honors they be) when tendered them."

Pointing out some of the defects of the existing pharmacy laws the President said that defects were more in evidence in some of the smaller towns than in the cities. He stated, "The keeping of drug stores by incompetent persons, the practice of pharmacy by proxy, and the collecting laws, are poor." He complained further that under existing law a physician no matter how limited his knowledge of medicine, who by some means has obtained a diploma from some medical college, and who could not stand the rigid examination of our State Board of Pharmacy, is granted a license as a pharmacist simply upon the presentation of his diploma from a medical school to the Pharmacy Examining Board.

The President pointed out that the law now permitted anyone to run and to own a drug store, simply by employing a licensed clerk, and that this condition brought men into the business who had no ambition higher than that of making money, and that they knew nothing about this profession and hence had no professional pride.

"The clerk is simply an employee, paid to do as they say, and is sometimes a physician, broken down, and a failure in his own profession, and employed simply because he can get a license upon his diploma."

The President pointed out another inequity of the law of that particular time when he called attention to the fact that the bill from a doctor is the first bill to be paid and has prior claim on the estate of a person, but that in the case of the pharmacist from whom the medicines were furnished during that same illness, the bill takes the place of ordinary accounts and has no priority. Thus, frequently, the druggist goes unpaid.

A human interest item occurs in the Minutes of the Association, as follows:

"When Mr. Kieffer's query was called for by the Secretary,

Mr. Shuptrine explained that Mr. Kieffer was absent due to the fact that he had been shot by a ruffian and was now quite ill. A motion was adopted expressing the sympathy of the Association for Mr. Kieffer." [Note: Mr. K. and Mr. S. were both retail pharmacists in Savannah.]

Mr. Schumann of Atlanta made some very critical remarks about the Board of Pharmaceutical Examiners and the "lax method now in vogue concerning the examinations." Following the discussion of this statement a motion was passed that the Association should recommend suitable men to the Governor for appointment as pharmaceutical examiners.

[Author's Note: It appears here that appointment on the Board was left entirely to the Governor up to that time.]

But, finally, instead of allowing the Association to recommend suitable men, the motion was amended to name the following— S. C. Durban and Charles H. Behre and M. H. Taylor, representing the Association—and that they should be responsible for recommending to the Governor suitable men to assume duties as pharmaceutical examiners. While this discussion was going on, Mr. Joerger pointed out that Laudanum and other items were being sold by grocerymen, and that "it is so weak in content, if any, that it probably could be drunk by the dozens without producing any effect."

It seems that the members of the Board of Examiners were not present at the Meeting at all. So, at this point, a motion was made instructing the Secretary to invite the Examiners to attend the meetings of the Association.

Under the heading of new business, Mr. Schumann of Atlanta moved that "three members and the President, ex-officio, of the Association be appointed to confer with the Commissioners of the School of Technology to see if a School of Pharmacy could be effected in connection with it." He made a strong argument in favor of the establishment of such a school in Atlanta. Mr. Slack, the Secretary, seconded the motion, and made a speech in which he showed that such a college in connection with the technological school would only necessitate the establishment of two Chairs; namely, that of Materia Medica and Pharmacy. It was his opinion that the School of Pharmacy would be self-sustaining. Other speeches were made in favor of the motion, and it was then unanimously passed. The chairman appointed on this committee Messrs. Schumann, Rankin, Stanford, and Case.

[Author's Note: This appears to be the first real, serious

℞ SUPPLEMENT D 345

thought on the part of the pharmacists of Georgia regarding the possibility of establishing a School of Pharmacy in the State, and this effort resulted in failure.]

Competing for a prize of $20.00 offered by Mr. Rankin, Mr. Ed. A. Abbott of Savannah and Mr. H. R. Slack of LaGrange submitted two papers contending for the prize on the subject, "How to deal with price cutting." Mr. Slack was awarded the prize because his paper involved a suggestion which was thought possible as being practicable. It was this: that the formation of a corporation in each town should open up a store near the "cutter," whoever he might be, and to undersell the "cutter."

13th Annual Meeting—1888

The 13th Annual Meeting of the GPA was held in Atlanta in 1888. The session was called to order by President George D. Case of Milledgeville. On roll call there were 45 members who answered to their names. But some 32 names were proposed as new members in the Association.

In his opening remarks, Mr. Case calls attention to the fact that in looking over the audience, he sees some present there who were among the organizers of the Association in 1875. Unfortunately, the names of these people do not occur in the Minutes.

The President calls attention to the progress that the organization has made in the 13 years of its life, among which items is the fact that "13 years ago, our profession was bound tight and fast to the doctors. Every sensible man knows, or ought to know, that the two are separate and distinct professions. Formerly, a druggist's license was to be obtained in Georgia only from a Medical Examining Board. We had no professional recognition whatever; while today we have our own Board of Pharmacy (although the law constituting it is defective). With no pharmacy school in our midst with which to gauge a respectable professional standard, our Pharmacy Board was a necessity, and is now no longer an appendage to the medical profession."

The names of the Board of Pharmacy members (which appears to be the first all-pharmacy Board) were as follows: Theo. Schumann of Atlanta, J. W. Goodwyn of Macon, S. C. Durban of Augusta, Geo. D. Case of Milledgeville, and Henry R. Slack, Junior, of LaGrange. This Board was appointed by His Excellency Governor John B. Gordon on November 12, 1887, on the recommendation of the GPA.

President Case makes an interesting statement when he states:

"I for one take the position that our Association work is not so much one of money matters as it is professional. Trade affairs regulate themselves. While we are here, we don't care whether the patent medicines are profitable or not. We do not clamor by petition and committees to be protected by law or otherwise in our commercial affairs. As merchants, we must take our places with all the other profit-seekers in the busy channels of trade. But, as pharmacists, with a love for our profession as noble as that of the physician, let us strive to elevate our standards, study, and search in the scientific fields, feel the importance of our philanthropic duties, and thus hold the respect and confidence of our fellow-man."

Mr. Case then states that the profession needs educational facilities in the State, since our young men must go every year to the Northern and Western colleges to be taught pharmacy because there is no place in Georgia to get this instruction. Then he asks the question: "Now what greater work could this Association take in hand than to try to establish such a school, and what better way can it be done than by cooperation? There are many ways in which this school can be established. And if, after attempting one, the Association should fail, let the Association collectively and individually persist until successful."

President Case points out some weaknesses in the laws, saying it is out of the power of the Board of Pharmacy promptly and directly to have violators stopped and punished. He complains that the State supports means and machinery for all other kinds of crimes to be suppressed directly; "but the Board of Pharmacy, the State's guardian of pure drugs and clean pharmacy haven't a single prompt prerogative in maintaining the evident intention of the pharmacy law."

In answer to the query, "What Effect Has Prohibition Had On Pharmacy?," Mr. Rankin of Atlanta prepared a paper which was read by Mr. R. H. Land of Augusta. He points out that they have not had much opportunity to judge of the value of prohibition. But during the short life of it, "the people were improved in morals, in dress, and in health." "And property in some localities has been enhanced, some 25% to 50% in value, this being especially true of Decatur and West Peters Street."

Secretary Slack inserts this note: "Mr. Rankin's paper excited no comment; not because it was incorrect, but because prohibition has now assumed a political aspect, and politics are not discussed in these meetings."

An interesting discussion occurred under the query, "Do Retail Druggists Prepare Their Tinctures and Syrups With Fluid Extracts?" Dr. G. C. Huss implied that this practice was being indulged in. He concludes his paper by saying: "Of all the swindling perpetrated and palmed off on our fellow-man, the greatest, the most damnable of all crimes is the falsity of one who would sell a spurious article of medicine—one who would sell a dilute for a full-strength medicine." There followed a bitter but enlightening discussion of this paper.

The Honorable Henry W. Grady, invited by the President to address the Association, came into the Hall, and stated before the group the following:

"Gentlemen, I will say, as a member of the Board of Trustees of the University of Georgia, that the petition of this Association through your committee, signed by Mr. Schumann, Slack, and others, was presented at the last meeting of our Board in Athens and was very favorably received. We could take no definite action on it because the Commissioners of the School of Technology were not present. I assure you that your efforts to establish a school of pharmacy at the technological school met with favor by the Board of Trustees, and we hope to take some definite action in that direction."

This speech by Mr. Grady was received with applause.

Mr. Theo. Schumann of Atlanta, Chairman of this committee to confer with the School of Technology with reference to the establishment of a school of pharmacy there, reported that the Commissioners of the School of Technology have requested a written statement from the Association. His communication addressed to the Commissioners of the School of Technology states:

"At various times the proposition has been made to establish a School of Pharmacy in Atlanta, in connection with a school of Medicine. *But it has always come from one or the other of those colleges of medicine, and was therefore not supported by the druggists. Medicine and pharmacy should never be taught in the same college, for pharmacy will come out short.* Therefore, a college of pharmacy merely appended to a college of medicine will not, and cannot, have the support of pharmacists and apothecaries, and such a college should always be under the direction, or at least under the advice, of pharmacists and apothecaries."

Later Mr. Schumann gives further arguments in favor of a state-supported school of pharmacy, calling attention in fact to the State of Michigan which has established a school of pharmacy in connection with the State University at Ann Arbor. He ends his statement by saying: "Whatever could be said in favor of a school of technology is certainly equally true as to the establishment of a school of pharmacy."

Dr. McMaster, however, moved that a School of Pharmacy be established in connection with the Medical Department of the University of Georgia at Augusta. Mr. Land seconded this motion. But Mr. Behre took the floor against this motion, and showed the advantages to be derived from having the School in connection with the School of Technology. Dr. McMaster, replying to Mr. Behre, said: "To have that school here in Atlanta would require four extra professors, while Augusta would require only one. Of course, you Atlanta men want the school in Atlanta, but we must have it where it would be most likely to succeed and to secure it by aid of the State."

Mr. Taylor, in replying to Mr. McMaster, said: "Mr. President, as a Ph.G., I know that three professors can do the work in any college of pharmacy, and it is simply absurd to say that we must have four."

Someone proposed that instead of having the school in Atlanta or in Augusta, it might be located in Macon. Then several other towns in the State were suggested as the location for the school. The result of this disagreement with regard to the location of the proposed school, which might have been established as a part of the Georgia School of Technology, discouraged the Board of Trustees, and the proposed School was not established anywhere.

In referring to the Pharmacy Law of 1881, Dr. Slack uses this expression: "Oh, folly of follies! In legislation to make a thing unlawful and yet not provide a penalty!"

At this Meeting some suggestions were made as to amendments for the existing pharmacy law, which if passed would be far-reaching in their effect. But these amendments proposed here did not become a part of the law for a number of years.

In the Proceedings for the year 1888, the following items were published: the Constitution; the Pharmacy and Poison Laws, as follows—The Law to Regulate the Sale of Poisons in the State (passed in 1876); the Establishment of the Board of Pharmaceutical Examiners (passed in 1881); the new Opium Law; and a List of Members of the Association, as well as a List of Persons Licensed By the State Board of Pharmacy for the Year 1887-1888, of which number there were 66.

℞ SUPPLEMENT D 349

This 13th Annual Meeting of the Association was referred to in later years as one of the most constructive in the history of the Association.

14th Annual Meeting—1889

The 14th Annual Meeting of the GPA, held at Sweetwater Park near Atlanta, July 23, 1889, was opened by its President, William S. Parks. It was reported that 16 new members had been elected to membership in the Association. Letters of regret for absence were read from quite a number of members, among them letters from George Case, Dr. W. M. Terrell, J. R. Gregory, and others, as well as a telegram from Mr. George A. Bradford.

In his address President Parks called attention to the fact that a Bill is now in the Legislature to incorporate the GPA, and that he has been assured by friends in that body that there is no doubt of its passage and that the House will act upon the Bill at this session of the Legislature. He states that the new Pharmacy Law as submitted by the committee appointed at the last Meeting might also receive favorable consideration. He suggests that the Secretary send copies of this proposed Law to every druggist in the State.

The President makes this comment:

"The time has come when as a corporate body, chartered by the Legislature of Georgia, we have the rights and privileges that must be respected. And if they are not, then go to that old mother and demand it. And, on the contrary, this Association must respect and help to enforce the laws which she has created for our good by aiding our most excellent Board of Pharmacy in their efforts in this direction. Otherwise, the State will have the right to repudiate any further claims we may make."

The Committee on Legislation reported as follows: "That an amendment to the existing Pharmacy Law had been introduced in the House which provided for a 'staggered term' for Board members. A total of five were to be named, one of whom would serve for one year, one for two years, one for three years, one for four years, and one for five. And that, thereafter, the Governor would appoint one new Board member each year on recommendation of the State Pharmaceutical Association. The duties of this Board were defined in the Act."

Another amendment provided for the prevention of the sale of any adulterated or misbranded product. A third amendment provided for the taking up of samples of drugs for analysis. The fourth amendment was to provide for the employment of an expert chemist or analyst who would examine the samples of drugs taken up.

In a discussion of the queries, Query Number 3 was, "What Is the Experience From Their Own, Or From Information of the Physicians, As To the Merits of Antipyrin, As Compared With Quinine in the Treatment of Fever?" Mr. Goodwyn said that he knew of a number of cases where the physicians had actually killed their patients by substituting Antipyrin for Quinine in the treatment of fever. All present expressing themselves agreed that "while Antipyrin is a splendid antipyretic, and antispasmodic, yet it could not be used with impunity in the treatment of fever."

In discussing the matter of fees for license, and the proposed annual renewal fee of $2.00, Mr. Slack, Secretary, stated: "There are now in Georgia 440 drug stores and 600 licensed druggists." This is the first time, as far as written records go, that any such figures have been available as a correct, official figure as to the number of drug stores in the State in 1889.

An interesting comment is to the effect that Mr. Goodwyn, in discussing the matter of fees, stated that at the last meeting of the Board in Atlanta, though it was thoroughly advertised, *not a single candidate appeared for examination for license to practice pharmacy in Georgia.*

The President was called on to make a statement in regard to the proposed college of pharmacy. The Minutes indicate that the President made a strong plea for the college, in which he showed the need for such an institution in Georgia and the proper method of procedure in order to secure the school. The druggists of our State must work in concert, and the best concert of action can be had through the State Association and the proper committees, he urged.

The Secretary of the Board of Pharmacy in giving his annual report showed that there had been three meetings during that year, and also a meeting to confer with the Legislative Committee. He stated: "We have examined 12 candidates, 8 of whom passed a successful examination, while 4 failed."

The Secretary also reported that one druggist had been prosecuted for selling adulterated drugs. But the Attorney General had said that the man could not be prosecuted for selling adulterated drugs as it was not a penal offense, but that the charge would have to be brought for cheating and swindling. The Grand Jury of the county in which the offense occurred found a

True Bill, but owing to a technical error, the indictment was quashed. The party referred to was expelled from the Association for adulterating drugs, such conduct being unbecoming and disgraceful to a pharmacist. (But it developed that the man could not be expelled from the Association because he had not paid his membership dues and therefore was not a member of the Association.)

The list of members for the year 1889 is given as 137 individuals, of whom 37 were present at this Meeting. And the list of those attending, along with those listed as members 1886-87-88-89 is attached in the *Proceedings*, including 131 names.

15th Annual Meeting—1890

The 15th Annual Meeting of the GPA was held in Macon, Georgia, July 15-16, 1890.

On February 14, 1890 an application for a charter for the Georgia Pharmaceutical Association was filed in the Court of Fulton County, Georgia. The application was signed by T. A. Cheatham, M. H. Taylor, R. H. Land, S. C. Durban, Theodore Schumann, J. W. Goodwyn, George D. Case, Harry Sharp, W. C. Kendrick, Osceola Butler, W. B. Shuptrine, E. M. Wheat, Geo. A. Bradford, Walter A. Taylor, and H. R. Slack. The Charter was granted on the 19th of March, 1890.

In his presidential address President Cheatham reviewed the history of the Association from its beginning in 1875.

Commenting about the need for a school of pharmacy in the State, Mr. Cheatham said:

"There is probably no subject of greater importance in our rising generation of pharmacists in the State than the formation of a school of pharmacy, either in connection with or separate from some chartered school or college."

He regretted that out of the large number of druggists in the State, so few were graduates in pharmacy and subscribed to or read any pharmaceutical literature of any kind, or manifested any interest whatsoever in the acquiring of any higher or more progressive knowledge.

Under the new Constitution, the matter before the Association was the election of officers. Mr. John W. Goodwyn, "a pharmacist and a gentleman," was named for the office of President. His nomination was seconded. There being no other nominations, Mr. Goodwyn was declared elected.

One of the wisest moves the Association had made up to that time was the election of Secretary Slack for a term of five years, instead of the one-year period that had prevailed before. Dr. Slack was very efficient and he is responsible for the fact that the *Proceedings* for the ten-year period just previous to this are available at this time.

A law had been passed calling for the election of members of the State Board of Pharmacy on a staggered-term basis. They were nominated as an entire Board for re-appointment. Mr. Slack was nominated for the long term of five years, and the others were elected for four, three, two, and one year.

Attention was called to the fact that now that the GPA was incorporated, the Association was entitled to representation in the United States Pharmacopoeial Convention. Mr. Goodwyn, Mr. Brunner, and Mr. Payne were named for this work.

[Author's Note: It will be recalled that in the first meeting of the Pharmacopoeial Convention, Dr. Joel Abbot and Dr. William Terrell were Georgia's representatives as charter members of the Convention.]

The Secretary of the State Board of Pharmacy, reporting for that year, (1890), called attention to the fact that 28 candidates had been examined and that 23 of them had passed. Five had failed. But the Board had noticed a marked improvement in the preparation that had been made by the young men coming up for examination. The fees paid in to the State Board for the year amounted to $192.50 and the expenses had been $102.70, leaving a net balance of $89.80, which divided equally among the five men, gave them $17.94 as their compensation for the year.

It was pointed out that under the Charter, the Pharmaceutical Association could now have honorary memberships. The following men were elected as honorary members, the first in the history of the Association.

Professor John Attfield
Professor William Simon
Professor D. M. R. Culbreth
Professor Charles F. Chandler
Professor P. W. Bedford
Professor J. P. Remington
Professor J. M. Maisch

The Secretary reported that this was the largest and best attended Meeting of the Association since *1885*.

16th Annual Meeting—1891

The 16th Annual Meeting of the GPA was held in Masonic Hall, Augusta, Georgia, on May 12-13, 1891. It was called to order by the President, J. W. Goodwyn, and new members numbering 24 were elected to the Association.

Secretary Slack reported also that he had attended a meeting in New Orleans recently, at which time 14 states had agreed to reciprocate licenses. These states were: Alabama, North Carolina, Georgia, Florida, Louisiana, Texas, Arkansas, Michigan, Wisconsin, Illinois, Kentucky, North and South Dakota, and Montana.

Mr. S. C. Durban, of Augusta, speaking on the subject, "Higher Standards For the Practice of Pharmacy," pointed out that a number of problems were involved, an important one of which was that physicians could get a license to practice pharmacy without having to take the examination. They are undesirable for the practice of pharmacy for "they have none of the heritage of pharmacy," he stated. He said further that "it is a gross injustice for the public as well as for the bona fide pharmaceutically trained people." He made one other strong statement, that there had been evidence that a person would actually go to a medical college to get the diploma so that he could practice pharmacy without having to undergo examination. This, he said, "is simply ridiculous."

At this Meeting, Dr. Slack resigned as Secretary of the Association because of his inability to carry the work longer. He had been licensed as a physician as well as a pharmacist, and he entered actively into the practice of medicine. Mr. H. H. Arrington, of Summerville, later of Rome, was elected to take Dr. Slack's place. Actually, the Association did not relieve Dr. Slack entirely because he was elected President of the Association for the coming year.

As Secretary of the State Board of Pharmacy, Dr. Slack reported that 20 applicants had come up for license during the year, and that 15 of them had passed. He stated: "We have issued this year 67 licenses, *a large majority of them being upon doctors' diplomas.*" He reported that each member of the Board received for his services that year $21.39.

Dr. Payne, discussing the tax situation confronting the druggists—and mentioning the city license tax, a state tax, a county tax, a city tax on medicines, a $25.00 tax to the U.S. Government for keeping alcohol, and a $50.00 state tax to the State on alcoholic stimulants, as well as a $30.00 city tax for putting any liquor in a prescription—points out that a physician can keep his own drugs and can prepare his own prescriptions. But if a druggist puts them up for him, the druggist has all these taxes to pay, whereas the physician pays none. He closes his remarks with the suggestion that the Pharmaceutical Association and the pharmacists in general demand the title of "Doctor of Pharmacy."

A vacancy in the State Board of Pharmacy existing, Dr. George F. Payne, who was also State Chemist at that time (1891), was nominated and elected to the Board of Pharmacy.

Secretary Slack, of the Board of Pharmacy, argued for "universal reciprocation" of licenses, so far as the U.S. was concerned. He stated: "Georgia leads with the oldest Board of Pharmacy in the United States." [Author's Note: Whether this statement can be substantiated is not known.]

Dr. Slack published an article in answer to the query, "Why Do Many Pharmacists Forsake Their Profession For the Study and Practice of Medicine?" It is interesting to note that Dr. Slack had done just this.

17th Annual Meeting—1892

The 17th Annual Meeting of the GPA was held in Columbus, Georgia, May 3-4, 1892.

President Slack, the presiding officer at this 17th Annual Meeting, had the meeting opened by prayer by the Rev. Robt. H. Harris, who offered a very fervent prayer. As far as can be determined, this is the first time an Annual Meeting of the GPA was opened with a prayer. In recent years this practice has been customary. But whether it has been customary every year since this beginning (in 1892) cannot be determined.

In his address Dr. Slack as President called attention to some progress that had been made over the years, mentioning particularly the fact that the State Board of Pharmacy and the Association, which had been separated by a feud, were now united; that the Board is now, under the law, subservient to the Pharmaceutical Association. He stated further that one of the "prime objects of our Association is to foster education" and that "steps have been taken to provide for a well-equipped college of pharmacy in the State." He says, meanwhile the Atlanta College of Pharmacy, prior to the establishment of a state college, "is a Georgia school in which pharmacy and its cognate sciences are ably taught."

The Committee on Trade Interests reports that though we have a number of pharmacy laws, covering the vending of drugs and medicines in the State, still they are violated in many sections, for there are "many stores not conducted by druggists which dealt wholesale in Laudanum, Paregoric, etc."

Dr. Slack, reporting again for the Committee on a School of

Pharmacy, stated that he had been in touch with the President of the Georgia School of Technology by letter, but that prior to his receiving an answer, a fire had destroyed one of the main buildings there, which probably took the mind of the President off the letter. He had in any case never received a reply. In the meantime, he had conferred with the Dean of the Faculty of the Atlanta College of Pharmacy, which had been established the previous year. He said that the Dean, George F. Payne, was afraid of some antagonism on the part of the Association to his college (which was associated with the Atlanta Medical College). He was assured by Dr. Slack that there was no such thought on the part of the Association, and that the Association had been working for a State institution but not fighting his.

Dr. Payne, Dean of the Faculty of the Atlanta College of Pharmacy, made the following statement: "I took this position with the Atlanta College of Pharmacy last year. Its charter empowers them to carry on a College of Medicine and a College of Pharmacy. Students in the College of Pharmacy have access to every lecture that goes on in the College. During the past year, the first of our existence, we had 15 students, which was a very creditable showing. Out of this 15, 4 came up for examination before this Board. One took a score of 95, two with 85, and the fourth was a man who had failed twice before the Board."

It was reported by the Legislative Committee that an amendment to the Pharmacy Law had been passed. It was no longer required to issue licenses to physicians or pharmacists simply on the basis of a diploma. All would be required to take the examination. It was agreed, however, that physicians who had graduated prior to 1887 and could prove continuous practice for five years were entitled to registration as pharmacists, without examination.

In the report of the Secretary of the Board of Pharmacy was the fact that the Board further "reports that the State provided $200.00 to be spent in enforcing the law against adulteration, and that the Board purchased the following items: suspected drugs—$25.00; apparatus for making assays, etc., the balance of the $200.00." These suspected drugs for examination were purchased in Augusta, Atlanta, Columbus, and LaGrange, from both druggists and doctors. Laudanum purchased from grocers in the first three cities was in every instance adultered, being but little over half-strength. There were no prosecutions because the grocers in each instance promised, and did stop handling drugs.

The Proceedings of this year (1892) carry a list of all persons licensed by the State Board of Pharmacy from 1887-1892. (The list of licensed pharmacists, as soon as it can be completed, will appear along with this material.) [Note: There is no record that this was done.]

A diligent search in the libraries of the State has not revealed any published Proceedings of the Georgia Pharmaceutical Association from 1892, the year of the 17th Annual Meeting, until 1903, when the 28th Annual Meeting of the GPA was held in Macon. Whether Proceedings were published for these intervening years we do not know at the present time. But it is recognized that it is unfortunate if carelessness has caused the importance of publishing the Proceedings to be overlooked, as well as of preserving them once they are published.

28th Annual Meeting—1903

The 28th Annual Meeting of the GPA was held in Macon, May 19-20, 1903.

The Meeting was called to order by President John A. Polhill, of Fitzgerald, Georgia. The Rev. W. N. Ainsworth (later to become Bishop Ainsworth) invoked the blessing of Almighty God upon the Convention.

Mr. J. B. Riley, of the wholesale firm in Macon, was Secretary at the time of this Meeting, and reported: "We have the largest list of applicants that I have ever known. We have 55 applications for membership." These names were read and elected unanimously. It so happens that the author was elected to membership in the Association at that time.

In his address President Polhill makes the following statement: "It is noted with pleasure that the cause of pharmaceutical education is advancing in the State." He is referring to the fact that a School of Pharmacy was opened that year at Mercer University in Macon, one at the University of Georgia at Athens, and a third at the Southern College at Atlanta, all these being in addition to the Atlanta College of Pharmacy, which had been operating since 1891.

The President also said that "Many pharmacists throughout the State are looking forward to the requirement of graduation from a school of pharmacy before one would be allowed to come before the State Board of Pharmacy for license. This is in line with the work being done in other professions and in fact is already being done in some of them. To these noble men throughout the State who have labored for the professional upbuilding of pharmacy we are under many obligations. Many of these men who were not graduates in pharmacy themselves have done much to support the graduation of younger pharmacists."

Since it was customary at that time to have three grades of pharmacy licenses, it may be well to describe them. The lowest grade license was called the "druggist license," the next in order was the "apothecary license" and the highest grade was the "pharmacist license." Mr. Polhill suggested here that this system should be discontinued, and have just one grade of "pharmacist" license. This did not take place, however, for a number of years.

The President called attention to the fact that Dr. George F. Payne a "Georgia Cracker" and prominent pharmacist of this State, Dean of the School of Pharmacy in Atlanta, former State Chemist, and member of the State Board of Pharmacy, had been elected as President of the American Pharmaceutical Association.

Various changes for the Pharmacy Law were discussed at length, and amendments were drawn, to be introduced in the Legislature, most of which were opposed by Dr. George F. Payne, even though he was a member of the Board of Pharmacy and Dean of the School at Atlanta. His objections to the proposed amendments were based primarily on the fact that the law provided that no person connected with a school of pharmacy could be a member of the State Board of Pharmacy. When the matter had come before the Legislature at the State Capital, Dr. Payne had brought a number of his students into the hearing in opposition to the proposed changes.

Some resolutions were adopted at that time:

1. Reaffirming the loyalty of this Association to N.A.R.D. and approving the "Direct Contract or Serial-Numbering Plan" authorized by the Cleveland Convention of that body and put into operation by the Miles Medical Company.

2. It is the consensus of this Association that all proprietary manufacturers claiming friendship for the Retail Drug Association should, at the earliest possible moment, adopt the Miles Plan.

It was reported that the State Board had licensed 97 persons in 1903.

29th Annual Meeting—1904

The 29th Annual Meeting of the GPA was held in Augusta, May 17-18, 1904.

President C. D. Jordan, in his presidential address, recommended that the Association consider the appointment of a Drug Inspector, whose duty shall not only be the inspection of drugs, but "the prosecution of those violating the pharmacy laws as regards the sale of Cocaine, and running drug stores without a license." This, he said, "could be accomplished by obtaining an appropriation from the State."

Mr. Jordan makes this statement referring to the new colleges of pharmacy recently organized in the State: "This is an actual demonstration that pharmacists are demanding higher education, and I hope these colleges will meet with your support." (Note: There were 4 such schools operating then.)

The report of the Secretary of the Georgia State Board of Pharmacy showed that there were a total of 80 licenses granted during the year 1904. Attention is called to the fact that for the first time Negroes came up for examination. The Secretary also calls attention to the fact that there have been 1600 men licensed according to the records of the Georgia State Board of Pharmacy. Many of these men, he warns, have died and others have moved from the State. He states that we have now in Georgia 1200 or more licensed men.

There is no record that a Proceedings was published for the year 1905.

31st Annual Meeting—1906

The 31st Annual Meeting of the GPA, held at Atlanta, was presided over by Mr. Max Morris of Macon.

President Morris makes the following statement:

"We have an excellent Pharmacy Law; yet it is null and void for lack of an enforcement clause with the necessary support behind it. Our Law should be so amended as to provide for the appointment of a Drug Inspector, whose duty it shall be to inspect every drug store once a year, give a certificate, collect a fee, and at the same time give a report of his work to the State Board of Pharmacy."

President Morris also comments that the N.A.R.D. has done much for the druggists of our State. "It has improved the condition of the retailers to such an extent that while heretofore the future has looked dark and unpromising, a ray of light has now appeared." He also reports that the N.A.R.D. will convene in Atlanta on October the fourth, 1906. He recommends that this Association appropriate a sum of money to be placed to the credit of the Atlanta Branch of the N.A.R.D., to be used for the entertainment of that body.

Thad Rice of Greensboro announced to the Meeting that the Southern Bell Telephone & Telegraph Company had offered free long-distance service from their long-distance lines before 10 o'clock each morning and after 4 o'clock each afternoon (from the Kimball House booth only).

The Secretary of the State Board of Pharmacy, Dr. G. F. Payne, reported that there were 139 examinations held that year, at $15.00 each, totalling $2,085.00. In addition to this, fees collected by the Board ran the total up to $2,599.00. This was divided among the five members of the Board, allowing for 10% to go to the Secretary's office for his expenses. The result was that each member of the Board received an average of $374.54 for the year's work.

Mr. W. S. Elkin, Junior, of Atlanta, Chairman of the Executive Committee, called attention to the fact that the previous year there had been passed a Bill imposing a tax of $1,000 by the Internal Revenue Department upon certain articles, among them Peruna. He stated that this matter was called to the attention of the Attorney-General of the State. The Attorney-General first ruled that this tax would have to be collected in Georgia, but later, that rule was rescinded and Georgia druggists did not have to pay this tax for that year to sell Peruna. It was charged that Peruna was not intended as a medicine, but was intended as an alcoholic beverage.

Mr. Jordan, Chairman of the Legislative Committee, reported that some funds had been raised for the purpose of prosecuting drug stores operating illegally, from druggists over the State. He reported that "we succeeded in stopping 14 drug stores in the State of Georgia which were operating without a license, and about 12 general stores. Most of these cases we were able to settle without prosecution; five we had to prosecute, two of which were still pending, and three were settled."

Attention was called to the fact that George D. Case, Narcotic Drug Inspector, had suggested that as a remedy for the enforcement of the pharmacy laws, "we have the next Legislature pass an Act requiring the judges of the various circuit courts in Georgia, in charging the Grand Juries, to read to them the pharmacy laws of the State and instruct the Grand Juries to see that every drug store operating has its license."

Dr. Henry P. Hinson, of Baltimore, appeared before the

Association and read a paper in which he recommended that the Doctorate Degree should be settled upon in pharmacy.

32nd Annual Meeting—1907

The 32nd Annual Meeting of the GPA met in the DeSoto Hotel in Savannah on May 21, 1907, and was called to order by the President, W. B. Freeman. The Rev. Bascom Anthony, Pastor of the Trinity Methodist Church of Savannah, gave the Invocation.

It seems that Mr. Max Morris of Macon was acting as Secretary at that time, and he reported 55 applications for membership at this Meeting.

President Freeman states that since the last Meeting "matters of the gravest concern to the drug trade have transpired." He goes on to say that the first item was the passage of the Pure Food and Drug Act, passed by the Federal Government, which became effective on January first of the present year. He states that Georgia was the first, or among the first, to pass a law similar to that of the Federal Government. And it was "due to the splendid work of our Legislature, whose work I now take occasion to compliment in the highest terms, that the objectionable features were largely eliminated and a satisfactory measure secured."

33rd Annual Meeting—1908

The 33rd Annual Meeting of the GPA met in the Mitchell Hotel in the City of Thomasville, May 19, 1908.

The Secretary of the Board of Pharmacy reported that there had been 130 applicants for license, 56 of these appearing to be re-examined. All told, there were 71 failures and 59 successful applicants. This is a significant statement: that at this meeting of the Board during the year 1907-08, there were *four women* applying for license, all four of them being successful. Two of them received the pharmacist's license, which was the highest degree license. There was one Negro man and one Negro woman, the Negro man receiving a druggist license. (Note: This appears to be the first time women applied for license.)

Mr. Rice, of Greensboro, Chairman of the Committee on Trade Interests, reported on the legislation that had been passed recently. He referred to the Narcotics Bill, which he says many druggists opposed, on account of the great number of remedies prohibited. But he states: "We believe that the law is gaining in favor since we are beginning to realize that its purposes are high, and, if enforced, will elevate humanity by practically stamping out the drug habit in the rising generation and prove a benefit instead of a hardship to these unfortunates who are already within its grip."

Mr. Rice said further, "Whenever a physician makes it a business to write Morphine and Cocaine prescriptions for so much per, that the druggists should turn him over to the authorities and see that he is prosecuted. For we believe that he is a menace to society and a disgrace to his profession."

Also he said that the Pure Food and Drug Laws are accepted as a fact and are operating as smoothly as possible so far as Georgia is concerned, and that their effect upon unmeritorious medicines has been wholesome, since the label must tell the truth."

The Laws referred to here will be commented upon under the heading, "The Pharmacy Laws of Georgia," in Supplement C of this volume.

34th Annual Meeting—1909

The 34th Annual Meeting of the GPA met in Macon on May 25, 1909, and was called to order by the President, Ben S. Persons. The Invocation was given by the Rev. T. D. Ellis, Pastor of the Mulberry Street Methodist Church.

President Ben Persons reported that the Legislative Committee had a busy year, and that they had succeeded in having passed at the last session of the Legislature, "our Bill creating the office of Drug Inspector" of the State of Georgia. This Bill had been before the House for three years but had been unsuccessful until this time when it was provided that the Drug Inspector should be appointed by the Commissioner of Agriculture, upon the recommendation of the Board of Pharmacy, who were to prescribe his duties: the report of all violations of the Pharmacy Laws of the State, and particularly, of anybody operating a drug store without a license, to be made to the Commissioner of Agriculture.

The necessity of putting the Drug Inspector under the Commissioner of Department of Agriculture was due to lack of appropriations for this purpose. But now the Commissioner of Agriculture had found it possible to pay his salary and expenses.

The State Drug Inspector, in making this the first of such reports, gave the following facts and figures: 923 inspections of drug stores and druggists licenses, 253 general stores, 103 grocery stores, and 55 wholesale grocery stores, and a few physicians' office suppliers and the manufacturing department of every wholesale druggist in the State. He stated: "I have found and reported to the Commissioner of Agriculture 33 druggists who were conducting drug stores without license, and of this number 14 remain to be proceeded against as the law directs. I have found 225 who kept no poison register, and 175 who did not have their licenses registered with the Ordinaries of the various counties as required by law. Of all the vexing and unsolved problems that I have had to contend with, the Narcotic Law is the most difficult and complicated. Not that the law is so complicated that it cannot be understood, but its enforcement is made difficult by the elasticity of the violators' consciences, and the far-reaching interpretations of the law as they interpret it. It is more difficult to secure evidence that will convict the violators, from the fact that when it becomes known, like it is among the moonshiners of the mountain sections of North Georgia, by a kind of wireless telegraphy that the Inspector is around, there immediately takes place a great moral upheaval, and a religious regard for the enforcement of the law to that extent. Assuming a look of (injured) innocence they will assure you that in their estimation a man who would under any circumstances violate this great and good law deserves a visit from the night riders, to be hung without trial by jury."

The Secretary of the Board of Pharmacy reported that 92 licenses were issued during the year. He stated: "Only one lady applied for a license. She received the highest grade. There were three Negro men applying for license, one of whom received the druggist license. Also, there was one Negro woman who received a druggist license."

The Chief Chemist of the Department of Agriculture reported as follows on samples of drugs taken up by the Drug Inspector: (The Assay processes of the U.S.P. and the N.F. were used.) — 25 samples of Fowler's Solution were all below standard; all samples of Syrup of Ferrous Iodide were below standard; of 56 samples of Tincture of Iodine, 45 were classed as illegal since they varied in strength from 17.9% of the proper strength to 129% of the proper strength.

It was pointed out at this Meeting that Mr. W. S. Elkin, Junior, of Atlanta had been elected President of N.A.R.D. for the year 1909.

℞ SUPPLEMENT D

35th Annual Meeting—1910

The 35th Annual Meeting of the GPA was held in Athens, June 8-9, 1910. The Rev. E. L. Hill, Pastor of the First Presbyterian Church, delivered the Invocation.

In his address President Thad Rice had this to say about the itinerant drug vendors: "These sharks have been driven from other states by wise laws, and are flocking to Georgia in large numbers; they prey upon the ignorant white people and strip them of their hard-earned dollars. Their methods are too well known to require any explanation from me, and I would recommend that every druggist in Georgia take this up with his Representative or Senator and get them interested in this subject, because they may not see this evil as we do."

State Drug Inspector Cheatham reported: "I have found *975* drug stores where licensed men were in charge of the store, as required by law. But I found 175 druggists who were exempt from the operation of the law, and 50 druggists who conducted their business in open violation of the law by not having licensed men in charge of same. Of these I have reported to the Commissioner of Agriculture and the State Board of Pharmacy. Since that time all of these violators have complied with the law by placing licensed men in charge of their stores except six (6), and these are now being looked after by the Commissioner and the State Board of Pharmacy."

The Secretary of the Board of Pharmacy reported for that year (1910) that there were *117* successful applicants for license. Included therein were 4 women, 3 of whom were successful. Seven Negro men applied for license, 4 of whom were successful.

A resolution was adopted by the Association, pledging the pharmacists of the State to favor the enactment of a law governing the practice of Optometry.

Professor Sellers (of Mercer University), Chairman of a committee to consider a resolution introduced by Mr. John Montgomery, having to do with the education of pharmacists in Georgia, made this recommendation:

That the Georgia law be changed as follows: "In lieu of Section 1496, Paragraphs 1 and 2, the GPA petitions the General Assembly of the State of Georgia to substitute the following: 1. That licenses be granted to such graduates of a reputable college of pharmacy who shall have passed a satisfactory examination before such Board of Pharmacy, and, in addition, shall have presented such certification sworn to by a Notary Public showing that they have also had two years' practical experience under the supervision of a licensed pharmacist, and 2. Licenses to such physicians and graduates of a regular medical college, as shall have passed a satisfactory examination before said Board of Pharmacy."

The members of this Committee on Educational Requirements were: Messrs. Jordan, Persons, Hood, Elkin, Montgomery, Wilson, and Sellers.

Secretary Max Morris of the Association and Mr. Herman Shuptrine of Savannah, who was a member of the Legislature at this time, opposed the resolution, with the argument that an equal chance was not given to the *poor boy who does not have the opportunity to go to college.*

36th Annual Meeting—1911

The 36th Annual Meeting of the GPA was held at Indian Springs, Georgia, on the 13th of May, 1911, and was called to order by President Joe P. Walker.

President Walker reported that "our Anti-Narcotic Law is defective in that it still permits the sale of teething powders and soothing syrups containing narcotic drugs." He therefore calls for a revision of that phase of the Narcotic Law.

He also calls attention to the fact that some manufacturers are paying physicians a commission or bonus on the sale of the "nostrums" which they prepare. He points out that these manufacturers do not sell to the jobbers, but direct to one or two retail druggists in a town or city to whom the subsidized physician sends his prescriptions.

Secretary Jordan of the Board of Pharmacy stated that the Georgia Board approved the principle of reciprocation of license from one state to another, under proper safeguards for all the states involved. During that year (1911) *61* licenses were interchanged involving the Georgia Board.

For the first time someone called attention to the fact that the Georgia Pharmaceutical Association should have representation on the State Board of Health. [Note: This did not result until a number of years later.]

A disturbed speaker wanted the following bill introduced: "That we take definite steps to make it a misdemeanor for a doctor who lives within three miles of a drug store operated by a licensed pharmacist to fill his own prescriptions unless he has a state license to practice pharmacy."

Dr. T. A. Cheatham, the State Chief Drug Inspector, was named Secretary at this Meeting, since Mr. Ben S. Persons of Macon resigned this office. Mr. Thad Rice of Greensboro was named Treasurer to succeed Mr. J. T. Shuptrine, who had resigned.

37th Annual Meeting—1912

The 37th Annual Meeting of the GPA assembled at the DeSoto Hotel Ballroom in Savannah, on the 11th of June, 1912 at 11 o'clock. The Meeting was called to order by the Second Vice-President of the Association, J. W. Ridout of Macon, the President, Mr. John Montgomery of Thomasville having removed from the State, and the First Vice-President E. W. Johnson of Carrollton having been providentially detained from the Meeting.

Dr. Brigham addressed the Association on the subject, "An Ideal Education For Druggists." He stated: "An education is not a fact of existence; it must become an accomplished thing. It is merely a process, and is a never-ending process; literally, a drawing out from the individual; a development of his various faculties."

He pointed out that the educated man is not the man who can quote various facts and figures, but one who knows where to find information and proceeds to find it.

It was reported at this Meeting that Mr. Herman Shuptrine of Savannah had been elected as President of the N.A.R.D. A resolution was read from the Association expressing recognition of "this high honor that had come to one of our pharmacists." Mr. W. S. Elkin of Atlanta had previously served as President. It appears from the record that these men are the only two from Georgia who have served in the N.A.R.D. in this capacity.

A further resolution was adopted calling on the newspapers of the State, in writing up cases of suicide from the taking of poisons, not to mention the name of the poison, due to the fact that it suggests itself to other people who might be tempted to try a like method of suicide.

Secretary Jordan of the Board of Pharmacy reported that there were 234 applicants for license, and that 153 were successful during the year (1912). One lady had applied for examination and was successful. Four Negroes had applied, three of whom were successful.

The State Drug Inspector reported that the State had just cause for congratulations on the improved drug conditions as they existed in 1912 "compared to what they were three years ago."

A rather startling resolution was presented to this effect: "That in our humble opinion it is not safe for physicians to make a practice of using the telephone in giving prescriptions to the busy druggist. While we deeply appreciate every effort of the doctor to help us in our arduous work, still we would urge that physicians use every effort to protect druggists against this universal practice."

38th Annual Meeting—1913

The 38th Annual Convention of the GPA was presided over by President J. W. Ridout, of Macon. The Meeting was held in the Superior Courtroom of the Muscogee County Court, Columbus, Georgia, on the 10th of June, 1913.

President Ridout reported that one of the most "important results in the way of legislation that has been accomplished in recent years is the Narcotic Law. And we must not shut our eyes to the responsibility for the enforcement of this Law."

Mr. Cheatham, as Secretary of the Association and also the Chief Drug Inspector, had this to say in his report:

"In the suppression of this evil (the Narcotic evil) I have invited the assistance of the Judges of the various courts, the Sheriff of each county of the State, and the Chiefs of Police in cities and towns where this damning traffic is carried on and to some extent the sale has been lessened. The sale of Narcotic drugs is the most serious problem which the State and Nation have to deal with today, and its solution will have to be worked out by laws not yet enacted and perhaps not yet devised."

[Author's Note: The Harrison Anti-Narcotic Act was soon to follow.]

An unusual feature of this particular Convention is indicated by the following item:

AN AUTOMOBILE RIDE FOR THE LADIES

[But the weather did not permit.]

℞ SUPPLEMENT D

39th Annual Meeting—1914

The 39th Annual Meeting of the GPA was held at Indian Springs on June 9-10, 1914, and was called to order by President R. C. Wilson.

President Wilson pointed out in his address that state and national bodies seemed to have been in "a regulative frame of mind" during the past year, endeavoring to regulate everything from the larger Trusts on down. "Pharmacy has not escaped, for there have been something over 20 measures introduced over the past year which directly or indirectly affect the retail drug business."

Pointing out that rumors were afloat that there was considerable criticism in the State about our system of drug inspection, the President made this observation: "The Drug Inspectors are powerless to carry on this work unsupported by us. They stand ready and willing to make drug inspection work real and efficient —just as real and just as efficient as is indicated by the support of the retail druggists of Georgia."

The President made a number of recommendations, among them a revision of the Pharmacy Laws, and some changes to be made which will keep the membership in the Association uniform from year to year, a change in the method of election of officers and Board members, and limiting the term of Board members to one term of five years each. Also, that Board members be paid on a per diem basis rather than on a fee basis as prevailed up to this time.

The Secretary of the Board of Pharmacy reported that there were 326 applicants during the year for license. Of this number 162 were successful. It will be borne in mind that during this period when so many were coming up for license the "Quiz Schools" were active in the State, and many applicants were coming into Georgia from other states to get a license and then to reciprocate out. At that time, it must be remembered, there were no educational requirements whatever as a preliminary to examination.

It was at this Meeting that the Traveling Men's Auxiliary was accepted as an affiliate of the GPA, and the Charter members of this Auxiliary were the following: John H. Vinson, Macon; W. R. Bell, Atlanta; T. B. Lewis, Atlanta; A. I. Jesup, Columbus; A. H. Walden, Atlanta; W. J. Deas, Augusta; J. J. Franz, Tampa; A. M. Hitt, Savannah; R. C. Head, Atlanta;

W. M. Meadows, Macon; C. C. Tunison, Macon; O. L. Johnson, Athens; J. T. Wages, Winder; T. A. Cheatham, Macon.

40th Annual Meeting—1915

The 40th Annual Convention of the GPA was held at Tybee Island, Georgia, June 8-9, 1915.

The Meeting was called to order by President W. A. Pigman.

Dr. W. F. Brunner, Health Officer of the City of Savannah, presented a brief address in which he criticized the indiscriminate prescribing of narcotic drugs, and the sale of these items by pharmacists of the State. He called upon the pharmacists of the State Association to begin some steps looking toward remedying this situation. Following his address, there was much discussion and criticism of his personal references. But eventually, it was recognized as being a wholesome, worthwhile address, with the final result that the drug (narcotic) situation in Georgia was very much improved.

Mr. A. O. Blalock, Collector of Internal Revenue for the State of Georgia, addressed the group, calling on the doctors and druggists of the State to do something about the narcotic situation in Georgia, and to formulate a State Law that would be strong enough to help carry out the National Law, which we now know as the Harrison Anti-Narcotic Act, passed in 1914.

Mr. George D. Case, the Narcotic Inspector in Mr. Blalock's office, reported many violations of the State Narcotic Law. "I think I have filed in Mr. Blalock's office as many as 5,000 prescriptions which showed a spirit of crookedness, which evidenced a desire to make money out of the sale of Narcotic drugs."

In discussing the Harrison Law, President Pigman stated that "this Law will lead to the *disenthrallment* of more dope victims than anything that has ever been done for them."

Mr. Case raised the question as to whether there were too many druggists in Georgia. He was convinced that "it is a fact."

Mr. Shuptrine, in discussing the matter of the Harrison Law, said: "Unless we can amend the Harrison Law so that a doctor cannot under any circumstances fill his own prescriptions for Narcotics, the Law will be ineffective."

41st Annual Meeting—1916

The 41st Annual Convention of the GPA met in Atlanta and was called to order by the President, Samuel E. Bayne, of Macon.

℞ SUPPLEMENT D 369

President Bayne called attention to the fact that there were more than 1500 druggists in Georgia, and there were less than 500 who were members of the Association, and he appealed to the present membership to devise some method of drawing a large membership.

In a discussion of the Harrison Anti-Narcotic Law, it was brought out that the sale of Godfrey's Cordial, Bateman's Drops and Paregoric, all of which contain Opium in small amounts, should be prohibited by law in stores other than drug stores.

Mr. Ivan Allen of Atlanta, a business man with a national reputation, addressed the Association, saying among other items the following:

"The things you read today and the things you think today are the things you will become tomorrow. You are a composite of the things you say, the books you read, the thoughts you think, the company you keep, and the things you aspire to become."

Secretary Cheatham, in his report, called attention to the fact that the Proceedings could not be published without funds arising from the sale of advertising space. (Note: This must not have been attended to at this Meeting, 1915, for there was a lapse of several years before printed Proceedings again appeared, and no record can be found of Proceedings during that interim.)

The Drug Inspector, Dr. Cheatham, reports an interesting item: "In the year 1915-16 there are still in the State 150 druggists who are exempt from having a license recorded." (This was probably a hang-over from the original law, when it was passed, which permitted those who had been in practice for a certain number of years to be automatically licensed.)

42nd Annual Meeting—1917

The 42nd Annual Meeting of the GPA convened in the City of Macon at the usual time in the Spring, H. D. Bell of Albany presiding as President. But no copies of the Proceedings of this Annual Convention have been found preserved, if any were published.

43rd Annual Meeting—1918

The 43rd Annual Meeting of the GPA convened in the Pavilion of the Hotel Tybee, Tybee Island, Georgia, on June 18, 1918. The Convention was called to order by President I. A. Solomons, Junior, of Savannah.

Mr. Case, the Narcotic Inspector of the State representing Mr. Blalock's office, made several statements before the Association which are worth recording: "If there is any species of temptation that affects humanity that is worse than addiction to Narcotic drugs, my God, I don't know what it is. My business as an officer in these investigations to attempt to enforce the provisions of this Act has thrown me in touch with this situation for the past three years. All of us who have read Bunyan's *Pilgrim's Progress* know that whenever you get into a hole and attempt to get out, and it seems impossible to get out, you are seized with utter despondency and despair. Narcotic addiction is just exactly what is described and portrayed in Bunyan's *Pilgrim's Progress*."

Dr. Cheatham, in reporting as Drug Inspector, says that in view of the War conditions, and in view of the fact that many of the younger men have been called into the Service, he fears that many of the drug stores will have to be closed for lack of licensed men to conduct them.

Mr. Persons, in reporting for the Board of Pharmacy, calls attention to the shortage of licensed personnel, and says that the Board of Pharmacy has been more lenient in the grading of examination papers in this period than ever before, in an effort to issue as many licenses as possible and still stay within proper limits of safety, so far as the public is concerned. He also states that he thinks it inadvisable to make any changes in the Pharmacy Law during this period, but to wait until after the War and things become normal again, and we begin to raise the educational standard for pharmacists in Georgia.

44th Annual Meeting—1919

The 44th Annual Convention of the GPA convened at the Hotel Tybee, Tybee Island, Georgia, on June 10, 1919 and was called to order by President T. F. Burbank, of Cedartown. The Invocation was delivered by the Rev. Dr. McLaurin, of Savannah.

Mr. Ben S. Persons of Macon, addressing the group, states that he comes not as a member of the Board of Pharmacy, and its Secretary, but as a druggist. He tells the group that "education for pharmacy in the State and in the United States is a 'must,' if pharmacy is ever to be recognized as a profession on a comparable basis to medicine and the other professions." He proposes that the Drug Inspector, (who then operated under the

Department of Agriculture) be placed under the Board of Pharmacy.

[Author's Note: Actually, it was 20 or more years before the pharmacists of the State were successful in pushing this matter through the Legislature. The failure to secure favorable legislation was due to the presence in the Legislature of several elderly physicians who opposed such legislation.]

Mr. Persons also proposed that the members of the Board of Pharmacy be paid on a per diem basis and not on a fee basis, as at present. This likewise was postponed for a number of years, but in the main Mr. Persons' recommendations were eventually carried out, and even exceeded in importance the objectives he had in mind at that time. Various persons present who were members of the organization endorsed what Mr. Persons had to say, including Mr. Case and Mr. E. L. Murray, of Americus, and Mr. D. G. Wise, of Atlanta. Mr. Wise, approving the suggestions that had been proposed, suggested that a committee composed of Messrs. Wilson, Persons, and Shuptrine be appointed to draft the changes in the legislation in accordance with the suggestions made by Mr. Persons.

[Author's Note: The recommendations of Mr. Persons, endorsed by so many of the others in the Association, regarding the matter of education, were the first concrete step toward improving educational conditions for the licensure and practice of pharmacy in Georgia.]

45th Annual Meeting—1920

The 45th Annual Convention of the GPA was held in Macon, Georgia, at the Dempsey Hotel, June 8, 1920.

The Secretary of the Board of Pharmacy reported the number of applicants for license for that year was 345. Of this number 229 were successful. The Board members were still operating on a fee basis. Each man received $791.00 for his services in holding three meetings of the Board of Pharmacy for that year.

In his presidential address, Mr. W. T. Knight, Senior, as President stated that in his opinion the dues in the Association ought to be raised from $2.00 to $25.00, and that a full-time field secretary of the Association should be employed, saying: "Let's pay him a salary for the work he can and will do." He was a number of years ahead of his time in making this recommendation.

46th Annual Meeting—1921

The 46th Annual Convention of the GPA assembled in the Auditorium of Atlanta, Georgia, on July 6, 1921. The Meeting was called to order by the President, D. G. Wise, of Atlanta.

At this time, it was decided that the Meeting would be opened by the singing of one verse of the song, "America," with Mr. Al Walden, of Atlanta, leading the singing. This was the first instance on record of the Georgia Pharmaceutical Association being opened with singing, and it came to be a custom which was to extend for many years thereafter.

In the welcoming address Mayor James L. Key, of Atlanta, stated that he had been acquainted with the drug business "from its almost prehistoric days, since my father was a country doctor and was his own pharmacist, and in that way I became acquainted with the drug business in its almost primeval state."

The Secretary of the Board of Pharmacy reported that there were 449 applicants before the Board during the year, and that 278 of these were successful.

At this 46th Meeting the proposed law written by Mr. Persons and his committee was read, and it was pointed out in the presentation of the Bill that it had not been drawn by the colleges but had been drawn primarily by the members of the Board of Pharmacy, and that no one could profit by the legislation. But that, on the other hand, each member of the Board of Pharmacy would sacrifice from the passage of the Bill because it was proposed in the Bill that each member of the Board would now be put on a per diem basis rather than on a fee basis. That for the past several years the Board members had received $900 each for a few days' work. But that, under the system provided in the new Bill, they would be on a per diem basis. Copies of the proposed law were passed out among the members and, since the law had to be voted on it was suggested that the law be read paragraph by paragraph. Mr. Jordan, of Monticello, suggested however, that since there was only one section of the Bill about which there was any controversy, that section only should be read. Mr. Cheatham, the Secretary, then read the section in question, which had to do with the qualifications for license. Mr. Jordan opposed the requirements, and made this statement: "I would rather have a man come out of Ben Persons' store and know that Ben stood over him and taught him prescription work than have a graduate from the Philadelphia College of Pharmacy. I would take him, and most of you would do the same thing. This is the man I'm trying to protect, the man who has not the money to get an education, and has gotten it from experience taught to him by an experienced man." Other druggists opposed that section, but Mr. Jones, Mr. Johnston, Mr. Wilson, Mr. Marshall, Mr. Murray, Mr. Williams of Macon, Mr. Billingslea, and Mr. Dunwoody, of Atlanta, favored the Bill. And when the vote was called, the section under discussion was carried overwhelmingly.

47th Annual Meeting—1922

The 47th Annual Convention of the GPA assembled on Tybee Island on June 20, 1922. The Meeting was called to order by the President, Mr. Jabe Stamps.

In his presidential address Mr. Stamps called attention to the fact that the law which had been introduced in the Legislature setting up new standards for licensure had been defeated because the country legislators felt that the education clause in the Bill was discriminating against the people from the country.

It was reported that the number of applicants for license this year (1922) was 530, and that 358 of these had been granted license, and that $1,125.25 had been paid to each of the Board of Pharmacy members as their portion of the receipts from the fees for this number of examinations. The report pointed out that the large number of persons who received their licenses included many coming from out of Georgia, and these had come up for Georgia license to get around the requirements in their own states. Then, getting a Georgia license, they hoped to reciprocate out.

It was reported at this Meeting by the Committee on Necrology that Dr. George D. Case, one of the founders of this Association, and one of the most active pharmacists in the State, had died during the year. The committee also reported the names of the following: Mr. H. R. Palmer, Athens; Mr. John S. Hoge, Macon; and Mr. Louis S. Dozier, LaGrange.

Mr. Tom Marshall, of Atlanta, discussing a legislative Bill on the subject of education, stated that in 1921 there were 488 applicants for license in Georgia; and at the same time there were only 42 in North Carolina, 16 in South Carolina, 63 in Tennessee, 63 in Florida, and 70 in Alabama. Mr. Marshall further stated: "That is the proportion they are running." He pointed out that these people would come to Georgia because of the low educational requirements, and that Georgia was coming to be the "dumping ground" for the poorly educated pharmacists of the nation, getting a license here and not being able to reciprocate out. That "in the State of Georgia there was said to be about 1 druggist for every 500 citizens, with the result that nobody can make a living."

A strong plea was made for the individual members of the Association, particularly those from the country counties, to try to influence their legislators to favor the pharmacy bill which was to raise the educational requirements.

48th Annual Meeting—1923

The 48th Annual Convention of the GPA met in the Ballroom of the Richmond Hotel, Augusta, Georgia, on the 12th of June, 1923. The Meeting was called to order by President H. C. Shuptrine, of Savannah.

There were 35 applicants for membership in the Association, including the name of Dr. Joseph Jacobs, of Atlanta, who had been a member of the Georgia Association, had withdrawn, and was reelected at this Meeting.

The Secretary of the Board of Pharmacy reported that there were 353 applicants for license that year, of which number 123 passed.

The Secretary of the Board of Pharmacy read the following resolution:

"WHEREAS the educational requirements of adjoining states to this State for admitting applicants to pharmacy had been raised to such a standard as to make reciprocity between the State and adjoining states undesirable to our sister states, and,

"WHEREAS this is due to low standards of educational requirements in this State, and is embarrassing to licentiates of this State and also to members of the Board of Pharmacy of this State;

"THEREFORE, BE IT RESOLVED by the members of the Board of Pharmacy in executive session, on this the second day of April, 1923, that on and after the 15th day of June, 1923, the Georgia Board of Pharmacy shall require all applicants for admission to the Pharmacy Examination an educational requirement equal to two years of high school training, and,

"RESOLVED further, that the applicant be required to file with the Secretary of the Georgia Board of Pharmacy proof of this high school work on or before date of examination, which proof shall be in the form of a certificate from principal of high school, or secretary of the Board of Education of the town or county school commissioner of the county in which the school is located;

"BE IT FURTHER RESOLVED, that a copy of this resolution be sent to the National Association of Boards of Pharmacy, the Secretaries of the Boards of Pharmacy of adjoining states, and to the interested Schools of Pharmacy; and,

"BE IT FURTHER RESOLVED, that a copy of this resolution shall be printed by the Secretary in his next annual report to the Georgia Pharmaceutical Association."

(Signed) Henry D. Bell, *President*
E. L. Murray, *Secretary*

(The Seal of the Association accompanied this resolution.)

Mr. D. G. Wise, of Atlanta, offered a motion that the Association endorse the resolution and the action of the Board of Pharmacy. But Mr. Cheatham raised the question as to whether the Board had the authority to pass such a resolution. Mr. Murray, the Secretary, stated that the Board did have that power. Mr. Cheatham stated that if they did not have the power he wanted to make a motion that the law be amended so that they would have the power.

There followed a heated discussion about the proposed two-year high school requirement, but Mr. Shuptrine took the floor as President and argued for a four-year course (or a minimum of 15 Carnegie units). This was supported by various members of the Board and by various other members of the Association. It was opposed by a very few. But on the standing vote, there were 32 who voted to raise the educational requirements to graduation from high school (or 15 units) and only 2 voted against it. The resolution voted by the Board of Pharmacy was then read, as amended, calling for four years instead of two years' high school work.

Mr. Wise reported that a questionnaire had been sent to the druggists of the State to get the amount of taxes they were paying, and that, of the 322 drug stores replying to the questionnaire, he estimated that the drug stores now paid in $925,000 in special taxes per year. And that, if all the thousand druggists in the State had reported, the amount of the taxes would run well over one million in these special taxes. This did not include the ad valorem tax.

Mr. Wise also reported that the Pharmacy Education Bill

had been killed on the last night of the last Session of the House, even though it had passed the Senate without opposition.

President Shuptrine made this observation: "One of the reasons why 75% to 90% of the druggists are not here at this Meeting is that 75% to 90% of the druggists of this State do not have even a high school education. That's the same proportion, that, when we raise the standards of men who are qualified to take the Board, we will at the same time raise the entire standard of the drug business throughout the State of Georgia." He argued: "This is the only way to keep progress going, to continue to raise the educational requirements."

Mr. A. R. Munn said that there should be something in the law that would make it impossible for a person to use the term "drug store," "pharmacy," "apothecary" or any other sign that would be misleading to the public, unless the store was operated by a licensed pharmacist. Several years thereafter such a law was passed, and the signs in drug-department stores, or department stores, or what-not, were taken down for lack of a licensed man in charge.

There was considerable discussion of the possibility of the passage of a law prohibiting chain drug store operations in Georgia, with the statement that very few of the chain stores operated in that period.

Discussing this whole matter of chain store operation, cut prices, et cetera, Mr. Mack Hodges of Marietta stated that in his town there were four drug stores, and never one item was cut in price. He said he believed that the answer to this problem is that Georgia needs a full-time competent Secretary on a full-time basis to keep the druggists in the Association posted about the various problems and how to meet them. But Mr. Marshall of Atlanta proposed that the Association discontinue fighting the chain stores, and get them to come in and join us and work with us in building our profession of pharmacy in the State.

50th Annual Meeting—1925

The 50th Annual Meeting of the GPA was held on Tybee Island, Georgia, June 15-16, 1925. The Session was called to order by the President, Jasper L. Brooks. The Invocation was given by the Rev. Silas Johnson of Tybee.

Secretary Cheatham reported that he as the official Secretary was "unable to have the Proceedings printed last year. The lowest price that I received from any printer was $625, and the largest amount that I had ever collected from advertisements in the Proceedings was $400. I didn't see where I could raise that deficit of $225." Therefore, there are no Proceedings for the year preceding, i. e., 1924.

Mr. H. C. Thompson, Manager of the Liggett chain of drug stores in Atlanta, addressed the group on the matter of organization. So far as can be determined from the records, this is the first time a representative of a national chain drug store had participated in the activities of the Association.

Mr. Walter D. Jones, of Savannah, addressing the Convention, stated that one trouble with the drug business was that too many people were being allowed to come into the drug store without any educational requirement. "Under the laws qualifying him for examination, a soda jerker can spend three years behind the fountain of a drug store and then qualify as a druggist. He then gets financed and opens up a store of his own, and becomes a competitor of his old employer." Later in the discussion, Mr. Jones pointed out that his remarks "were more particularly directed at the 'three months school' (or the man who comes from the three months' school of pharmacy)."

Unfortunately, there seem to be no printed Proceedings of the 51st Annual Meeting of the GPA.

52nd Annual Meeting—1927

The Proceedings of this 52nd Annual Meeting were not published, but there is a typewritten account of the Minutes by Mr. Cruselle, Stenographer and Reporter, who took the following notes in shorthand and then transcribed them.

The 52nd Annual Meeting of the GPA was held in the Opera House in the City of Athens, May 23-25, 1927. The Meeting was called to order by President A. R. Munn. The Invocation was given by the Rev. W. P. King, of the First Methodist Church, Athens.

The address of welcome was given by Dean R. C. Wilson, of the School of Pharmacy at the University of Georgia, and also by Mayor A. G. Dudley, Athens, and by Chancellor Charles M. Snelling on behalf of the University, and by Dr. A. M. Soule of the State College of Agriculture.

Mr. Fred Bridges had been elected Secretary of the Association, succeeding Mr. Hohenstein, who had served for one year. Like Mr. Hohenstein, Mr. Bridges was not a pharmacist but a public relations man.

As Secretary, Mr. Bridges reported that "we have 600 to 700 new members," stating that in the City of Augusta every druggist belongs to the Association and the same is true of Savannah.

Mr. A. R. Munn, serving his second term as President, stated in his annual address: "At the time of our Savannah Meeting in 1925 our membership totalled around 100 members, dues paid. In Macon the total membership reached 250. And today, my friends, your Association can proudly boast of more than 800 dues-paid members. And I challenge any man, in or out of this great State, to doubt the sincerity, aggressiveness, and enthusiasm of this body of high-toned gentlemen."

Mr. Munn also proposed that for the Association to render its full measure of usefulness, it should function the year round. To carry this into effect, he recommended the creation of a Board of Directors, who would be empowered to act for the Association between meetings. This Board would meet at stated intervals or at the call of the President for the transaction of Association business. He stated further that the success of the Association for this year, and the large membership, was due to the untiring efforts of Mr. Bridges, Secretary-Treasurer. He recommended that Mr. Bridges be employed on a full-time basis as Secretary-Business Manager of the Association.

Mr. Munn called attention to the work of the Women's Auxiliary under the leadership of Miss Rose Grier, who was one of the first licensed woman proprietors of a drug store, and the work of the Traveling Men's Association also. He stated that plans were to be completed at this Meeting for the permanency of the Women's Auxiliary.

President Munn proposed that congratulations and encouragement be extended to the School of Pharmacy at the University of Georgia for its advancement of the cause of pharmacy throughout the State of Georgia, for the School had abolished its short-term courses and gone exclusively to the four-year requirement for graduation. He pointed out that this School was the first in the United States to adopt the minimum four-year requirement.

The Secretary of the Board of Pharmacy, Mr. Claude Rountree, reported that up to this time the Board had required only two years of high school work. But that beginning in January of this next year a new procedure would prevail:

"A person who had three years of actual work under the supervision of a licensed pharmacist, and who had the equivalent of 15 Carnegie Units of high school training, would be entitled to examination by the Georgia Board. But in the event he cannot supply the practical end of it, and is coming to the Board with a college diploma, it is required that he be graduated from a recognized college that has a required course of not less than 3 years."

The Resolutions Committee proposed that, following a suggestion from the President, the Constitution and By-Laws of the Association be amended to include the naming of a Board of Directors, one from each Congressional District. That an Executive Committee of five, quorum of which might act for or on behalf of the Board in emergencies, be formed. The Board of Directors were directed to redraft the Constitution and By-Laws of the Association to conform to the changes which have been made or may be made in the form of organization, and that the Association should have a full-time paid Secretary. That the Board of Directors shall consider any changes needed in the Pharmacy Law, and that these changes be embodied in a proposed Pharmacy Law, to be passed at the next Session of the General Assembly. Also, that the Law be amended so that all pharmacists in the State pay an annual registration of $10.00, which would include dues in the Association. That the payment of this fee of $10.00 automatically would give all the rights and privileges in the Association. Failure to pay this fee would automatically forfeit the right to practice pharmacy in the State.

[Author's Note: This law, as stated, was considered but was declared unconstitutional.]

As regards the Secretaryship of the Association, it was pointed out that the Secretary of the Association was to be employed by the Board of Directors and not elected by the Association.

53rd Annual Meeting—1928

The 53rd Annual Meeting of the GPA was convened in the Court House in Columbus, on Wednesday, June 6, 1928. The Meeting was called to order by President A. R. Munn, and was promptly led in the song "America" by Al Walden.

In his presidential address, President Munn set up five objectives:

1. A sensible and clearly defined method for pharmacists to show their allegiance to the Association and to the profession.

2. Encouragement toward increased membership.
3. Provision for full secretarial service.
4. A definite legal protection for registered pharmacists.
5. Provisions for adequate financing.

The President pointed out that the pharmacists of Georgia "have kept faith with the founders of the Association, who 53 years ago banded together as the Georgia Pharmaceutical Association for the noble purpose of advancing the science and the art of pharmacy, and for the development of pharmacy as a profession."

In his recommendation regarding the Board of Pharmacy, President Munn stated the following:

1. That members of the Board of Pharmacy be compensated for their work on an ample per diem basis, rather than on the fee basis which had prevailed.
2. That the enforcement of the Pharmacy Law, as well as those Sections of the Food and Drug Law as relate to the practice of pharmacy, be transferred from the Food and Drug Division of the Department of Agriculture to the Board of Pharmacy where it rightfully belongs.
3. That in the Pharmacy Law which was proposed for passage, any balance in the Treasury of the Board of Pharmacy be automatically transferred to the Treasury of the State Association so that it may render better service to the State, and to pharmacists.
4. He further pointed out that under the new Law, it was a misdemeanor to practice pharmacy in the State of Georgia under a license which is not registered annually.

The report of the Legislative Committee by Mr. T. C. Marshall showed that the drug law which had been proposed the year before had been passed, but that in the process of passage through the Legislature, the Bill was secretly amended so as to eliminate all the educational requirements which the State Board of Pharmacy had recently established. That in 1929, it would be necessary to amend the present law to restore the educational requirements.

Under the new system of election of Board members whereby the Association was to nominate only one man for the Board (under the law which specified that the Governor had to appoint the nominee), Mr. W. T. Edmunds of Augusta was the person this year (1928) who received the highest number of votes. His name was passed on to the Governor for appointment.

℞ SUPPLEMENT D

54th Annual Meeting—1929

The 54th Annual Convention of the GPA was held at the Court House in the City of Valdosta, April 17-18-19, 1929. The Convention was called to order by President A. R. Munn.

It was pointed out that during the year Secretary Bridges had resigned and R. C. Wilson, of Athens, was named Secretary and Treasurer by the Board of Directors.

The next item on the Program was the presidential address by President A. R. Munn. This was the fourth consecutive year in which Mr. Munn had been President, the only time in the Association's history that a man had been named for consecutive terms, nor has it happened since that a man should succeed himself as President.

Mr. Claude Rountree of Thomasville reported that his representative in the Legislature had notified him that the Governor had called a meeting of various officials to meet in Atlanta to discuss a number of matters. Among these was a movement to transfer the Drug Inspection work from the Department of Agriculture to the Department of State Board of Health. Mr. Rountree argued that "now is the logical time for us to push for a 'Department of Pharmacy,' rather than to remain in the Department of Agriculture or go into the State Board of Health."

Mr. J. B. Pendergrast, of Atlanta, Secretary of the Board of Pharmacy, reported to the Association that Georgia was having trouble with reciprocation of licenses. That 37 of the other states do not recognize the Georgia license; that, of the 16 who passed the Board recently, only 5 were able to reciprocate into other states. And, in answer to what the trouble was (question by Mr. Munn), Mr. Pendergrast stated that it was "the low requirements of the Georgia Board." President Munn then asked what the remedy was. Mr. Pendergrast replied that the remedy was "to make the applicant a graduate in pharmacy." Then, in discussing this same matter, Mr. Rountree stated the following: "Out of 65 who came up, 60 came from foreign states, and it is true that Pharmacy Laws should be strengthened, or we'll be the dumping ground, the one with the lowest standards in the whole United States. That is the proposition in a nut-shell. Why, we have applicants from Puerto Rico and Cuba and other such states because they cannot take examinations anywhere else. Our requirements are so low that they cannot reciprocate and are dumped off on us. 75% of those who took the last Board were foreigners."

It was promptly moved that the Legislative Committee be requested to attempt to pass the revision of the existing Law, and to incorporate graduation from a college of pharmacy.

55th Annual Meeting—1930

The 55th Annual Session of the GPA convened in the Dempsey Hotel in Macon, April 23, 1930, under the call of President W. D. Jones.

The President's address included several recommendations: The first item was the need for a Field or Assistant Secretary, whose duty would be to sell memberships in the Association, insurance in the Druggists' Group Policy, the compensation of this person being on a percentage basis. He insisted that according to his prediction the dues would never be gotten if the mails are depended on, but that some person must call on individuals to collect dues. Next, he stated that in his conviction membership in the Association ought to be required by law, and that, finally, he must compliment Mr. Marshall, Chairman of the Legislative Committee, who "has done a wonderful job on defense, there being no offensive legislation proposed at this Session."

Mr. J. B. Pendergrast, reporting as Delegate to the N.A.R.D., came back and reported that "there are only four states in the Union that will acknowledge the Georgia license, now secured on experience alone." He stated further that, while attending a meeting of the Boards of Pharmacy of the United States in which he believed every state was represented, "they all laughed at the low standards that prevailed in Georgia."

Mr. Stead, the Drug Inspector, estimated that the number of legal drug stores in the State of Georgia in 1930 was 1,022. That the number of pharmacists registered with the Board was 1,141.

Mr. Stead called attention also to the fact that Mr. R. B. Beedles was now Assistant Drug Inspector. This is the first mention of the office of "Assistant Drug Inspector" in the State.

Mr. Marshall, reporting for the Legislative Committee, said that a Bill had been introduced into the Legislature to the effect that "regular drug stores manned by licensed pharmacists" were to be termed "pharmacies" but that the term "druggist" was to apply to grocery stores or any other such places operated without a licensed pharmacist.

℞ SUPPLEMENT D

56th Annual Meeting—1931

The 56th Annual Convention of the GPA met in Macon, April 22, 1931, and was called to order by President T. C. Marshall.

In the presidential address Mr. Marshall called attention to the fact that the Board of Pharmacy had for many years been trying to convince the druggists of Georgia of the low position they had in rank among the other Boards of Pharmacy in the United States. Up until the last few years Georgia had been next to the last, but now they were at the very bottom. Mr. Marshall also called attention to the fact that the Legislature was in session while the Pharmaceutical Association was also in session this year. He pointed out an arrangement between the Association and the *SE Drug Journal* where the Journal was to be the official publication of the Association, and whereby the Journal was to receive fifty cents from all dues-paid members. In turn all members of the Association were to receive a subscription to the Journal for a period of one year.

Mr. H. C. Christensen, President of the A.Ph.A., and Secretary of the National Association of Boards of Pharmacy, addressed the Association. He pointed out the importance of a "collegiate educational requirement for the practice of pharmacy;" that already 38 states have such a provision; that is, one requiring a college education. He cautioned Georgia that as long as they have no standards, the State will continue to be a dumping ground for those who cannot meet the standards in other states: "This is an undesirable class of applicants that want to secure a license, but are not willing to put in the time and the effort to earn it. All the Southern states with the exception of Georgia and Tennessee are now on a college pre-requisite basis. And, as Tennessee is now working for such a Bill, you can readily appreciate why Georgia must take immediate steps for her own protection." He points to the fact that the University of Georgia had already gone to a four-year course, anticipating that it would eventually be required in all states, and that the State University was the first of such universities to pass a four-year requirement.

Mr. Marshall, reporting for the Legislative Committee, said that a Bill had been introduced into the Legislature to the effect that "regular drug stores manned by licensed pharmacists" were to be termed "pharmacies" but that the term "druggist" was to apply to grocery stores or any other such place operated without a licensed pharmacist.

Dr. Robert L. Swain, the Chief Food and Drug Inspector from Baltimore, Maryland, was introduced. This was the first of a number of visits Dr. Swain was to pay to the GPA.

Mr. W. S. Elkin moved that the Board of Pharmacy and the Legislative Committee be instructed to get the passage of such laws through the legislative body as would put Georgia on an educational basis comparable to the other states. He also offered a resolution to change the Constitution and By-Laws by amendment, to call for a mail ballot for voting for officers of the Association.

57th Annual Meeting—1932

The 57th Annual Convention of the GPA was called to order by the President, R. C. Coleman. The Meeting convened in the City of Atlanta.

In giving his report the Secretary mentioned among other items the fact that Mr. R. C. Coleman had been appointed Joint Secretary of the State Examining Boards under the Governor's reorganization plan.

It was stated that it was regrettable that the amendments to the Pharmacy Law failed to pass the Legislature.

The Secretary reported on the meetings of the Board of Directors, at the Macon meeting of which Board, 14 Directors and officers were present.

The Secretary also reported that he had tried to secure Gov. Franklin Roosevelt of New York as the main speaker for the next Meeting of our Association. But, unfortunately, Gov. Roosevelt was not available.

Secretary E. F. Kelly, of the American Pharmaceutical Association, addressed the group, his main topic being a discussion of the work that had been done on medical care, in which the cost of medicines was a feature. He gave some figures from the U.S. Department of the Census, in which it was estimated that the volume of business in the average drug store in America was in 1932 about $29,000, on an annual basis.

Governor Richard Russell addressed the Association, saying:

"It has been said of drug stores in the cities that they sell everything but drugs, but that in the small rural areas they sell not only drugs, but everything else. The druggist is the one source of information about all that pertains to the activities and life of the town. He and the Chief of Police know exactly where every citizen lives, know everything about his family, and know the names of every man, woman, and child in the community, and he holds the esteem of the people of his community. And, in company with the doctor, he holds the position of high priest and prophet, and confessor and friend."

Secretary Wilson gave a list of the taxes carried by the druggists of the State, which totalled 45 in all. This list of taxes was printed and distributed to all the druggists of the State and to all the legislators.

58th Annual Meeting—1933

The 58th Annual Convention of the GPA was called to order by President Claude Rountree, of Thomasville, on May 31, 1933, in Augusta, Georgia.

Mr. H. L. Chichester, First Vice-President, presiding, the President delivered his annual address. He stated:

"In order to put this dream through, I realize the necessity to answer my call at all times, men who will be willing to make a sacrificial service to their Association, that the interests of their fellow druggists might be taken care of. I immediately appointed one outstanding druggist from each Congressional District and selected five from the State at Large, placing them on my Board of Directors, and calling them together at Atlanta."

President Rountree referred to a little booklet that was entitled, "The Georgia Plan." This was a little booklet prepared by the Secretary, aided by Mr. Roy Dorsey, of The Coca-Cola Company. It outlined a plan of organization for a state pharmaceutical association on a district basis, and even on down to the county level. It contained a program outlined for protection, particularly in the matter of taxes. Large numbers of these little booklets were published and were sent from one end of the United States to the other, and a number of states adopted the plan as outlined in this Georgia booklet.

Mr. Rountree called attention to the fact that "we now have a Pharmacy Law that puts Georgia pharmacy on a level with any in the United States from an educational standpoint, and Georgia, under the new system, will never again be the dumping ground of all of the States of the United States." He does regret that we failed to get through the Legislature at that time the uniform "Narcotic Act," which was designed to conform in some measure to the Federal Narcotic Act.

Mr. Rountree also reports that he is glad to inform the group that, in the reorganization of the state government, the State

Board of Health was reorganized. And that, due to the activities of Secretary Wilson of the Association, pharmacists were able to get the medical and other groups composing the State Board of Health to agree that pharmacy should have a minimum of two members on the State Board of Health, and that they were to be elected by the Association on the same basis as the State Board of Pharmacy members were elected. Except that, in the case of the Board of Pharmacy, the Association named only one person to the Governor, and he, according to the law, was compelled to appoint that person. But when it came to the matter of the State Board of Health, the Governor argued that the Association should send at least four names up to him, and he was to select two from that number (because he said that the Association might name someone who was personally objectionable to him). This was agreed upon, and the law provides that four from the Association are to be named, and he is to select two from that number for appointment on the State Board of Health.

Mr. Rountree, who is from the Second Congressional District, calls attention to the fact that it seems to him desirable to have women in the pharmaceutical organization, where there are licensed women available, and that Miss Rose Grier of Baconton had served as Secretary of the District Association, and had performed a most useful and valuable service. Therefore, he recommends that this be done in other districts where possible.

Secretary Wilson stated among other items in his report:

"This Association can never properly compensate President Claude Rountree for the tremendous amount of time, thought, and energy he has given to this Association during this year. He has at all times held himself available for any call, and has rendered a service of such character that his name should be enshrined in our memories for all time. And I would point to him as an example for others in the State to follow in rendering unselfish service to the cause. Every druggist in the State is due him a debt of gratitude."

The Secretary lays particular stress on the fact that "all pharmaceutical legislation has been sought on the basis of its being in the interest of the public health and welfare, and not for purposes of monopoly." He also reported that Mr. W. S. Elkin had been appointed Chief Drug Inspector, and that under his guidance splendid progress was being reported, in the matter of putting "drugs back into the drug store."

At this time the By-Laws of the Association specified that in the selection of members of the State Board of Health, they must be actively engaged in the retail drug business. This change was made in the Constitution and By-Laws and became an integral part of it.

Dr. W. A. Mulherrin, of Augusta, a Fraternal Delegate from the Medical Association of Georgia, complimented the Association on the stand they had taken on the raising of educational requirements for the study and practice of pharmacy, stating:

"I think this is the one big move that you have made to put a cultural and educational background in your profession. It will gradually go upwards, and you will get better men there and will serve your State better. We also want to commend you for the stand you have taken in demanding recognition for your profession. I refer especially to the stand you have taken in your State activities. We are glad to see that you will have representation on the State Board of Health. You should have representation there: medicine will be there, the dentists will be there, *and you should be there!*"

Mr. Tom Oliver, a retail druggist in South Georgia, and before that a representative of one of the pharmaceutical houses, was in the State Senate, in 1933. He was active in the interest of pharmaceutical legislation there, and it was due to him that the Association was successful in getting through the educational requirement previously referred to. Though also interested in the Uniform Narcotic Law, Mr. Oliver was unable to get it through the Senate. But at the next Session of the Senate, the Uniform Narcotic Law was passed, largely as a tribute to the respect that the Senate and House had for Mr. Oliver.

59th Annual Meeting—1934

The 59th Annual Convention of the GPA was held at the DeSoto Hotel in Savannah on June 12, 1934, and the Meeting was called to order by President H. L. Chichester.

Mr. Chichester, in his presidential address, chides the Association of druggists for the fact that there are only 69 dues-paid members in the Association at the present. He states:

"Your Association has been carried on, dictated to, and run by a small group of pharmacy politicians. This is the reason you haven't had an Association in the State of Georgia up until now." He also criticizes the fact that politics plays too large a part in the affairs of the Association in the record of past years. He recommends that the Constitution and By-Laws be changed, to make it possible for the presidents of each Congressional District to be elected by the District rather than to be appointed by the President. Also, that the District Presidents would constitute the Board of Directors of the Association, except that the President might have the privilege of appointing five from the State-at-Large. He suggests also that the Board of Directors constitute the Nominating Committee for officers in the Association. He asks for a joint meeting of professional people to be arranged, such as pharmacists, physicians, dentists, and nurses, in order to discuss the matter of "state medicine."

The Secretary called attention to the fact that the Georgia Association is being recognized nationally; as witnessed by the fact that President Chichester is First Vice-President of the N.A.R.D. for the current year, Mr. Charles H. Evans is President of the National Association of Boards of Pharmacy, Mr. W. S. Elkin is Chairman of one of the important committees of N.A.R.D. Various others in the Association are members of the National Drug Trade Conference, and the Secretary has been President of the Association of State Association Secretaries, and a member of various committees on a national level.

The Secretary also proposed a mail ballot system for the election of officers and Board members. He also pointed out the necessity for planning to operate a full-time Secretary or Business Manager. He stated that a full-time Business Manager, traveling over the State in the interest of the State Association could eventually get a one hundred percent membership from all districts.

There was a resolution unanimously adopted that the GPA oppose the sale of alcoholic beverages in the drug stores of Georgia. This motion was unanimously carried.

60th Annual Meeting—1935

The 60th Annual Convention of the GPA met in Albany, Georgia, on May 22, 1935, and was called to order by President W. T. Knight, Junior.

President Knight called attention to the fact that when a Director comes to a meeting of the Board, he should come there instructed by his District how to vote, and not just to express his personal opinion. He should express the opinion that represents his District on any subject.

The report of Secretary Wilson indicated that his resignation had been tendered to the Board at their last meeting (of the

Association). But since no one has been elected to fill the vacancy, he has continued to serve for this year (1935). Mr. W. S. Elkin, who was scheduled to take the place, was named to the National Retail Drug Code Authority, as Secretary, and has moved to Washington.

The Secretary stated that he had traveled over the State, attending District Meetings, legislative meetings, and in addition to the above trips, had attended the N.A.R.D. Meeting in New Orleans, in September, and a joint committee meeting in Washington City, composed of representatives of the Conference of State Association Secretaries, the N.A.R.D., and the A.Ph.A., to discuss means whereby a closer tie between State Associations might be made, so as to insure closer cooperation and better understanding between the state associations and the two national organizations, and further to develop a national program covering all phases of pharmacy.

There having been some criticism of the State Board of Health for dispensing large quantities of yeast and serums free in the State, Dr. Abercrombie, the Director of the State Board of Health, was invited to attend the Association Meeting and discuss the matter. He defended the Board of Health in saying that the people needed that service, drawing a distinction between *needing* a service and *demanding* a service. He stated that in the year 1931 the State Board of Health bought 50 tons of yeast and distributed it, but that in 1934 it ran down to about 18 tons, and in 1935 was going to be about 4 tons.

Mr. Charles H. Evans, Chairman of the Legislative Committee, reported that some amendments had been passed to the Pharmacy Law. The first, a fee of $2.00 upon each licensed pharmacist and a fee of $1.00 for each store operated in the State for the sale of medicinal supplies and medicines. That amendment was introduced in the Legislature. Next, an amendment to empower the Board of Pharmacy with authority to name home remedies to be sold in stores other than licensed drug stores. These amendments were unanimously passed at the December meeting of the Board of Directors, and were drafted and presented to the Committee on Agriculture. A vigorous attack on the proposed legislation was made by the Chatham County Pharmaceutical Association, who had also introduced a pharmacy bill, and there remained the possibility of a veto on the part of the Governor because of the additional tax imposed in the first amendment. Neither of the measures passed, but the committee does not feel that the work was in vain, as contacts were made that will be of much value in the next session of the Legislature.

It is to be recalled that at this time the members of the Board of Pharmacy were now on a per diem basis and not on a commission basis, as previously reported. The expenses of the Board of Pharmacy were reported as $698.00.

The officers for the ensuing year were elected by the mail ballot.

Again there is a long lapse between the Proceedings of the GPA. For a period of 11 years, from 1935 to 1946, the Proceedings either were not printed or, if they were printed, no copies have been preserved.

71st Annual Meeting—1946

The 71st Annual Convention of the GPA met in the Dempsey Hotel in Macon, April 15-16-17, 1946.

President Avera expressed thanks to the Almighty for the end of "this horrible conflict, the Second World War." He announced that a Committee with Dean R. C. Wilson as Chairman had been set up to make an exhaustive study of the need of amending the pharmacy laws, and stated that the officers and the Board of Directors met with the officers of the Georgia Medical Society, and discussed matters of unusual interest. He reported that at the various District Meetings, unusual enthusiasm prevailed, and that he attended quite a number of them at which the attendance had been between 20 and 75.

The President called attention to these matters:

First, the matter of raising the membership fee, which had been recommended by Mr. Rainey.

Second, that the Association adopt the recommendation of Mr. Evans that all students of pharmacy be made members of the Association free of charge until they become graduate pharmacists.

For the first time in the history of the Association, so far as the printed Proceedings are available, the Association now had a balance in the bank, after all expenses were paid, a balance of $4,537.38. In addition, the Association had War Bonds in the amount of $2,220.00, a Savings Account of $458.00, and a Scholarship Fund of $2,206.00, making a total net worth of the Association of $9,422.00.

Mr. P. D. Horkan had been appointed Chief Drug Inspector

during this interval of 11 years. He gives his report as follows:

Pharmacists registered with the Secretary	1500
" actively engaged in practice	1408
" employed in retail stores	1323
" employed in hospitals	24
" employed in wholesale houses	59
Number of women pharmacists included in above	31
" of veterans included in above	94
Pharmacists now in Service in Armed Forces	58
Total number of drug stores in State	942

The Secretary called attention to the fact that 22 more pharmacists left the State that year than came in by reciprocity. Mr. Coleman, the Joint Secretary, gives these interesting figures: 1935-1940, Licenses by examination and reciprocity were 363; 1940-1945, Licenses by examination and reciprocity were 232. He estimates this represents about a 50% loss in that five-year period. Whereas, he claims, over the same period, the medical and dental professions' figures show that they had an increase in the number of licenses issued for the same period.

Secretary Rainey reported among other items that at the annual Meeting of the Board of Directors held in Atlanta on April 15, 1945, the Secretary was authorized to prepare resolutions to be mailed to the National Association of Retail Druggists and the American Pharmaceutical Association, demanding "immediate action to curb and restrict the sale and use of barbiturates, barbituric acid derivatives, and dangerous drugs." The resolutions brought before the National Association brought favorable response from the respective Secretaries of the other states, and similar resolutions from other sections of the country resulted in a National Conference held in Washington in October, in which all health groups participated. Further, Mr. Rainey reported: "At a subsequent meeting of the Board of Directors, held May 2, further discussion of the barbiturate problem developed into plans for a joint meeting of the GPA, the Georgia Medical Society, the State Board of Health, the U.S. Narcotics Bureau and the State Board of Pharmacy." The purpose of the meeting was "to more fully consider the problems and difficulties involved, and to arrange for some definite conclusion or solution." "On July 19," Mr. Rainey said, "a joint dinner meeting of the groups previously referred to was held at the Biltmore Hotel. Dr. R. C. Wilson presided as Chairman, and every phase of the barbiturate problem was discussed. It was generally agreed that Federal legislation would be the most effective means of curbing the sale and use of these drugs."

"Upon the invitation of Dr. R. P. Fischelis, Secretary of the A.Ph.A., Dr. Wilson was delegated by the Association to attend the Washington Conference on Barbiturates. Upon his return, Dr. Wilson made a most comprehensive report to the Board of Directors. He reported that it was the consensus of opinion of the group assembled in Washington that the solution rested with the State enforcement rather than with Federal supervision, and that uniform state laws would be prepared for adoption by the State."

"Meanwhile," Mr. Rainey stated, "the abuse continues; and almost daily the newspapers report headlines of suicides from overdose of barbiturates and other hypnotic drugs."

In another section of his report Mr. Rainey stated:

"Pharmacy for some reason is a favorite target for each and every Session of the Legislature; for in the five-day Session of the 1945 Legislature, and in the fifteen-day Session early in 1946, it developed some real headaches and some real work for your officers and those delegated with the responsibilities of looking after the legislative interests of druggists in these legislative halls. In each of the Sessions, efforts to lower the educational standards of pharmacy in Georgia were initiated by members of our own rank, desiring to secure licenses for some member of the family or for an employee."

"Such individuals fail to realize that any deviation from the present standards would place in jeopardy the license of every man practicing pharmacy in Georgia. Doubtless, we will be confronted with similar efforts in future sessions of the Legislature, and we must be prepared to protect the interest of our members and to defeat the efforts of a few individuals who would sacrifice the entire profession to achieve their selfish and personal aims."

Mr. Rainey reports further that "the volume of business done by the retail drug stores of Georgia (931 of them) is $43,000,-000 for 1945-46."

72nd Annual Meeting—1947

The 72nd Annual Convention of the GPA was called to order by President Charles H. Evans, in the Bon Air Hotel at Augusta, Georgia, on April 14, 1947.

Fraternal Delegates were: Dr. Ralph Cheney from the Medical Association of Georgia, Mrs. Olive Barton from the Georgia

State Nurses Association, and Dr. Clyde Maxwell, from the Georgia Dental Association.

President Evans pointed out in his presidential address:—

(1) That the pharmacists of America "on the corner of the main street in every town and hamlet are in a better position than the average citizen to visualize the far-reaching efforts in atomic research." He pointed out the possibilities of danger, and the important part which the druggists of America may be called upon to play in the Atomic Era. He stated that "it behooves America to heed the admonition of the Master Scientist, who laid down 2000 years ago the principle upon which all material and moral forces should be governed."

(2) Pride in "our educational standards in Georgia as being high and in keeping with other health professions." He said that now Georgia, along with 46 of the other 48 states, requires college graduation from a recognized college of pharmacy, and that our pharmacy laws are adequate to protect the profession of pharmacy, as well as the health and welfare of the people of the State. Also, that "our four-year college graduates are fast taking their places in the stores of our State, adding materially to the prestige pharmacy is getting for itself as a public health profession, with the drug store in every community a recognized health center."

(3) That the membership in the Association is the largest in the history of the Association, with 1075 dues-paid members. This is one of the largest memberships of any state association in America. He gives credit for this to the Chief Drug Inspector, Mr. Pat Horkan, and his two assistants, Jack Bush and Gus Parkerson.

(4) Presented to the Association the oldest living Past President of the Association, Mr. Thad B. Rice, of Greensboro. Mr. Rice pointed out some members of the group who were "not so bald and not so gray then as Bob Wilson is now." Mr. Rice stated that he had "abandoned the drug business, and am now President of a bank and will lend the druggists money."

(5) Pointed out the fact that the Women's Auxiliary had accumulated $2300 for a scholarship fund, and that the income of this fund had been loaned to worthy boys and girls, and never one dollar of it lost.

(6) President Evans recommended that a Professional Relations Council be formed in the State, to include representatives of the various health professions.

(7) Suggested some changes in the manner of nomination of the State Board members. Mr. Evans pointed to a new feature of the law which was recently passed by the Legislature, that the law puts a new responsibility and a new authority in the Board of Pharmacy which never existed before. This included giving the Board authority to pass any rule or regulation it sees fit to pass, within the Constitution of the State, which would govern not only the practice of the Board, but the practice of pharmacy in the State. While speaking of legislative matters, Mr. Evans pointed especially to the fact that Mrs. Iris Blitch, a member of the Senate and the wife of a druggist, was very helpful in getting our Bill passed by the House and the Senate.

In his report, Mr. Horkan, Chief Drug Inspector, stated the Bill No. 184-185 before the Legislature is "an accomplishment that shall go down in history as the greatest legislative achievement in the annals of pharmacy in Georgia." He expressed the belief that the Dangerous Drugs Act, which was passed by the Legislature, and the amendment added to it, had made inspections easier, and that better enforcement of the law was taking place.

His report also showed 30 women engaged in the practice of pharmacy, 24 pharmacists engaged in hospital pharmacy, and a total of 975 drug stores in the State of Georgia.

Secretary Rainey called attention to the fact that all students in the two Schools of Pharmacy in Georgia had been initiated into the Association as non-voting members. A special dinner meeting was held in Athens for the University of Georgia students, and a similar one in Atlanta for the Southern College of Pharmacy students. In all, 352 students received membership cards.

Dean E. R. Serles, President of the A.Ph.A., called special attention at this Meeting to the fact that Dr. Cheney, the Fraternal Delegate for the Medical Association, had asked the help of the Pharmaceutical Association in the matter of socialized medicine. He said that this was the first time in the history of the GPA that the medical association had ever asked a favor of pharmacy. He said: "You are to be congratulated for the establishment of legislation, the text of which, and the import of which, does not exist in any other state of the Union as of the present date." Then Dean Serles reviews some of the advances in medical products and practices in recent years, including vaccines, sulfa drugs, the antibiotics, micro-chemical determinations, new methods, parenteral solutions, new means of diagnosis, et cetera. He states that the part pharmacy is playing in the development, distribution, and handling of these drugs is an important feature.

Dean R. C. Wilson, Chairman of the Legislative Committee, reported to the group and discussed some of the important changes in the new Law whereby amendments had been made to cover some weaknesses. Conceivably, the most important change made in the Law is the fact that the new Law gives to the Board of Pharmacy the power to set up any rule or regulation it sees fit for the conduct of pharmacy in Georgia, and that these regulations will have the full effect and status of law, thus putting on the Board of Pharmacy the full power to enforce any rule or regulation it sees fit to pass. He calls attention to the fact that the chief difficulty so far lies in the fact that no appropriation Bill was passed providing funds for the Pharmacy Board and inspection and enforcement of the Law. Such funds as have been available heretofore have come from the Governor's Incidental Fund. This matter should be borne in mind when the next Legislature convenes, and proper efforts should be made to see that a proper appropriation is made directly for the operation of the Drug Enforcement Law.

73rd Annual Meeting—1948

The 73rd Annual Meeting of the GPA was held at the Oglethorpe Hotel, Savannah, May 3-4-5, 1948, and was called to order by President J. L. Hawk.

Secretary Rainey reported that in cooperation with the Board of Pharmacy a Digest of the new laws was printed and distributed to doctors, dentists, veterinarians and druggists throughout the State of Georgia. He called attention to the fact that Mr. Charles H. Evans had been named Chairman of the House of Delegates of the A.Ph.A. He also reported that there had been a keen interest taken in the affairs of the Association, and in each of the District Meetings throughout the year they had dealt with problems relating to drug-store operations on the retail level. He called attention to the dangers confronting Fair Trade Laws. Commenting on this matter, he stated: "Fair Trade can never hope to receive consideration from a Press no longer interested in fair play, but looking only to the source of its revenue, the advertiser's dollar." He made three recommendations to the Association: 1—That the annual membership dues be increased from $5.00 to $10.00. 2—He suggested that consideration be given to the development of a training program for employers and employees to promote modern merchandising and operating methods. 3—That the GPA unanimously support the N.A.R.D.'s Objective Number One, which reads as follows: "To combat with all the facilities at our command the organized effort to destroy Fair Trade."

The Drug Inspector, in his report for the year 1948, gave the following figures: Number of women in Georgia licensed as pharmacists was 50; number of hospital pharmacists had grown to be 22; and the number of retail pharmacies in the State he gave as 976.

74th Annual Meeting—1949

The 74th Annual Meeting of the GPA was held at the Dempsey Hotel in Macon, April 4-5-6, 1949. The Meeting was presided over by President J. E. Massey.

The Treasurer's report showed something over $15,000 cash balance (counting securities) at the year's end.

President Massey called attention to the fact that there were still places in the State being operated under the name of "drug stores" without licensed pharmacists in the store. He called on the Board of Pharmacy to prosecute efforts to clear this up. He also called attention to the disregard for the law in the handling of paregoric, barbiturates, and other dangerous drugs.

Mr. Rainey called attention to the passing of Mr. T. C. Marshall, prominent member of the Association, Secretary-Treasurer for a number of years, a member of the Board of Pharmacy, and of the State Board of Health, and prominent and active in many other activities in the profession of pharmacy.

Mr. Charles Evans stated that he had presided as Chairman of the House of Delegates of the A.Ph.A., and that Mrs. Evans presided as President of the Women's Auxiliary of the A.Ph.A., and had been re-elected for a third term.

The Necrology Committee reported the passing of 20 of the members. A Memorial to Thomas Callaway Marshall was read and made a part of the Minutes, the Memorial being written by Dean R. C. Wilson, long-time friend and co-worker of Mr. Marshall.

Mr. Chichester, as President of the Board of Pharmacy, made a very serious appeal to the members of the Association for the individual support of the druggists of the State in strengthening the pharmacy laws.

75th Annual Meeting—1950

The 75th Annual Meeting and Diamond Jubilee Convention of the GPA was called into session by President W. A. Blasingame at the Biltmore Hotel in Atlanta, April 3-4-5, 1950.

At this time the official Historian of the Pharmaceutical Association, Dean R. C. Wilson, gave a brief summary of the History of the Pharmaceutical Association from 1875 to 1950. The full text of this story is published in the *Southeastern Drug Journal* of that year.

President Blasingame reviewed briefly the background and the activities of the Association through the years, and he used this statement:

"All the achievements in science, all executive ability and organization, all modernization, all improvement in drugs, all eloquence in the calibre of pharmacists personally, all elevation of the educational standards of our trade, all extension of the life span of our people, and all joys of radiant health on this Continent today, is simply a suggestion of the recognized progress of our profession in the last two generations and a suggestion of the unmeasured possibilities yet ahead of us."

Mr. Horkan, as Drug Inspector, stated that pharmacists registered with the Secretary for the year 1950 was 1,744, that pharmacists actually engaged was 1,570. Of this number, 52 were women, 26 were in hospital pharmacies, and 68 in wholesale houses and pharmaceutical concerns. There were 1,039 retail drug stores, actively in business, in the year 1950.

At this point Bishop Arthur Moore of the Methodist Church addressed the Association on some of the things we need in America. He concluded by saying, "What we desperately need is a revival of religion." He called attention to the dangers of Communism and suggested how it may be confined.

The Past Presidents of the Association were honored, and beautiful pins were given in recognition of their service. The following Past Presidents received pins: D. G. Wise, J. P. Walker, R. C. Wilson, I. A. Solomons, Junior, R. C. Coleman, Jasper Brooks, Claude Rountree, H. L. Chichester, H. S. Peters, J. W. Brinson, W. W. Fincher, Bonnie Brown, M. Z. Claxton, T. S. Deen, H. J. Avera, C. H. Evans, J. L. Hawk, J. E. Massey.

And, since Mr. Blasingame was presiding, he was presented with a Past President's pin at the final session.

Mr. Charles H. Evans, reporting for the legislative committee, told about a Bill which was introduced in the Legislature to lower the educational requirements, or rather to cut them out entirely, so that any person who had worked in a drug store could come up before the Board for examination. Mr. Evans reported that the committee tried to have the Bill withdrawn, but without success. The Bill was given a number (H. B. 909) and referred to the Committee on the State of the Republic. This was supposed to be the Administration's greediest committee for quick and favorable action. A copy of the Bill had been furnished the Chairman of the Legislative Committee of the Association by Chief Inspector Horkan; copies were made, and members of the State of the Republic Committee were listed; and a bulletin with a copy of the Bill and complete information went out that night in the mail to every drug store in the State. "Then it happened," he reported. All over the State phone calls, letters, telegrams, personal contacts, and a roused student body at the University of Georgia swarmed into action. Too much credit for action cannot be given to the student bodies of the two schools of pharmacy. In years past, with a handful of students in our two pharmacy schools, student strength in political scraps was negligible. But now, with around 500 students, the old sayings, "In unity there is strength," and "It takes numbers to make an organization strong" meant something. These students literally camped on the Capitol steps and in the legislative halls. The opposition meanwhile saw the handwriting on the wall, and the legislation was killed completely.

Shortly after the adjournment of the Meeting, Mr. Rainey, who had exhausted his strength in the many preparations for this Jubilee Convention, passed away.

76th Annual Meeting—1951

The 76th Annual Convention of the GPA met at Augusta on April 10-11-12, 1951, with President M. T. Anderson presiding.

In his report, Mr. Horkan, Chief Drug Inspector, called attention to the fact that there were now (1951) 70 women licensed as pharmacists and engaged in practice in Georgia. There was a total of 1,100 drug stores, 1,073 of these being retail pharmacies, and 27 of them hospital pharmacies.

Mrs. Regina Baird, as Secretary, reported on several items, since she had been asked to complete Mr. Rainey's unexpired term. She called attention to a considerable drop-off in the number of dues-paid members during the year. Mrs. Baird stated that the number of dues-paid members for the current year is 851, just 50% of the registered druggists of Georgia. She also cautioned the Association that a number of legislative items on the Federal level, as well as on the State level, are jeopardized, including Fair Trade, particularly on the State level. She warned Georgia to be prepared to fight for it.

Relative to the matter of officers for the next year, Mr. Carlton Fite, who had been elected President, had left the drug business and had left the State. There was no By-Law covering this particular situation; therefore Mr. Robert Belcher, of Valdosta, being Second Vice-President, was elevated directly to the presidency, without going through the routine of serving as First Vice-President.

77th Annual Meeting—1952

The 77th Annual Meeting of the GPA convened on April 28-29-30, 1952, in Savannah, Georgia, and was called to order by President Robert Belcher.

Dr. M. Fernand Nunez, Chief of the Laboratory Service, U.S. Veterans Hospital, in Dublin, Georgia, was introduced to the group. He was born in Savannah, and is a direct descendant of the original Dr. Nunez, who came over with Oglethorpe to Georgia as a settler, who practiced medicine, who opened the first apothecary shop in Savannah, and who delivered the first male white child to be born in the colony of Georgia.

President Belcher stated that the goal for the year was 1000 members, and he was happy to report a "total paid membership of 1,135." He said: "We have continued our fight for Fair Trade, and hope that in the very near future we shall see it again in force."

Chief Drug Inspector Horkan reported that there were now (1952) 80 women practicing pharmacy in the State. The number of drug stores operated by 1 pharmacist was 623, the number of stores with 2 pharmacists was 350, the number served by 3 pharmacists was 80, by 4 pharmacists, 12 stores, and by 5 pharmacists, 5 stores. There were now 28 hospital pharmacies.

78th Annual Meeting—1953

The 78th Annual Convention of the GPA was held in Macon, April 6-7-8, 1953, with President Stacy Jones presiding.

Secretary Baird reported that the volume of business done in

Veterans Administration prescriptions for the year was $55,-209.00, and that there were 269 drug stores in Georgia qualified to fill VA prescriptions.

Mr. Horkan reported that there were now 85 women practicing pharmacy in the State.

President Jones called attention to the fact that the Georgia Supreme Court had decided that the Fair Trade Act of 1937 was unconstitutional.

Mr. Morris Mermy, Director of the Bureau of Education on Fair Trade, in addressing the Association, stated:

"I am not here to criticize the decision of any Court, and I am not a lawyer. But I am interested in this clause which the Supreme Court considered applicable here, known as the 'Due Process Clause.'" He issued an appeal to the Association to rewrite the Fair Trade Law, reintroduce it in the Legislature in the hope that it could meet the criticism of the Court and be ruled constitutional.

79th Annual Meeting—1954

The 79th Annual Convention of the GPA met in Atlanta on April 19-20-21, 1954, with President Bill Lee presiding.

A panel discussion was held on the topic, "Drug Law Enforcement," with Hoke Peters as Moderator, along with the following panel members: Mr. McGeever, U.S. Narcotic Bureau; James C. Pearson, District Chief, Food and Drug Administration; Asbury Baldwin, President of the Georgia State Board of Pharmacy; P. D. Horkan, Georgia Chief Drug Inspector.

The Fair Trade Law under which Georgia had been operating for a number of years having been declared unconstitutional, a committee composed of R. C. Wilson, H. L. Chichester, and C. H. Evans was formed to raise funds and to get the Fair Trade Law restored by legislative enactment. The committee reported that the Bill passed the Senate with only one dissenting vote, and passed the House with only two dissenting votes, and the Law had been signed by the Governor.

Thomas R. Luck, Chairman of the Board for that year, stated that Mr. L. M. Roberts, Senior, had been elected Treasurer, and that Felton Gordon, Secretary and Public Relations Director, was named, with Regina Baird as Executive Secretary, and R. C. Wilson as Secretary of the Fair Trade Committee.

President Lee presented as his objectives for the year the following:

℞ SUPPLEMENT D 401

1. To restore Fair Trade.
2. A vocational guidance in the high schools of the State, emphasizing choosing pharmacy as your vocation.
3. A united Georgia Pharmaceutical Association.
4. Professional pharmacy as a theme for district meetings.

Dr. Allen H. Bunce, President of the U.S. Pharmacopoeial Convention, addressed the Association on the subject of "Interprofessional Relations." This address was distributed among the members but not printed in the Minutes.

80th Annual Meeting—1955

The 80th Annual Convention of the GPA met at Augusta, Georgia, April 18-19-20, 1955, with President Thomas R. Luck presiding.

Mr. P. A. Whatley, of Gainesville, Chairman of the Board of Directors, stated that there had been four meetings of the Board during the year, and that Mrs. Regina Baird had been approved as Executive Secretary, and H. S. Peters, as Treasurer. The Directors approved an appropriation of $3,000 for attorneys' fees to carry the N.A.R.D. appeal case through the Supreme Court of Georgia; that is, the Fair Trade Law, which later was declared unconstitutional for the second time.

It was pointed out that the life of the Association Charter had expired, and that the President was authorized to petition for a new Charter, which was done.

The Treasurer's report, given by H. S. Peters, showed that the total assets of the Association for the year 1955 were $33,664.22.

Chief Drug Inspector Horkan pointed out in his report that there were 97 women included in the total of 2,097 active pharmacists in Georgia.

He also gave the total number of drug stores in the State as 1,139.

81st Annual Meeting—1956

The 81st Annual Meeting of the GPA was held in Savannah, April 23-24-25, 1956, with President W. H. Dunaway presiding.

In his comments President Dunaway reported that "we have been successful in preventing the passage of some Bills in the Legislature which were detrimental to pharmacy, and, in aiding the passage of other Bills, like the old Codeine Bill, and the Act preventing the sale of medicines via vending machines.

Some of the Problems pointed to by Mr. Dunaway, as they were brought to his attention, were the following:

1. There is great complaint and concern over the filling of prescriptions by non-registered men.

2. There is great confusion and uncertainty over the re-filling of prescriptions containing so-called "dangerous drugs," and "prescription-legend" drugs.

He calls on the Board of Pharmacy to critically review its responsibilities under the Law, and then make any necessary recommendations to the Association as soon as possible, for a better enforcement program. He also advised the employment of an attorney on a retainer basis, so that he would be available at all times for advice and counsel to the GPA on state pharmaceutical matters.

Inspector Horkan reported that for the first time in Georgia history the number of women pharmacists had passed above the 100 mark.

Mr. R. C. Coleman having retired, Mr. Cecil Clifton had been named to be Joint Secretary of Examining Boards.

The Board of Directors reported that they had provided for a committee to study the existing laws and to hire an attorney for advice and counsel, to draw up new legislation, and to present it at the 1957 Session of the Legislature.

82nd Annual Meeting—1957

The 82nd Annual Convention of the GPA was held in Atlanta on April 15-16-17, 1957.

Mr. P. D. Horkan, Drug Inspector, reported as follows:

Pharmacists registered with Joint Secretary	2,716
Pharmacists actually engaged	2,305
In retail stores	1,990
As owners	762
As partners	240
As employees	979
In hospital pharmacies	65
In wholesale houses or pharmaceutical firms	77
As field representatives of manufacturers or wholesalers	98
In teaching or governmental positions	40
In miscellaneous positions	35

Mr. Horkan reported that the number of women pharmacists included in the above had reached 110. One of the outstanding items in the progress of the work of the Association has been the fact that an increasing number of women have been attracted into the profession of pharmacy, on a progressive basis; as witnessed by the following data.

1946	31 women actively engaged in pharmacy
1948	50 women actively engaged in pharmacy
1950	52 women actively engaged in pharmacy
1952	80 women actively engaged in pharmacy
1955	97 women actively engaged in pharmacy
1957	110 women actively engaged in pharmacy

Mr. Horkan also reported the following facts for the year 1957:

Total number of drug stores in Georgia	1,083
Number of stores served by 1 pharmacist	655
Number of stores served by 2 pharmacists	261
Number of stores served by 3 pharmacists	135
Number of stores served by 4 pharmacists	22
Number of stores served by 5 pharmacists	10
Number of hospital pharmacies	38

Officers of the Georgia Pharmaceutical Association*
(1875-1959)

Presidents

1875-1876	John W. Clarke	Milledgeville
1876-1877	L. W. Hunt	Macon
1877-1878	R. H. Land	Augusta
1878-1879	Osceola Butler	Savannah
1879-1880	John Ingalls	Macon
1880-1882	Theo. Schuman	Atlanta
1882-1883	J. W. Rankin	Atlanta
1883-1885	S. C. Durban	Augusta
1885-1886	H. C. Hutchinson	Atlanta
1886-1887	J. W. Stanford	Cuthbert
1887-1888	George D. Case	Milledgeville
1888-1889	William S. Parks	Atlanta
1889-1890	T. A. Cheatham	Atlanta-Macon
1890-1891	John W. Goodwyn	Macon
1891-1892	H. R. Slack	LaGrange
1892-1893	E. M. Wheat	Columbus
1893-1894	C. M. Crosby	Marietta

*Any omission in this List of Officers is due to the fact that records are not complete over the years.

Presidents

1894-1895	John P. Turner	Columbus
1895-1896	D. W. Curry	Rome
1896-1897	I. A. Solomons, Sr.	Savannah
1897-1898	H. H. Arrington	Rome
1898-1899	Chas. O. Tyner	Atlanta
1899-1900	Ralph O. Howard	Columbus
1900-1901	Mallory H. Taylor	Macon
1901-1902	W. S. Elkin, Jr.	Atlanta
1902-1903	John H. Polhill	Brunswick
1903-1904	Charles D. Jordan	Monticello
1904-1905	James E. Kidd	Milledgeville
1905-1906	Max Morris	Macon
1906-1907	W. B. Freeman	Atlanta
1907-1908	J. D. Persse	Savannah
1908-1909	Ben S. Persons	Macon
1909-1910	T. B. Rice	Greensboro
1910-1911	J. P. Walker	Montezuma
1911-1912	John Montgomery	Thomasville
1912-1913	J. W. Ridout	Macon
1913-1914	R. C. Wilson	Athens
1914-1915	W. A. Pigman	Savannah
1915-1916	S. E. Bayne	Macon
1916-1917	H. D. Bell	Albany
1917-1918	I. A. Solomons, Jr.	Savannah
1918-1919	T. F. Burbank	Cedartown
1919-1920	W. T. Knight	Savannah
1920-1921	David G. Wise	Atlanta
1921-1922	Jabe Stamps	Thomaston
1922-1923	H. C. Shuptrine	Savannah
1923-1924	T. H. Brannen	Atlanta
1924-1925	Jasper Brooks	Tifton
1925-1929	A. R. Munn	Atlanta
1929-1930	W. D. Jones	Savannah
1930-1931	T. C. Marshall	Atlanta
1931-1932	R. C. Coleman	Dublin
1932-1933	C. Rountree	Thomasville
1933-1934	H. L. Chichester	Macon
1934-1935	W. T. Knight, II	Savannah
1935-1936	R. Lee Olive	Augusta
1936-1937	H. S. Peters	Manchester
1937-1938	J. W. Brinson	Wrightsville

Presidents

1938-1939	W. W. Fincher	Canton
1939-1940	Bonnie Brown	Lyons
1940-1941	J. W. White	Thomasville
1941-1942	M. Z. Claxton	Dublin
1942-1943-1944	T. S. Deen	Douglas
1944-1945-1946	H. J. Avera	Fort Valley
1946-1947	C. H. Evans	Warrenton
1947-1948	J. L. Hawk	Atlanta
1948-1949	J. E. Massey	Hahira
1949-1950	W. A. Blasingame	Moultrie
1950-1951	M. T. Anderson	College Park
1951-1952	Robert Belcher	Valdosta
1952-1953	Stacey Jones, Sr.	Atlanta
1953-1954	Bill Lee	Newnan
1954-1955	Thomas R. Luck	Carrollton
1955-1956	W. H. Dunaway	Marietta
1956-1957	Malcom W. Fort	Columbus
1957-1958	William Berry	Villa Rica
1958-1959	Ralph S. Tilly	Rome

Secretaries

1875-1877	Fred King	Atlanta
1877-1880	W. A. Taylor	Atlanta
1880-1881	T. A. Cheatham	Macon
1881-1883	J. T. Shuptrine	Savannah
1883-1885	I. Zacharias	Columbus
1885-1886	W. S. Park	Atlanta
1886-1891	H. R. Slack	LaGrange
1891-1896	Campbell T. King	Macon
1896-1902	H. H. Arrington	Rome
1902-1905	J. B. Riley	Macon
1905-1910	Max Morris	Macon
1910-1911	Ben S. Persons	Macon
1911-1924	T. A. Cheatham	Macon
1925-1926	C. V. Hohenstein	Atlanta
1927-1929	Fred T. Bridges	Atlanta
1929-1935	R. C. Wilson	Athens
1935-1942	Z. O. Moore	Atlanta
1942-1950	R. D. Rainey	Atlanta
1951-1953	J. T. Selman	Atlanta

Secretaries

1953-1954	Felton H. Gordon	Atlanta
1954-	Regina Baird	Atlanta

Treasurers

1875-1876	L. W. Hunt	Macon
1876-1879	John Ingalls	Macon
1879-1887	T. L. Massenburg	Macon
1887-1900	Mallory H. Taylor	Macon
1905-1910	J. T. Shuptrine	Savannah
1911-1912	T. B. Rice	Greensboro
1912-1916	D. G. Wise	Atlanta
1916-1925	T. C. Marshall	Atlanta
1927-1928	Fred Bridges	Atlanta
1928-1935	R. C. Wilson	Athens
1935-1949	T. C. Marshall	Atlanta
1949-1953	J. L. Hawk	Atlanta
1953-1954	L. M. Roberts, Sr.	Atlanta
1954-1959	H. S. Peters	Manchester

First Vice-Presidents

1875-1876	John Ingalls	Macon
1876-1877	Osceola Butler	Savannah
1877-1878	E. H. W. Hunter	Louisville
1878-1879	H. P. Tarrant	Augusta
1879-1880	I. A. Solomons	Savannah
1880-1881	M. D. Hood	Columbus
1881-1882	L. W. Hunt	Macon
1882-1883	I. A. Solomons	Savannah
1883-1884	S. C. Durban	Augusta
1884-1885	J. W. Stanford	Cuthbert
1886-1887	P. C. Magnus	Atlanta
1887-1888	T. A. Cheatham	Macon
1888-1889	John S. Goodwyn	Macon
1889-1890	T. F. Burbank	Cedartown
1890-1892	E. M. Wheat	Columbus
1892-1893	C. M. Crosby	Marietta
1893-1894	George F. Payne	Atlanta
1894-1895	D. W. Curry	Rome
1895-1896	I. A. Solomons	Savannah
1896-1897	Charles O. Tyner	Atlanta

SUPPLEMENT D

First Vice-Presidents

1897-1898	John S. Hoge	Macon
1898-1899	R. O. Howard	Columbus
1899-1900	Nathan J. Gillespie	Savannah
1900-1902	J. H. Polhill	Brunswick
1902-1903	Charles D. Jordan	Monticello
1903-1904	James E. Kidd	Milledgeville
1904-1905	Max Morris	Macon
1905-1906	W. B. Freeman	Atlanta
1906-1907	J. D. Persse	Savannah
1907-1908	L. S. Brigham	Columbus
1908-1909	John Montgomery	Thomasville
1909-1910	Jos. P. Walker	Montezuma
1910-1911	E. W. Johnson	Carrollton
1911-1912	J. W. Ridout	Savannah
1912-1913	R. C. Wilson	Athens
1913-1914	W. A. Pigman	Macon
1914-1915	S. E. Bayne	Macon
1915-1916	J. T. Wages	Winder
1916-1917	I. A. Solomons, Jr.	Savannah
1917-1918	T. F. Burbank	Cedartown
1918-1919	W. T. Knight	Savannah
1919-1920	D. G. Wise	Atlanta
1920-1921	R. E. Perry	Savannah
1921-1922	H. C. Shuptrine	Savannah
1922-1923	T. H. Brannen	Atlanta
1923-1924	R. H. Land	Augusta
1924-1925	C. D. Robinson	Albany
1927-1928-1929	Walter D. Jones	Savannah
1929-1930	T. C. Marshall	Atlanta
1930-1931	Claude Rountree	Thomasville
1931-1932	J. B. Pendergrast	Atlanta
1932-1933	H. L. Chichester	Macon
1934-1935	R. Lee Olive	Augusta
1935-1936	Homer J. Avera	Fort Valley
1945-1946	C. H. Evans	Warrenton
1948-1949	Walter Blasingame	Moultrie
1949-1950	Mel T. Anderson	College Park
1950-1951	Robert Belcher	Valdosta
1951-1952	Stacey Jones, Sr.	Atlanta
1952-1953	Bill Lee	Newnan

First Vice-Presidents

1953-1954	T. R. Luck	Carrollton
1954-1955	W. H. Dunaway	Marietta
1955-1956	Malcom W. Fort	Columbus

Second Vice-Presidents

1875-1876	Theo. Schuman	Atlanta
1876-1877	A. W. Smith	Americus
1877-1878	R. B. Hall	Macon
1878-1879	J. M. Madden	Brunswick
1879-1880	W. K. Root	Marietta
1880-1881	N. B. Drewery	Griffin
1881-1882	R. E. Carter	Columbus
1882-1883	G. H. Howard	Atlanta
1883-1884	J. W. Stanford	Cuthbert
1884-1885	S. J. Cassels	Thomasville
1885-1886	P. A. West	Milledgeville
1886-1887	F. J. Moses	Augusta
1887-1888	W. B. Shuptrine	Savannah
1888-1889	H. K. Main	Dalton
1889-1890	E. M. Wheat	Columbus
1890-1891	D. B. Stauffacher	Atlanta
1891-1892	C. M. Crosby	Marietta
1892-1893	C. S. Bondurant	Valdosta
1893-1894	D. W. Curry	Rome
1894-1895	R. C. Dickinson	Thomasville
1895-1896	Campbell T. King	Macon
1896-1897	W. S. Elkin	Atlanta
1897-1898	R. O. Howard	Columbus
1898-1899	N. J. Gillespie	Savannah
1899-1900	J. H. Polhill	Brunswick
1901-1902	Chas. D. Jordan	Monticello
1902-1903	James E. Kidd	Milledgeville
1903-1905	Campbell T. King	Macon
1905-1906	J. D. Persse	Savannah
1906-1907	L. S. Brigham	Savannah
1907-1908	Ben S. Persons	Macon
1908-1909	T. B. Rice	Greensboro
1909-1910	John S. Montgomery	Thomasville
1910-1911	T. H. Brannen	Atlanta
1911-1912	J. W. Ridout	Macon
1912-1913	W. A. Pigman	Savannah

Second Vice-Presidents

1913-1914	S. E. Bayne	Macon
1914-1915	B. W. Mills	Tifton
1915-1916	H. D. Bell	Albany
1916-1917	L. S. Brigham	Columbus
1917-1918	H. C. Shuptrine	Savannah
1918-1919	David G. Wise	Atlanta
1919-1920	Robt. E. Perry	Savannah
1920-1921	Jabe Stamps	Thomaston
1921-1922	F. T. Bergstrom	
1922-1923	Mack D. Hodges	Marietta
1923-1925	A. R. Munn	Atlanta
1927-1929	George Wheat	Columbus
1930-1931	J. L. Hawk	Atlanta
1931-1932	Walter West	Sandersville
1932-1933	W. T. Knight, Jr.	Savannah
1934-1935	Walter West	Sandersville
1935-1936	J. W. Brinson	Wrightsville
1945-1946	Walter West	Sandersville
1946-1947	J. L. Hawk	Atlanta
1947-1948	W. A. Blasingame	Moultrie
1952-1953	T. R. Luck	Carrollton
1954-1955	Malcom W. Fort	Columbus
1955-1956	Henry A. King	Atlanta
1956-1957	Ralph S. Tilly	Rome

Third Vice-Presidents

1875-1876	J. R. Janes	Dawson
1876-1877	Theo. Schuman	Atlanta
1877-1878	Osceola Butler	Savannah
1878-1879	J. W. Jones	Rome
1879-1880	L. E. Welch	Albany
1880-1881	G. M. Heidt	Savannah
1881-1882	Harry Sharp	Atlanta
1882-1883	A. M. Brannon	Columbus
1883-1884	E. S. Lyndon	Athens
1884-1885	H. K. Main	Dalton
1885-1886	J. B. Davenport	Augusta
1886-1887	L. C. Strong	Blakely
1887-1888	C. H. Behre	Atlanta
1888-1889	D. E. McMaster	Tennille
1889-1890	C. D. Jones	Atlanta

Third Vice-Presidents

1890-1891	G. R. Butler	Savannah
1891-1892	James P. Smith	Augusta
1892-1893	J. P. Miller	West Point
1893-1894	W. F. Mims	Atlanta
1894-1895	Lynn Fort	Atlanta
1895-1896	B. J. Smith	Waycross
1896-1897	F. Joerger	Brunswick
1897-1898	J. P. Smith	Augusta
1898-1899	J. H. Polhill	Brunswick
1899-1900	Chas. D. Jordan	Monticello
1901-1902	Jas. E. Kidd	Milledgeville
1902-1903	Campbell T. King	Macon
1903-1904	R. L. Palmer	Atlanta
1904-1905	J. D. Persse	Savannah
1905-1906	L. S. Brigham	Columbus
1906-1907	Mack D. Hodges	Marietta
1907-1908	Thad B. Rice	Greensboro
1908-1909	H. W. Head	Macon
1909-1910	Miss Nenva Straughn	Atlanta
1910-1911	T. H. Brannen	Atlanta
1911-1912	W. A. Pigman	Savannah
1912-1913	S. E. Bayne	Macon
1913-1914	B. W. Mills	Tifton
1914-1915	J. T. Wages	Winder
1915-1916	I. A. Solomons, Jr.	Savannah
1916-1917	T. F. Burbank	Cedartown
1917-1918	D. G. Wise	Atlanta
1918-1919	Robert E. Perry	Sylvania
1919-1920	Jabe Stamps	Thomaston
1920-1921	J. H. Shuptrine	Savannah
1921-1922	J. T. Selman	Atlanta
1922-1923	J. L. Brooks	Tifton
1923-1924	C. D. Robinson	Albany
1924-1925	A. H. Walden	Atlanta
1927-1928	J. C. Ramsay	Louisville
1928-1929	John Montgomery	Thomasville
1930-1931	Mack D. Hodges	Marietta
1931-1932	H. L. Chichester	Macon
1932-1933	Mack D. Hodges	Marietta
1934-1935	H. S. Peters	Manchester
1935-1936	W. W. Fincher	Canton

SUPPLEMENT D

Third Vice-Presidents

1945-1946	J. L. Hawk	Atlanta
1946-1947	W. A. Blasingame	Moultrie
1947-1948	Mel T. Anderson	College Park
1952-1953	W. H. Dunaway	Marietta
1953-1954		
1954-1955	Henry A. King	Atlanta
1955-1956	Ralph Tilly	Rome
1956-1957	C. E. Hallman	Lakeland

GEORGIA PHARMACISTS SERVING AS OFFICERS OF NATIONAL PHARMACEUTICAL ORGANIZATIONS

AMERICAN PHARMACEUTICAL ASSOCIATION

Presidents: 1884—John Ingalls, Macon; 1902—George F. Payne, Atlanta; 1940—Charles H. Evans, Warrenton
Honorary President: 1949—Robert C. Wilson, Athens
Vice President: 1858—Robert Battey, Rome; 1870—Fleming Grieve, Milledgeville; 1877—John Ingalls, Macon; 1896-97, 1898-99, 1901—George F. Payne, Atlanta; 1927—Joseph Jacobs, Atlanta
Chairman of House of Delegates: 1936—Robert C. Wilson, Athens; 1947—Charles H. Evans, Warrenton
Member of Council: 1942-48—Charles H. Evans, Warrenton; 1936—Robert C. Wilson, Athens (ex officio)

NATIONAL ASSOCIATION OF BOARDS OF PHARMACY

President: Charles H. Evans, Warrenton

AMERICAN ASSOCIATION OF COLLEGES OF PHARMACY

President: Robert C. Wilson, Athens

NATIONAL CONFERENCE STATE ASSOCIATION SECRETARIES

President: Robert C. Wilson, Athens

NATIONAL ASSOCIATION OF RETAIL DRUGGISTS

President: W. S. Elkin, Jr., Atlanta; H. C. Shuptrine, Savannah
Vice President: H. L. Chichester, Macon
Treasurer: H. L. Chichester, Macon

WOMEN'S AUXILIARY AMERICAN PHARMACEUTICAL ASSOCIATION
President: Mrs. Charles H. Evans, Warrenton

THE WOMEN'S AUXILIARY
OF THE GEORGIA PHARMACEUTICAL ASSOCIATION

For a number of years prior to 1927, the desirability of having a Women's Auxiliary of the Georgia Pharmaceutical Association was recognized, but its birth awaited the spark which seems to have been supplied by Miss Rose Greer who owned and operated a drug store in the town of Baconton.

"Miss Rose," as she was affectionately known, was the first woman, or at least among the first women, to own and operate a drug store as a licensed pharmacist in Georgia. She was likewise the first woman to hold an official position in the Georgia Pharmaceutical Association as a District President. It was therefore fitting and proper that she should have initiated the idea of forming the Women's Auxiliary and become its first President.

The annual meeting of the Georgia Pharmaceutical Association for 1927 was held in Athens. The Association for that year was operated under the virile leadership of A. R. Munn as President, and Fred T. Bridges as Secretary. The membership for the year was said to be the largest in the history of the Association, totaling approximately 700 members.

With the enthusiasm existing in the parent organization at that time, it proved to be the proper time for the organization of a Women's Auxiliary since there were probably more women present at this meeting than at any previous meeting of the Association.

The following 18 women constituted the Charter Members of the Auxiliary:

Miss Rose Greer, Baconton; Mrs. E. C. Kidd, Milledgeville; Miss Dorcas Greer, Atlanta; Mrs. L. C. Waldrop, Tallapoosa; Miss Mildred Brannen, Atlanta; Mrs. W. T. Knight, Savannah; Mrs. T. H. Brannen, Atlanta; Mrs. W. A. McRae, Valdosta; Mrs. A. R. Munn, Atlanta; Mrs. A. T. Salter, Bartow; Mrs. Fred T. Bridges, Atlanta; Mrs. L. B. Waltham, Newnan; Mrs. H. G. Martin, Uvalda; Mrs. I. H. Reid, Athens; Mrs. Eta Mobley, Uvalda; Mrs. Claude Rountree, Thomasville; Mrs. Charles H. Evans, Warrenton; Mrs. Walter West, Sandersville.

℞ SUPPLEMENT D 413

At this organizational meeting, the following officers were elected: President, Miss Rose Greer of Baconton; Vice President, Mrs. I. H. Reid of Athens; Secretary, Mrs. Claude Rountree of Thomasville. A complete roll of all succeeding officers, 1927-1959, is attached.

There have been many contributions at the hands of the Auxiliary in the life of pharmacy in Georgia, but, in the opinion of the writer, there are three contributions of particularly outstanding value to the cause of pharmacy in Georgia:

1. There is no doubt in this writer's mind but that the Auxiliary, through its own activities, has popularized the parent organization with the men of the profession to the point that today there is the largest dues paid membership in the history of the Association, and the annual meetings of the Association continue to show a larger and larger attendance from year to year with constructive interest more apparent with the passing years.

2. With the sponsorship of the Auxiliary in the movement to raise funds for the establishment of student loan funds and scholarships, there was created throughout the state an appreciation of the values of education as a factor in building a profession.

3. Stimulated and guided by the State Auxiliary, a number of local and district auxiliaries have been formed, thus bringing all members of the profession, both men and women, closer together and centering their aims and objectives toward a higher and more efficient service to the people of Georgia.

With the exception of the War-Year, 1945, the auxiliary has held annual meetings with varying numbers of dues-paid members and attendance. The high point in membership and attendance seems to be at the Augusta meeting, 1951, with 322 members.

Mrs. J. J. Glynn of Savannah, one of the stalwarts of the Auxiliary from 1927-1959, has prepared a summary of the Minutes of the Auxiliary covering these years, from which data come the following notes:

1927—Organizational Meeting at Athens. Annual dues set at 50¢.
1928—Meeting at Columbus—35 members. Talks: "Pharmacy and Literature," and "Lessening the Burdens of Our Husbands at Home."
1929—Meeting at Valdosta—13 members. Talks: "Sharing Our

Husbands' Responsibility," and "Women of All Ages." Dues now $1.00.

1930—Meeting at Macon—13 members. Plans were made to build membership.

1931—Meeting at Macon—43 members. Mrs. Evans proposes establishment of student loan and scholarship fund.

1932—Meeting at Atlanta—63 members. Voted to establish student loan and scholarship fund. Wives of traveling men invited to join Auxiliary.

1933—Meeting at Augusta—41 members. Committee proposed details of plan to raise money for scholarship fund.

1934—Meeting at Savannah—114 members. Plans adopted for scholarship loan fund. Districts asked to raise funds by giving entertainments.

1935—Meeting at Albany—67 members. Two student loans reported amounting to $457.46 and repayments amounting to $235.00.

1936—Meeting at Macon—82 members. Three loans amounting to $335.00 and $342.00 paid back.

1937—Meeting at Atlanta—113 members. $195.95 paid back on loans. Gave $50 to University of Georgia Library.

1938—Meeting at Augusta—115 members. Two student loans made in amount of $162.00; $70.00 paid back.

1939—Meeting at Savannah—110 members. Three student loans amounting to $437.50, and $53.59 paid back. "Benefits Provided by Auxiliary Loans."

1940—Meeting at Valdosta—150 members. Two loans made amounting to $295.00 and $196.91 paid back. Total loans out $772.59. Augusta Auxiliary gave $100 to University of Georgia Library.

1941—Meeting at Macon—163 members. $322.66 paid back on loans. Total amount out in loans $382.00. Atlanta Auxiliary gave $100 to Southern College of Pharmacy Library. 4th District Auxiliary organized.

1942—Meeting at Atlanta—196 members. 15th Anniversary of Auxiliary. Two Loans to students $150.00 reported and $298.40 paid back. Total loans out $382.00. Atlanta Auxiliary gave $100 to Southern College of Pharmacy Library. Balance on hand in bank $1082.49.

1943—Meeting at Macon—124 members. Two student loans made $222.50; $95.25 paid on loans. Balance on hand in bank $1,161.71. A $1000 War Bond was purchased.

SUPPLEMENT D 415

1944—Meeting at Atlanta—$303.30 reported paid on loans. Total amount out in loans $322.50. A second $1000 War Bond purchased.

1945—No meeting held due to War—62 members. Financial statement showed cash on hand in bank $494.46—two $1000 War Bonds.

1946—Meeting at Macon—62 members. One loan of $343.00 with $374.82 paid on loans. All Senior Women Pharmacy students made members of Auxiliary. All outstanding loans paid up with interest. Twelve students having benefitted from student loans.

1947—Meeting at Augusta—140 members. One loan of $414.00 reported. This was 20th Anniversary. 790 letters sent out in membership drive.

1948—Meeting held in Savannah—235 members. No report recorded in minutes.

1949—Meeting in Macon—144 members. One student loan reported and $250.00 paid on outstanding loan.

1950—Meeting in Atlanta—265 members. $623.16 paid on loans. All loans paid in full with interest. This was the Diamond Jubilee Meeting of Ga. Phar. Assoc'n. Pins were purchased for all Past-Presidents of Women's Auxiliary.

1951—Meeting in Augusta—322 members. The financial statement showed cash in bank $1,152.00 and two $1000 War Bonds. A Gavel was presented by Savannah Auxiliary. The Columbus Auxiliary reported organized with 37 members. Pharmacy Dames, Student Wives Auxiliary at U. of Ga. organized with 35 members. This was first organization of its kind in America.

1952—Meeting held in Savannah—246 members. This was Silver Anniversary of Auxiliary. Phy-Wys, Student Wives Auxiliary organized at Southern. $25.00 contributed to APHA Auxiliary Student Loan Fund. Records of Auxiliary 1927-1952 ordered put in permanent form. Revised Constitution and By-Laws was accepted. Past Presidents presented with orchids.

1953—Meeting in Macon—274 members. Student loan fund bonds cashed and funds placed in savings account. Constitution and By-Laws ordered printed for distribution to members.

1954—Meeting in Atlanta—281 members. Constitution and By-Laws distributed to members.

1955—Meeting in Augusta—220 members. Auxiliary Award

established—not to exceed $100 annually to one student University of Georgia and one student at Southern College. The Atlanta Auxiliary gave $1,750 to Southern College.

1956—Meeting in Savannah. Auxiliary awards $100 each to W. O. McMahan of Southern College and John Williams of University of Georgia.

1957—Meeting in Atlanta. Two student awards were made.

1958—Meeting in Atlanta. Two loans were reported.

1959—Meeting in Augusta. Application reported for an additional loan. Dues were increased to $2.00 annually.

MORE POWER TO YOU, WOMEN OF THE AUXILIARY: You have achieved much in the thirty-two years of your existence, but there are many more worthwhile and worthy contributions you can make on the knowledge of pharmacy's needs you have gained through the years. These will come to you as a challenge which we believe will be accepted with your usual enthusiasm and handled with your usual efficiency and good will.

OFFICERS OF THE WOMEN'S AUXILIARY
TO THE GEORGIA PHARMACEUTICAL ASSOCIATION
1927-1959

1927—Athens, Georgia, May 24

Organizational meeting presided over by Miss Rose Greer, Chairman.

1927-28

President . . . . Miss Rose Greer, Baconton
Vice-President . . . . Mrs. I. H. Reid, Athens
Secretary-Treasurer . . Mrs. Claude Rountree, Thomasville

1928—Columbus, Ga., June 7
1928-29

President . . . . Miss Rose Greer, Baconton
Vice-President . . . . . Mrs. George Wheat, Columbus
Secretary-Treasurer . . Mrs. Claude Rountree, Thomasville

1929—Valdosta, Ga., Daniel Ashley Hotel, April 18
1929-30

President . . . . Mrs. R. C. Wilson, Athens
Vice-President . . . . . . Mrs. V. A. McRae, Valdosta
Secretary-Treasurer . . Mrs. Charles H. Evans, Warrenton

1930—Macon, Ga., April 24
1930-31

President . . . . . Mrs. Charles H. Evans, Warrenton
Vice-President . . . . . . Mrs. Nelson Arthur, Athens
Secretary-Treasurer . . . . Mrs. J. L. Williams, Macon

1931—Macon, Ga., Macon Woman's Club, April 23
1931-32

President . . . . . Mrs. Charles H. Evans, Warrenton
Vice-President . . . . . . Mrs. Nelson Arthur, Athens
Secretary-Treasurer . . . . Mrs. J. L. Williams, Macon

1932—Atlanta, Ga., Biltmore Hotel, May 18
1932-33

President . . . . . Mrs. Charles H. Evans, Warrenton
Vice-President . . . . . . Mrs. Nelson Arthur, Athens
Secretary-Treasurer . . . . Mrs. J. L. Williams, Macon

1933—Augusta, Ga., May 23 and 24
1933-34

President . . . . Mrs. W. T. Edmunds, Augusta
Vice-President . . . . . . Mrs. Homer Burson, Macon
Secretary . . . . Mrs. J. K. Patrick, Athens
Treasurer . . . . . Mrs. Claude Rountree, Thomasville
Scholarship Loan Fund Committee:
                       Mrs. W. T. Edmunds, Chairman
                       Mrs. W. S. Elkin, Decatur
                       Mrs. R. C. Wilson, Athens

1934—Savannah, Ga., June 12
1934-35

President . . . . Mrs. W. T. Edmunds, Augusta
Vice-President . . . . . . Mrs. John Taylor, Davisboro
Recording Secretary . . . Mrs. W. L. West, Sandersville
Treasurer . . . . Mrs. H. C. Frech, Savannah

1935—Albany, Ga., May 22 in Minor Auditorium, and May 23 at New Albany Hotel
1935-36

President . . . . Mrs. W. T. Edmunds, Augusta

Vice-President . . . . Mrs. John Taylor, Davisboro
Recording-Secretary . . . Mrs. W. L. West, Sandersville
Treasurer . . . . Mrs. H. C. Frech, Savannah

1936—Macon, Ga., May
1936-37

President . . . . Mrs. John Taylor, Davisboro
First Vice-President . . . . . Mrs. R. L. Olive, Augusta
Second Vice-President . . . . Mrs. J. L. Vaught, Atlanta
Secretary . . . . Mrs. R. C. Wilson, Athens
Treasurer . . . . Mrs. H. C. Frech, Savannah

1937—Atlanta, Ga., Biltmore Hotel, May 11
1937-38

President . . . . Mrs. R. L. Olive, Augusta
First Vice-President . . . . . Mrs. J. L. Vaught, Atlanta
Second Vice-President . . . Mrs. J. E. Gilmore, Savannah
Secretary . . . . Mrs. R. C. Wilson, Athens
Treasurer . . . . . Mrs. William V. Pentecost, Atlanta

1938—Augusta, Ga., Bon Air Hotel, April 26 and 27
1938-39

President . . . . Mrs. J. L. Vaught, Atlanta
First Vice-President . . . . Mrs. J. E. Gilmore, Savannah
Second Vice-President . . . . Mrs. R. M. Mitchell, Griffin
Secretary . . . . . . Mrs. W. T. Edmunds, Augusta
Treasurer . . . . Mrs. W. V. Pentecost, Atlanta

1939—Savannah, Ga., DeSoto Hotel, June 20 and 21
1939-40

President . . . . Mrs. J. E. Gilmore, Savannah
First Vice-President . . . . Mrs. R. M. Mitchell, Griffin
Second Vice-President . . . . Mrs. W. J. Gower, Atlanta
Secretary . . . . . . Mrs. W. T. Edmunds, Augusta
Treasurer . . . . Mrs. W. V. Pentecost, Atlanta

1940—Valdosta, Ga., Daniel Ashley Hotel, April 24 and 25
1940-41

President . . . . Mrs. R. M. Mitchell, Griffin

SUPPLEMENT D

First Vice-President . . . . . Mrs. W. J. Gower, Atlanta
Second Vice-President . . . . . Mrs. Dan Smith, Valdosa
Secretary . . . . Mrs. W. T. Edmunds, Augusta
Treasurer . . . . Mrs. W. V. Pentecost, Atlanta

1941—Macon, Ga., Dempsey Hotel, April 23 and 24
1941-42

President . . . . Mrs. W. J. Gower, Atlanta
First Vice-President . . . . . Mrs. Dan Smith, Valdosta
Second Vice-President . . . . Mrs. C. B. Smith, Newnan
Treasurer . . . . Mrs. W. V. Pentecost, Atlanta
Secretary . . . . Mrs. J. C. Jackson, Augusta

1942—Atlanta, Ga., Piedmont Driving Club, April 14;
  Biltmore Hotel, April 15
1942-43

President . . . . Mrs. Dan Smith, Valdosta
First Vice-President . . . . . Mrs. C. B. Smith, Newnan
Second Vice-President . . . Mrs. T. M. McClesky, Atlanta
Secretary . . . . Mrs. J. C. Jackson, Augusta
Treasurer . . . . Mrs. F. F. Walker, Atlanta

1943—Macon, Ga., Lanier Hotel, April 15
1943-44

President . . . . Mrs. T. O. McClesky, Atlanta
First Vice-President . . . . . Mrs. J. J. Glynn, Savannah
Second Vice-President . Mrs. C. M. Hilderbrand, Tallapoosa
Secretary . . . . Mrs. J. C. Jackson, Augusta
Treasurer . . . . Mrs. F. F. Walker, Atlanta

1944—Atlanta, Ga., Biltmore Hotel, April 20
1944-45

President . . . . Mrs. J. J. Glynn, Savannah
First Vice-President . Mrs. C. M. Hilderbrand, Tallapoosa
Second Vice-President . . . Miss Hyta Plowden, Valdosta
Treasurer . . . . Mrs. J. C. Crumbley, Savannah
Secretary . . . . Mrs. W. B. Chandler, Atlanta

Meeting to be held April, 1945, in Atlanta cancelled due to war conditions

1946—Macon, Ga., Dempsey Hotel, April 15, 16 and 17
1946-47

President . . . . . . Mrs. C. M. Hilderbrand, Tallapoosa
First Vice-President . . . Mrs. W. V. Pentecost, Atlanta
Second Vice-President . . . Mrs. Homer Avera, Ft. Valley
Secretary . . . . Mrs. W. T. Edmunds, Augusta
Treasurer . . . . Mrs. T. C. Marshall, Atlanta

1947—Augusta, Ga., Sheraton Bon Air, April 15 and 16
1947-48

President . . . . Mrs. W. T. Edmunds, Augusta
First Vice-President . . . . Mrs. Homer Avera, Ft. Valley
Second Vice-President . . . . Mrs. J. H. Butler, Atlanta
Secretary . . . . Mrs. Gus Sanders, Augusta
Treasurer . . . . Mrs. T. C. Marshall, Atlanta

1948—Savannah, Ga., General Oglethorpe Hotel, May 4 and 5
1948-49

President . . . . Mrs. Homer Avera, Ft. Valley
First Vice-President . . . . . Mrs. J. H. Butler, Atlanta
Second Vice-President . . . Mrs. W. W. Cowart, Savannah
Secretary . . . . Mrs. Bert Stewart, Augusta
Treasurer . . . . Mrs. T. C. Marshall, Atlanta

1949—Macon, Ga., Dempsey Hotel, April 5 and 6
1949-50

President . . . . Mrs. J. H. Butler, Atlanta
First Vice-President . . . Mrs. W. W. Cowart, Savannah
Second Vice-President . . . . Mrs. Carlton Fite, Calhoun
Secretary . . . . Mrs. Bert Stewart, Augusta
Treasurer . . . . Mrs. W. V. Pentecost, Atlanta

1950—Atlanta, Ga., Biltmore Hotel, April 4 and 5
1950-51

President . . . . Mrs. W. W. Cowart, Savannah
First Vice-President . . . . . Mrs. Carlton Fite, Calhoun
Second Vice-President . . . Mrs. J. M. Goldman, Atlanta
Secretary . . . . Mrs. Bert Stewart, Augusta
Treasurer . . . . Mrs. W. V. Pentecost, Atlanta

1951—Augusta, Ga., Bon Air Hotel, April 11 and 12
1951-52

President	Mrs. W. V. Pentecost, Atlanta
First Vice-President	Mrs. J. M. Goldman, Atlanta
Second Vice-President	Mrs. M. W. Williamson, Soperton
Secretary	Mrs. Harold Hamlet, Augusta
Treasurer	Mrs. Chas. H. Evans, Warrenton

1952—Savannah, Ga., DeSoto Hotel, April 29 and 30.
 Twenty-fifth anniversary
1952-53

President	Mrs. J. M. Goldman, Atlanta
First Vice-President	Mrs. M. W. Williamson, Soperton
Second Vice-President	Mrs. J. M. Monts, Americus
Secretary	Mrs. Harold Hamlet, Augusta
Treasurer	Mrs. Carl Jacobs, Columbus

1953—Macon, Ga., Dempsey Hotel, April 7 and 8
1953-54

President	Mrs. M. W. Williamson, Soperton
First Vice-President	Mrs. Harold Hamlet, Augusta
Second Vice-President	Mrs. C. M. Waldrop, Jr., Savannah
Secretary	Mrs. Charles L. Mundy, Atlanta
Treasurer	Mrs. Carl Jacobs, Columbus

1954—Atlanta, Ga., Biltmore Hotel, April 20 and 21
1954-55

President	Mrs. Harold Hamlet, Augusta
First Vice-President	Mrs. C. M. Waldrop, Jr., Savannah
Second Vice-President	Mrs. R. H. Hogg, Macon
Secretary	Mrs. Charles L. Mundy, Atlanta
Treasurer	Mrs. Leon Brown, Atlanta

1955—Augusta, Ga., Bon Air Hotel, April 19 and 20
1955-56

President	Mrs. C. M. Waldrop, Jr., Savannah
First Vice-President	Mrs. R. H. Hogg, Macon
Second Vice-President	Mrs. Charles L. Mundy, Atlanta
Secretary	Mrs. J. M. Monts, Jr., Americus
Treasurer	Mrs. Leon Brown, Atlanta

1956—Savannah, Ga., DeSoto Hotel, April 24 and 25

1956-57

President	Mrs. R. H. Hogg, Macon
First Vice-President	Mrs. Charles L. Mundy, Atlanta
Second Vice-President	Mrs. Leon Brown, Atlanta
Secretary	Mrs. Cal Hopkins, Augusta
Treasurer	Mrs. H. M. Kennedy, Savannah

1957—Atlanta, Ga., Capital City Club, April 16, and Biltmore Hotel, April 17

1957-58

President	Mrs. Charles Mundy, Atlanta
First Vice-President	Mrs. Leon Brown, Atlanta
Second Vice-President	Mrs. H. M. Kennedy, Savannah
Secretary	Mrs. Malcolm Forte, Columbus
Treasurer	Mrs. Allen Casey, Atlanta

1958—Atlanta, Ga., Piedmont Driving Club, April 15; Biltmore Hotel, April 16

1958-59

President	Mrs. Leon Brown, Atlanta
First Vice-President	Mrs. H. M. Kennedy, Savannah
Second Vice-President	Mrs. H. D. Moseley, Dawson
Secretary	Mrs. Ben F. Boutwell, Macon
Treasurer	Mrs. Allen Casey, Atlanta

1959—Augusta, Ga., Bon Air Hotel, April 28; Partridge Inn, April 29

1959-60

President	Mrs. Leon Brown, Atlanta
First Vice-President	Mrs. H. D. Moseley, Dawson
Second Vice-President	Mrs. Allen Casey, Atlanta
Secretary	Mrs. W. H. Black, Swainsboro
Treasurer	Mrs. Ben F. Boutwell, Macon

1960—Savannah, Ga.

APPENDICES

APPENDIX 1

Glossary of Terms and Formulas of the Period, 1733-1800

AGRIMONY—Eupatoria, Cocklebur, Stickwort
ALL-HEAL—Valerian, Brunella (Prunella)
AQUA SULFURATA—Hydrogen Sulphide Water
AQUA VITAE—Brandy, Whiskey
BALM OF GILEAD—Poplar Buds
BARK—Cinchona
BLACK ALDER—Ilex, Prinoa, Winterberry
BLACK HELLEBORE—Veratrum
BRAMBLE LEAVES—Blackberry
BRIMSTONE—Crude Sulfur
BURDOCK ROOT—Lappa
BUTCHER'S BROOM—Rusci
CARDUUS BENEDICTUS—Blessed Thistle
CHAMOMILE—Matricaria
CELANDINE—Chelidonium
CICHORY—Wild Succory
CINQUEFOIL—Tormentil
COLUMBO—Calumba. A Bitter
CONFRY LEAVES—Comfrey, Symphytum, Black Wort
CONSERVE OF ROSES—A complex formula based on Rose Petals and Sugar
DOCK LEAVES—Rumex, Lappa
DR. PAPA'S REMEDY—Remedy for "Yaws" (Sumac, Pine and Oak Barks)
ELIXIR OF VITRIOL—Aromatic Sulphuric Acid
ELM BARK—Slippery Elm, Ulmus
EMETIC TARTAR—Antimony and Potassium Tartrate
EYEBRIGHT—Euphrasia
FLAX SEED—Linseed
FLOWERS OF SULPHUR—Ordinary Sulfur
FRANKINCENSE—Asiatic: Olibanum, American: Turpentine
GROUND IVY—Glechoma, Nepeta, Cat-Foot
HARTSHORN—The Horn of the Hart
HEMLOCK LEAVES—Fool's Parsley
HIERA PICRA—A Powder of Aloes and Canella
HONEYSUCKLE LEAVES—Caprifolii
HUNGARY WATER—Spirit of Rosemary
HYSSOP—Evidently not the Biblical product. Possibly Skullcap, or Hedge Hyssop
INDIAN PHYSIC—American Ipecac, Gillenia Stipulata
JERUSALEM OAK—Wormseed, Chenopodium
LAPIS CALIMINARIS—Calamine
LAUREL LEAVES—Probably Cherry Laurel
LEEKS—Leek; Allium Parvum

LIVERWORT—Hepatica
LOGWOOD—Haematoxylon. A Dye
MADDER ROOT—A Dye
MALLOW LEAVES—Malvia, emollient, demulcent
MISTLETOE—(American) probably from the Oak. Various medicinal uses
MULLEIN LEAVES—Thapsus Verbascus
NETTLES—Probably Urtica or Stinging Nettles. A decoction used as diuretic
NITRE OR NITER—Potassium Nitrate
NORWAY TAR—Probably Tar from Norway Spruce
OIL OF AMBER—The Oil from the fossil resin
PELLITORY OF THE WALL—Probably Anthemis Pyrethrum
PIONY—Peony. For Convulsions in Children
PLANTANE SEED—Psyllium
POKEBERRY BOUNCE—Pokeroot; Phytolacca
POMATUM—A Pomade or Cosmetic
PRIMROSE—Primula, Cowslip, Lady's Fingers
QUICKSILVER—Metallic Mercury
ROSEMARY—The ordinary garden variety
RUE—Garden Rue, Ruta Graveolens
SAFFRON—Crocus. Dye and medicinal
SAL AMMONIAC—Ammonium Chloride
SAL PRUNELLA—Mixture Fused Potassium Nitrate and Sulphate
SALT OF TARTAR—Potassium Carbonate
SCURVY GRASS—Perhaps Horseradish or Cochlearia
SNAKEROOT—Virginia Snakeroot, Serpentaria
SOLOMON'S SEAL—Polygonatum
SORREL LEAVES—Perhaps Rumex, Yellow Dock
SPIRIT OF VITRIOL—Sulphuric Acid and Wine or Spirit of Ether
SPIRITS OF HARTSHORN—Spirit of Ammonia
TAR WATER—Wood Tar solution in water
TREACLE—Molasses
VALERIAN—All-heal, Brunella (Prunella)
VENICE TREACLE—See Formula
VERDIGRIS—Cupric Subacetate
VERJUICE—Crabapple Juice
WHITE COPPERAS—Zinc Sulphate
WHITE HELLEBORE—Veratrum Album, Sneezewort
WORMWOOD—Absinthium
YARROW—Milfoil
ZIBETHUM—A secretion from the Civet

FORMULAS OF THE PERIOD, 1733-1800

In checking the literature on these obsolete or almost obsolete products, we find that the formulas varied in different countries of the world and at various periods, since there were no law enforcement agencies to detect or prevent substitution, deletion or other change.

DAFFY'S ELIXIR. Known as THE ELIXIR OF HEALTH. Primarily a laxative depending on the presence of Senna, and, in some formulas, Jalap.

SQUIRE'S ELIXIR. Used indiscriminately in the treatment of diarrhoeas and

℞ APPENDIX 1

dysenteries, or intestinal disturbances, depending primarily upon the presence of Opium for its medicinal value.

GODFREY'S CORDIAL, BATEMAN'S PECTORAL DROPS, AND PAREGORIC. All of these products contain Opium in approximately the same amounts, but were aromatized with different volatile oils. All, however, are dependent for any medicinal value on the presence of Opium. They were introduced as a milder form of Laudanum and made more palatable by the introduction of flavoring agents. Godfrey's Cordial is flavored with Sassafras; Bateman's Pectoral Drops with Anise and Gambir; and Paregoric with Camphor, Anise and Benzoic Acid. They were specifically designed for administration to children as mild opiates, and were indiscriminately prescribed, sold, and used.

LANCASHIRE or VINEGAR OF OPIUM. Commonly called "Black Drop" because of its color and the fact that it was given in drops. It contained about 10% of Opium, and the formularies of 1800 called for the use of Verjuice (Crabapple Juice), Nutmeg to disguise the odor of Opium, Saffron for color, and sugar.

LAUDANUM. An unflavored hydro-alcoholic liquid commonly called Tincture of Opium. Said to have been originated by Paracelsus 1658. Contains 10% Opium.

SYDENHAM'S LAUDANUM. Commonly called Wine of Opium. Aromatized with spices. Contains 10% Opium.

DOVER'S POWDER. Said to have been originated by the Buccaneer, Dover, for administration to his sailors. The original formula is said to have contained, in addition to Opium and Ipecac, Potassium Nitrate and Potassium Sulphate and Licorice.

DALBY'S CARMINATIVE. An antacid and carminative to be given to infants and children. Contained Magnesium Carbonate, Potassium Carbonate, AND OPIUM, flavored with Caraway, Fennel, Peppermint, and Syrup.

DEWEE'S CARMINATIVE. An antacid and carminative for colic in children. Contained Magnesium Carbonate, Asafoetida, AND OPIUM. (The author is informed that, but for Dewee's Carminative, he may not have survived childhood.)

DUTCH DROPS or HARLEM OIL. Long known and used on the European Continent under various formulas but always as a "panacea." A product under this name is still available.

ELIXIR OF VITRIOL. Originally a secret formula under the name of Mynsicht's Elixir. In addition to the active constituent, Sulphuric Acid, the 1721 formula is said to have called for eleven vegetable drugs.

HUXHAM'S TINCTURE OF BARK. Prepared under a secret formula and very popular as a remedy for malaria prior to 1800. Huxham is reported to have exploited various proprietary products some of which were said to contain 400 different ingredients.

TURLINGTON'S or FRIAR'S BALSAM. Originated in the 15th or 16th century as a secret remedy and is said to have had during its life more different names than any other one product. The formula has changed from generation to generation and is popular today under the title, "Compound Tincture of Benzoin." Among the various names given to it over the years are the following: Balsamum Equitis Sancti Victoria; Balsamum Commendatoris; Balsamum Catholicum; Balsamum Traumaticum; Balsamum Vulnerarium; Guttae Mader; Guttae Hesuitarium; Tinctura Balsamica; Commander's Balsam; Turlington's Drops; Persian Balsam; Swedish Balsam; Vervain Balsam; Balsam of the Holy Victorious Knight; Turlington's Balsam of Life; Balsamum de Maltha; Ward's Balsam; Jerusalem Balsam; Wade's Drops; Wound Elixir; Saint Victor's Balsam; Balsamic Tincture.

VENICE TREACLE. This was a popular product in its day and the formula evidently varied with time, conscience, and conditions. This formula is taken from *The Edinburgh Dispensatory,* London, 1786, page 620, and represents polypharmacy at its worst.

Squill	Wild Valerian Root
Long Pepper	Gentian Root
Opium	Celtic Nard
Dried Vipers	Spignet
Cinnamon	St. John's Wort
Oil Nutmeg	Ground Pine
Agaric	Germander Tops
Orris Root	Carpobalsam or Cubeb
Scordium	Anise Seed
Red Roses	Sweet Fennel Seed
Navew Seeds	Lesser Cardamon Seed
Ext Licorice	Seeds of Bishop's Weed
Indian Nard	Hartwort
Saffron	Treacle Mustard
Amomum	Hypocistis
Myrrh	Acacia
Zedoary	Storax
Camel's Hay	Sagapenum
Cinquefoil	Terra Lamnia
Rhubarb	Green Vitriol
Ginger	Small Birthwort Root
Dittany of Crete	Lesser Centaury Tops
Horehound Leaves	Candy Carrot Seed
Calamint Leaves	Opoponax
Stechas	Galbanum
Black Pepper	Russian Castor
Macedonian Parsley Seed	White Amber
Olibanum	Calamus
Chio Turpentine	Clarified Honey

℞ APPENDIX 1 427

CONFECTION DAMOCRATES. Formula is from *The Edinburgh Dispensatory,* London, 1786, page 619.

Cinnamon
Myrrh
Agaric
Indian Nard
Ginger
Saffron
Mustard Seed
Frankincense
Chio Turpentine
Camel's Hay
Zedoary
Indian Leaf or Mace
Stechas
Long Pepper
Hartwort
Storax
Opoponax
Galbanum
Oil Nutmeg
Acacia
Bellies of Skinks
Russian Castor

Poley Mountain
Scordium
Cubebs
White Pepper
Candy Carrot Seed
Bellium
Celtic Nard
Gentian Root
Dittany of Crete
Red Roses
Macedonian Parsley Seed
Lesser Cardamon Seed
Sweet Fennel Seed
Gum Arabic
Opium
Calamus
Valerian
Anise Seed
Sagapenum
St. John's Wort
Clarified Honey

APPENDIX 2

Some Drugs Used by the American Indians
(As reported by Youngken, Kremers, Urdang, and Corlett)

* * Aletris
* * American Ipecac
* * American Wormseed
* * Anemone
*   Angelica
* * Arbor Vitae
*   Artemisia
* * Balm of Gilead (Poplar Buds)
*   Balsam of Fir
*   Bearberry
* * Beth Root
* * Black Cherry (Wild)
* * Black Cohosh
* * Black Snake Root
* * Black Walnut
* * Blackberry Root Bark
*   Blue Cohosh
* * Blue Flag
*   Blue Vervain (Verbena)
* * Boneset-Eupatorium
*   Butternut Bark and Sap
*   Button Snake Root
*   Canada Fleabane
* * Canada Snake Root
*   Canadium Hemp
*   Cascara
* * Cassina
* * Common Beggar Lice
* * Corn Smut
* * Cranesbill
* * Culver's Root
* * Dandelion
*   Dogbane—Apocynum
*   Echinacea—Purple Cone Flower
* * Elder Flowers
* * Elderberry
* * Flowering Dogwood
* * Garlic
* * Ginseng
* * Gold Thread—Coptis
* * Golden Ragwort
* * Green Hellebore
*   Grindelia or Gum Plant
* * Hemlock
*   Hepatica
* * Hops
* * Indian Tobacco
*   Jack-in-the-pulpit
*   Jalap—Wild
* * Jimson Weed
* * Juniper—Virginia
* * Ladies Slipper
* * Lobelia (Cardinalis)
*   Maiden Hair Fern
* * Mandrake—May Apple
* * Milkweed
* * Mitchella (Partridge Berry)
* * Mullein
* * Ordinary Tobacco
*   Pasque Flower
* * Pennyroyal
* * Pipsissewa
* * Pleurisy Root
* * Pokeberry—Pokeroot
* * Prickly Ash
* * Pumpkin Seed
* * Raspberry Wild
* * Red Cedar
*   Rhatany
* * Sanguinaria (Blood Root)
*   Sarsaparilla
* * Sassafras
* * Seneca Snake Root
* * Slippery Elm
* * Spikenard

*Reported found in Georgia.

* Sumach
  Sweet Birch
* Sweet Flag
* Turpentine
* Viburnum
* Virginia Snake Root
  Wahoo
* White Oak Bark
  White Pine Bark
* Wild Bergamot
* Wild Cherry
* Wild Indigo
* Wild Licorice
* Wild Mint
* Wintergreen
* Witchhazel
* Yarrow
* Yellow Dock
* Yellow Puccoon—Hydrastis
  Yerba Santa

APPENDIX 3

List of Drugs for Filling Medicine Chests or Boxes*

Allspice
Almonds, Oil of
Almonds, Sweet
Alum
Amber, Oil of
Anderson's Pills
Anise, Oil
Antimony
Aqua Fortis
Arabic, Gum
Arsenic
Asafoetida
Balsam Capivi
Balsam Peru
Balsam Tolu
Bark, Peruvian
Bark, Red
Barley Candy
Barley, Pearl
Bateman's Drops
Beaume de Vie
Benzoin
Bergamot
Blue Flag
Blue Stone
Borax
Brimstone, Flowers
Brimstone, Roll
British Oil
Burgundy Pitch
Calomel
Camphor or Camphire
Cannella alb.
Cantharides
Capers
Caraway Seeds
Cassiae fistulae
Castor Oil
Caustic, Lunar

Caustic, Common
Centaury
Chamomile
Cinnamon
Cloves
Cochineal
Columbo Root
Conserve of Roses
Contrayerva
Copperas
Coriander Seed
Corrosive Sublimate
Cream of Tartar
Currants
Daffy's Elixir
Diachylon, Gum
Diachylon, Plaster
Durham Mustard
Eau de Luce
Elemi, Gum
Elixir Bardana
Elixir of Vitriol
English Saffron
Epsom Salts
Essence of Peppermint
Fennel, Sweet
Figs, Turkey
Fine Salt
Foenugreek Bark
Foenugreek Seeds
Gamboge
Gentian Extract
Gentian Root
Ginger
Glauber Salts
Godfrey's Cordial
Guaiac, Gum
Guaiac, Shavings
Hartshorn

*From advertisements in Georgia newspapers, 1763-1800.

℞ APPENDIX 3

Hellebore
Hepatic, Aloes
Hiera Picra
Honey Water
Hooper's Female Pills
Hungary Water
Huxham's Tincture Bark
Ipecac
Isinglass
Jackson's Bitters
Jalap
James's Powders
James's Powders, Mild For Children
Japan Earth
Jesuit's Bark (See Peruvian Bark)
Juniper Berries
Kino
Laudanum
Lavender, Oil
Lavender, Spirits
Lavender Water
Lead, White
Lemon, Oil of
Licorice
Linseed
Mace
Magnesia
Manna
Marshmallow Roots
Melilot
Mercury
Mint, Oil of
Mint Water
Mezereum
Musk
Myrrh, Gum
Nitre, Sweet Spirit
Nutmeg
Nux Vomica
Oil, Olive
Oil, Sweet
Opium
Orange Flower Water
Paregoric

Pepper
Peppermint
Plaster
Pomatum
Precipitate, Red
Precipitate, White
Prunes
Quicksilver
Raisins
Ratsbane
Resina Flav.
Rectified Spirit of Wine
Rhenish Wine
Rhodium, Oil of
Rhubarb
Rochelle Salts
Saffron
Sage
Sal Ammoniac
Saltpeter
Sal Volatile
Sarsaparilla
Sassafras, Oil of
Scammony
Scurvy Grass, Spirit of
Seneka Snake Root
Senna
Spermaceti
Spike, Oil of
Spleenworth, Tincture
Squire's Elixir
Stoughton's Bitters
Sugar-candy
Sulphur, Flowers ("Brimstone")
Tapioca
Tartar Emetic
Tartar, Salt of
Tartar, Vitriolated
Tea
Thyme
Tolu, Balsam of
Tragacanth
Turlington's Balsam
Turmeric
Turpentine
Valerian

Venice Treacle
Verdigris
Vinegar, Distilled
Vitriol, Blue
Vitriol, Green
Vitriol, White
Vitriolic Ether
Water-Dock, Essence of
White Wax
Wine, Spirits of
Zedoary

APPENDIX 4

Diseases Transmittable from Certain Domestic Animals to Man*

Diseases Transmitted From Dog To Man

VIRUS DISEASES: Lymphocytic choriomeningitis; Rabies.
RICKETTSIAL DISEASES: Boutonneuse fever; Brazilian typhus; Colombian typhus; Kenya typhus; Rocky Mountain Spotted fever; South African tick fever; Q fever; Tsutsugamushi disease.
BACTERIAL DISEASES: Anthrax; *Brucellosis, Br. abortus; Brucellosis, Br. melitensis; Brucellosis, Br. suis;* Diphtheria; Hemorrhagic septicemia; Leptospirosis; Salmonellosis; Scarlet fever; Tuberculosis, bovine type; Tuberculosis, human type; Tularemia.
FUNGOUS DISEASES: Blastomycosis; Coccidioidomycosis; Cryptococcosis; Histoplasmosis; Ringworm, *Microsporum* canis; Sporotrichosis.
PROTOZOAN PARASITES: Amebiasis; Leishmaniasis, Espundia; Leishmaniasis, Kala-azar; Leishmaniasis, Oriental sore; Trypanosomiosis, American; Sarcocystitis.
NEMATODE DISEASES: Creeping eruption; Dirofilaria infection; Dracontiasis; Gnathostomiasis; Strongyloidiasis; Thelaziasis, *Th. californicus;* Thelaziasis, *Th. Callipaeda;* Trichinosis.
CESTODE DISEASES: Dog tapeworm infection; Fish tapeworm infection; Hydatid disease.
TREMATODE DISEASES: Echinochasmus infection; Fasciolopsis infection; Heterophydiasis; Lung fluke disease; Opisthorchiasis, *Clonorchis sinensis;* Opisthorchiasis, *Opis. felineus;* Opisthorchiasis, *Opis. viverrini;* Schistosomiasis, *Sch. japonicum.*
ARTHROPOD DISEASES: *Chigoe* dermatitis; Dog mite dermatitis.

Diseases Transmitted From Cat To Man

VIRUS DISEASES: Cat-scratch disease; Newcastle disease; Rabies.
BACTERIAL DISEASES: Anthrax; Brucellosis, *Br. melitensis;* Diphtheria; Hemorrhagic septicemia; Leptospirosis; Plague; Pseudotuberculosis; Rat bite fever (Sodoku); Salmonella infections; Tuberculosis, bovine type; Tularemia.
FUNGOUS DISEASES: Cryptococcosis; Favus; Histoplasmosis; Ringworm.
PROTOZOAN PARASITES: Amebiasis; Leishmaniasis, Kala-azar; Leishmaniasis, Oriental sore; Trypanosomiosis, American.
NEMATODE DISEASES: Creeping eruption; Gnathostomiasis; Thelaziasis; Trichinosis.

*Taken from Hull, Thomas G., *Diseases Transmitted from Animals to Man.* Springfield (Illinois): Charles C. Thomas, 4th ed., pp. 680-683.

CESTODE DISEASES: Dog Tapeworm infection; Fish Tapeworm infection.
TREMATODE DISEASES: Heterophydiasis; Lung fluke disease; Opisthorchiasis, *Clonorchis sinensis;* Opisthorchiasis, *Opis. felineus;* Opisthorchiasis, *Opis. viverrini;* Schistosomiasis, Sch. japonicum.
ARTHROPOD DISEASES: Dog mite dermatitis.

DISEASES TRANSMITTED FROM HOG TO MAN

VIRUS DISEASES: Foot-and-Mouth disease; Rabies; Vesicular stomatitis.
BACTERIAL DISEASES: Anthrax; Brucellosis, *Br. melitensis;* Brucellosis, *Br. suis;* Hemorrhagic septicemia; Leptospirosis (Swineherd disease); Listeriosis; Pseudotuberculosis; Salmonella food infections; Swine erysipelas; Tuberculosis, bovine type; Tuberculosis, human type; Tularemia.
FUNGOUS DISEASES: Actinomycosis; Aspergillosis.
PROTOZOAN DISEASES: Amebiasis *E. histolytica;* Amebiasis *E. polecki;* Balantidiosis; Trypanosomiasis, African.
NEMATODE DISEASES: Gongylonemiasis; Metastrongyliasis; Trichinosis.
CESTODE DISEASES: Hydatid disease; Pork tapeworm infection.
TREMATODE DISEASES: Fasciolopsis infection; Gastrodiscoides infection; Lung fluke disease; Opisthorchiasis.
ARTHROPOD DISEASES: Chigoe dermatitis.

DISEASES TRANSMITTED FROM SHEEP TO MAN

VIRUS DISEASES: Foot-and-mouth disease; Rabies; Rift Valley fever; Sore mouth of sheep (contagious ecthyma).
RICKETTSIAL DISEASES: Q fever; Rocky Mountain spotted fever.
BACTERIAL DISEASES: Anthrax; Brucellosis, *Br. abortus;* Brucellosis, *Br. melitensis;* Brucellosis, *Br. suis;* Hemorrhagic septicemia; Listeriosis; Pseudotuberculosis; Salmonella infection; Tularemia; Vibriosis.
FUNGOUS DISEASES: Actinomycosis, Coccidiodomycosis; Ringworm, *Trichophyton sp.*
PROTOZOAN DISEASES: Sarcocystitis; Trypanosomiasis, African.
NEMATODE DISEASES: Metastrongyliasis; Ostertagia infection; Sheep wireworm infection; Trichostrongylus infection.
CESTODE DISEASES: Hydatid disease.
TREMATODE DISEASES: Fascioliasis; Schistosomiasis, *Sch. bovis.*
ARTHROPOD DISEASES: Mange.

DISEASES TRANSMITTED FROM HORSE TO MAN

VIRUS DISEASES: Encephalomyelitis, Eastern; Encephalomyelitis, Western; Encephalomyelitis, Venezuelan; Encephalitis, Japanese B; Encephalitis, Murray Valley; Rabies; Vesicular stomatitis.
BACTERIAL DISEASES: Anthrax; Brucellosis, *Br. abortus;* Brucellosis, *Br. suis;* Glanders; Hemorrhagic septicemia; Leptospirosis; Pseudotuber-

culosis; Relapsing fever, endemic; Salmonellosis; Swine erysipelas; Tuberculosis, bovine type.

FUNGOUS DISEASES: Actinomycosis; Aspergillosis; Cryptococcosis; Epizootic lymphangitis; Rhinosporidiosis; Ringworm, *Trichophyton faviforme;* Ringworm, *T. mentagrophytes;* Sporotrichosis.

PROTOZOAN DISEASES: Sarcocystitis; Trypanosomiasis, African.

TREMATODE DISEASES: Schistosomiasis, *Schistosoma japonicum.*

ARTHROPOD DISEASES: Mange, *Sarcoptes sp.*

Diseases Transmitted From Cow To Man

VIRUS DISEASES: Cowpox; Foot-and-mouth disease; Milkers nodules; Newcastle disease; Rabies; Rift Valley fever; Vesicular stomatitis.

RICKETTSIAL DISEASES: Anthrax; Brucellosis, *Br. abortus;* Brucellosis, *Br. Melitensis;* Brucellosis, *Br. suis;* Diphtheria; Hemorrhagic septicemia; Leptospirosis; Listeriosis; Pseudotuberculosis; Relapsing fever, endemic; Salmonella infection; Scarlet fever; Septic sore throat; Tuberculosis, bovine type; Vibriosis.

FUNGOUS DISEASES: Actinomycosis; Aspergillosis; Coccidioidomycosis; Cryptococcosis; Nocardiosis; Rhinosporidiosis; Ringworm, *Microsporum canis;* Ringworm, *Trichophyton sp.*

PROTOZOAN DISEASES: Sarcocystitis; Trypanosomiasis, African.

NEMATODE DISEASES: Creeping eruption; Gongylonemiasis; Metastrongyliasis; Ostertagia infection; Sheep wireworm infection; Syngamosis; Trichostrongylus infection.

CESTODE DISEASES: Beef tapeworm infection; Hydatid disease.

TREMATODE DISEASES: Fascioliasis; Schistosomiasis, *Sch. bovis;* Schistosomiasis, *Sch. japonicum.*

ARTHROPOD DISEASES: Mange.

CHEMICAL POISONING: Milk Sickness.

APPENDIX 5

MEMBERS OF GEORGIA STATE BOARD OF PHARMACY, 1881-1958

Avera, Homer J.	Fort Valley	1954-1959
Baldwin, Asbury Q.	Madison	1950-1955
Barry, E.	Augusta	1881-1887
Bayne, S. E.	Macon	1904-1914
Bell, H. D.	Albany	1920-1923
Blasingame, W. A.	Moultrie	1938-1943
Brewer, Lester R.	Atlanta	1941-1946
Bridges, W. G.	Columbus	1933-1938
Bush, J. E.	Barnesville	1923-1928
Butler, Osceola	Savannah	1881-1887
Camp, L. N.	Atlanta	1936-1941
Case, Geo. D.	Milledgeville	1887-1890
Chichester, H. L.	Macon	1946-1951
Davis, B. D., Jr.	Douglas	1955-
Deen, H. A.	Vidalia	1930-1935
Deen, Tom S.	Douglas	1945-1950
Dodson, J. G.	Americus	1900-1903
Dunaway, W. H.	Marietta	1948-1953
Durban, S. C.	Augusta	1887-1903
Edmunds, W. T.	Augusta	1928-1933
Elkin, W. S., Jr.	Atlanta	1906-1911
Enloe, Van P.	Rome	1937-1942
Evans, Charles H.	Warrenton	1929-1934
Forte, Malcom W.	Columbus	1944-1949
Goodwyn, John W.	Macon	1887-1895
Hardman, S. L.	Covington	1958-
Hawk, Judson L.	Atlanta	1931-1936
Herrin, H. M.	Winder	1932-1937
Hodges, M. D.	Marietta	1923-1928
Ingalls, John	Macon	1881-1887
Joerger, F.	Brunswick	1890-1895
Johnstone, F. E.	Savannah	1920-1925
Jones, Walter D.	Savannah	1914-1919
Jordan, C. D.	Monticello	1900-1915
Land, R. H., Jr.	Augusta	1904-1914
Lyndon, E. S.	Athens	1885-1887
Marshall, T. C.	Atlanta	1916-1921
Massey, J. E.	Hahira	1939-1944
McCleskey, T. M.	Atlanta	1951-1956
Meadows, W. H.	Columbus	1914-1919
Mitchell, Jesse	Macon	1925-1930

℞   APPENDIX 5

Mitchell, R. M.	Griffin	1934-1939
Morris, Max	Macon	1899-1904
Murray, E. L.	Americus	1915-1925
Oatts, Ernest W.	Dublin	1956-
Olive, R. L.	Augusta	1940-1945
Oliver, E. C.	Thomasville	1952-1957
Payne, George F.	Macon	1891-1906
Pemberton, John S.	Atlanta	1881-1887
Pendergrast, J. B.	Atlanta	1926-1931
Persons, Ben S.	Macon	1913-1923
Peters, Hoke S.	Manchester	1947-1952
Rountree, C. L.	Thomasville	1924-1929
Schumann, Theo.	Atlanta	1887-1890
Selman, J. T.	Atlanta	1921-1926
Shackelford, B. H.	Atlanta	1957-
Sharp, Harry	Atlanta	1890-1902
Shuptrine, H. E.	Savannah	1908-1913
Slack, Henry R., Jr.	LaGrange	1887-1899
Turner, John P.	Columbus	1895-1900
Waldrop, L. C.	Tallapoosa	1927-1932
West, Walter L.	Sandersville	1935-1940
Whatley, P. A.	Gainesville	1942-1947
Williams, Everett	Statesboro	1949-1954
Woodcock, J. B.	Gainesville	1953-1958
Zacharias, Isidore	Columbus	1881-1885

Chief Drug Inspectors of Georgia

T. A. Cheatham	1907-1927
A. M. Stead	1927-1932
H. A. Deen	1932-1935
W. S. Elkin	1935-1937
J. E. Bush	1937-1941
M. M. Yearty	1941-1942
L. N. Camp	1942-1944
G. M. Parkerson	1944-1946
P. D. Horkan	1946-

APPENDIX 6
A Medical Fee Bill of Vintage 1865
From the *Southern Banner* (Athens), February 22, 1865

PHYSICIANS' FEES.

ATHENS, Jan. 18, 1865

A meeting of the physicians was held this morning at the office of Drs. C. W. & H. R. J. Long, and was organized by the nomination of Dr. G. L. McCleskey as Chairman, and Dr. R. M. Smith as Secretary.

The Chairman explained the object of the meeting to take into consideration the prices to be assessed for professional services, and if possible to arrive at a just and equitable schedule for the same.

Upon consultation, it was unanimously agreed that the fees should be—

Single visit, day light,	$15 00
" " night,	25 00
Mileage, in day time,	5 00
" night,	10 00
Fee for accouchment, simple,	200 00
" " complicated, 250 00 to	350 00
Extracting teeth,	5 00
Cupping and phlebotomy,	5 00
Opening abcesses,	5 00
Examination and prescription,	10 00
Consultation fee,	25 00
Cases of small pox per visit,	150 00

It is with regret that we are compelled to advance the fees, but the necessity for it is sufficiently obvious to need no comment.

The sentiments of the meeting are, that professional services should be at the old standard prices, if payment is made in produce or the necessary articles of life at old prices.

On motion, it was resolved, That all bills are due when the case is dismissed, and settlements required every three months.

R. D. MOORE,   G. L. McCLESKEY,
C. W. LONG,   J. B. CARLTON,
R. M. SMITH,   H. R. J. LONG,
              CICERO HOLT.

Feb. 22

NOTE: This Fee Bill illustrates the fact that "produce," consisting of food and other "necessities of life," was more valuable than the deflated paper currency of the period.

BIBLIOGRAPHY

Ackernecht, Erwin H., *Malaria in the Upper Mississippi Valley, 1760-1900*. Baltimore: The Johns Hopkins Press, 1945.
American Association of Colleges of Pharmacy, Proceedings of, 1900-1935.
American Druggist, July, 1956.
American Journal of Pharmaceutical Education, 1937-1957.
American Pharmaceutical Association, Journal of the, 1912-1957.
American Pharmaceutical Association, Proceedings of, 1852-1911.
Anderson, J. Randolph, "The Spanish Era in Georgia History," *Georgia Historical Quarterly,* Vols. 20-21, 1936-1937.
Athens Gazette, Athens, Georgia, Vol. IV, April 10, 1817.
Augusta Business Directory, Augusta, Georgia, 1859-1866.
Augusta Chronicle, Augusta, Georgia, 1784-1820.
Augusta Herald, Augusta, Georgia, 1799-1821.
Bassett, Victor H., "Voices of the Past," *Bulletin of The Georgia Medical Society,* Vol. I, Nos. 5, 6, 7, 8, and 9, 1936.
Battey, F. A., *Biographical Souvenir of the States of Georgia and Florida.* Chicago: F. A. Battey and Co., 1889.
Beasley, Henry, *The Druggist's General Receipt Book.* Philadelphia: Lindsay and Blakiston, 1863.
Blanton, Wyndham B., *Medicine in Virginia in the 17th Century.* Richmond: The William Byrd Press, Inc., 1930.
Blanton, Wyndham B., *Medicine in Virginia in the 18th Century.* Richmond: Garrett and Massie, Inc., 1931.
Boland, Frank Kells, *The First Anesthetic: The Story of Crawford W. Long.* Athens: University of Georgia Press, 1950.
British Pharmaceutical Codex, 1949-1954.
British Pharmacopoeia, 1953.
Brooks, R. P., *The University of Georgia Under Sixteen Administrations, 1785-1955.* Athens: University of Georgia Press, 1956.
Buchan's Physician (15th edition), 1797.
Bullock, Henry Morton, *A History of Emory University.* Nashville: Parthenon Press, 1936.
Buzzell, Frank M., "Origin and Development of the Ice Cream Industry," *Ice Cream Trade Journal,* Vol. 53, 1909.

Candler, Allen D., ed., *The Colonial Records of the State of Georgia,* 26 vols. Atlanta: Franklin Printing and Publishing Co., 1904-1916.

Candler, Allen D., ed., *Revolutionary Records of Georgia,* 3 vols. Atlanta: Franklin-Turner Co., 1908.

Candler, Charles Howard, *Asa Griggs Candler.* Atlanta: Emory University, 1950.

Candler, Charles Howard, *Asa Griggs Candler—Coca-Cola and Emory College, 1888.* Emory University Library Publications, Series VII, No. 2. Atlanta: Emory University, 1953.

Census of Business, U. S. Department of Commerce Bureau of the Census: 1929-1930; 1939-1940; 1954, Vol. II.

Centennial Meeting of the Medical Association of Georgia (Pamphlet), 1949.

Columbian Museum & Savannah Advertiser, Savannah, Georgia, 1797-1804.

Coulter, E. Merton, *College Life in the Old South.* Athens: University of Georgia Press, 1951.

Coulter, E. Merton, *Georgia: A Short History.* Chapel Hill: University of North Carolina Press, 1933.

Coulter, E. Merton, and Albert B. Saye, *A List of the Early Settlers of Georgia.* Athens: University of Georgia Press, 1949.

Cramp, Arthur J., *Nostrums and Quackery and Pseudo-Medicine,* Vol. III. Chicago: Press of the American Medical Association, 1936.

Culbreth, David Marvel Reynolds, *Materia Medica and Pharmacology* (3rd, 4th, 5th, 6th and 7th editions). Philadelphia: Lea and Febiger, 1927.

Ewell, James, *Planters and Mariners Medical Companions.* Philadelphia: John Bioren, 1807.

Farmer's Gazette, Sparta, Georgia, Vol. IV, May, 1807.

Faust, Ernest Carroll, "Clinical and Public Health Aspects of Malaria in the United States from an Historical Perspective," *American Journal of Tropical Medicine,* 1944-1945.

Fort, Tomlinson. *A Dissertation on the Practice of Medicine.* Milledgeville, Georgia: Printed at the Federal Union Office, 1849.

Franke, Norman H., "Pharmacy and Pharmacists in the Confederacy," *Georgia Historical Quarterly,* Vols. 37-38, 1953-1954.

Garrett, Franklin, *Atlanta and Environs,* Vol. II. New York: Lewis Historical Publishing Co., 1954.

Garrett, Franklin, "Coca-Cola and the Soda Fountain," c. 1949.

Gathercoal, Edmund Norris and Elmer H. Wirth, *Pharmacognosy.* Philadelphia: Lea and Febiger, 1949.

Georgia Express, Athens, Georgia, 1808-1815.

Georgia Gazette, Savannah, Georgia, 1763-1769.

Georgia Historical Collections, Vols. 1-9. Collections of the Georgia Historical Society, Savannah, Georgia.

BIBLIOGRAPHY

Georgia Historical Quarterly, Vols. 1-40, 1917-1956.
Georgia Journal, Milledgeville, Georgia, c. 1810-1815.
Georgia Pharmaceutical Association, Proceedings of, 1875-1958.
Georgia Republican and State Intelligencer, Savannah, Georgia, 1803-1805.
Georgia Royal Gazette, Savannah, Georgia, c. 1770-1783.
Gilmer, George R., *Sketches of Some of the Early Settlers of Upper Georgia.* New York: Appleton and Co., 1885.
Goodrich, W. H., "History of the Medical Department of the University of Georgia, 1828-1928," *Georgia Historical Quarterly,* Vol. 24, 1940.
Gordon, Maurice Bear, *Aesculapius Comes to the Colonies.* Ventnor, N. J.: Ventnor Publishing Co., 1949.
Graves, Robert, *Pocket Conspectus of the London and Edinburgh Pharmacopoeia.* Philadelphia, 1803.
Haggard, Howard W., *Devils, Drugs and Doctors.* New York: Harper & Brothers, 1929.
Harral, George, *Medicine Book.* Savannah, Georgia: T. G. Collier, 1807.
Hindle, Brooke, *The Pursuit of Science in Revolutionary America.*
Jacobs, Joseph, "How I Won and Lost an Interest in Coca-Cola," *Drug Topics,* 1929.
Jacobs, Joseph, "Some of the Drug Conditions During the War Between the States, 1861-1865," *Proceedings of The American Pharmaceutical Association,* Vol. 46: 192ff, 1898.
Jacobs, Joseph, "Soda Water in the 70's."
Jacobs, Joseph, "Some Personal Recollections of a Georgia Boy in a Georgia Drug Store," *Drug Topics,* 1926.
Jacobs, Sinclair, "Joseph Jacobs, Master of Pharmacy."
Jones, Charles E., *Education in Georgia.* Washington: Government Printing Office, 1889.
Justice, R. S., "Some Medicinal and Poisonous Plants of Georgia," *Bulletin of The University of Georgia School of Pharmacy,* Vol. XXXIX, No. 9, July, 1939.
Knight, Lucian Lamar, *Georgia's Landmarks, Memorials and Legends,* Vols. 1, 2. Atlanta, 1913.
Krafka, Joseph, "Medicine in Colonial Georgia," *Georgia Historical Quarterly,* Vols. 20-21, 1936-1937.
Kraemer, Henry, *Scientific and Applied Pharmacognosy.* Philadelphia: The Author, 1915.
Kremers, Edward, and George Urdang, *History of Pharmacy: A Guide* (2nd edition). New York: J. B. Lippincott, 1951.
LaWall, Charles H., *The Curious Lore of Drugs and Medicines.* Garden City, N. Y.: Garden City Publishing Company, 1921.
LaWall, Charles H., *Four Thousand Years of Pharmacy.* Philadelphia: J. B. Lippincott, 1927.
Legislative Acts of the State of Georgia (Medicine and Pharmacy), 1825-1958.

Lucas, P. S., "Ice Cream Manufacture," *Journal of Dairy Science,* June, 1956.
Macon Business Directory, Macon, Georgia, 1878-1879, 1919-1920, 1922, 1946.
Massengill, S. E., *A Sketch of Medicine and Pharmacy.*
Meadows, John C., *Modern Georgia.* Athens: University of Georgia Press, 1954.
Mortensen, Martin, "Means By Which the Ice Cream Industry Has Been Developed in the U. S.," *Proceedings: World Dairy Congress.* Vol. I: 446, 1923.
Merck Index (6th edition). Merck and Company, 1952.
National Formulary (10 editions). Distributed by J. B. Lippincott Co., Philadelphia, 1955.
National Formulary of Unofficinal Preparations (First Issue). American Pharmaceutical Association, 1888.
National Standard Dispensatory, Hare, Caspari, and Rusby. Philadelphia: Lea Brothers & Co., 1907.
New Dispensatory, Gentlemen and Faculty at University of Edinburgh, 1786.
Palmer, Carl J., *History of the Soda Fountain Industry* (Booklet).
Pemberton, J. S., "Essay on Guarana, Caffeine, and Coca." Paper given before 12th Annual Meeting of the Georgia Pharmaceutical Association, Cumberland Island, Georgia, April, 1887.
Pharmaceutical Recipe Book (1st, 2nd, and 3rd editions). Publication of the American Pharmaceutical Association.
Pharmacologia (Paris'), J. A. Paris (4th American edition), 1831.
Pharmacopoeia Officinalis and Extemporanea, John Quincy. London, 1719.
Pharmacopoeia of the United States (13 revisions), 1820.
Philadelphia College of Pharmacy 1821-1921, The First Century of. Philadelphia: Philadelphia College of Pharmacy, 1922. (Also First Decennial Supplement, 1931).
Phillipps Collection, "Egmont Manuscripts," Vol. 14204, 32-36. University of Georgia Library, Athens.
Pierson, George M., ed., and Edward L. Bortz, mgr. ed., *Cyclopedia of Medicine, Surgery and Specialties,* Vols. 1-15. Philadelphia: F. A. Davis Co., 1939-1943. (Service Volumes, 1943-1957).
Porcher, Francis P., *Resources of the Southern Fields and Forests* . . . . Charleston, S. C.: Steampower Press of Evans & Cogwell, 1863.
Prince's Digest of Laws, 1787-1837. University of Georgia Library, Athens.
Proctor, William, Jr., ed., *Practical Pharmacy* (By Mohr and Redwood). Philadelphia: Lea and Blanchard, 1849.
"Professional Education in the United States, *"Bulletin of The University of the State of New York,* No. 10, March 1900.
Ross, Mary, *Spanish Days in Glynn County. A Story of "The Virtuous Sassafras."* (Pamphlet).

BIBLIOGRAPHY

Savannah City Directory, Savannah, Georgia, 1859, 1866-1867, 1871-1872, 1875.
Saye, Albert B., *Georgia Government and History.* Evanston, Illinois: Row Peterson and Co., 1957.
Sollmann, Torald, *A Manual of Pharmacology* (5th edition). Philadelphia: W. B. Saunders Co., 1936.
System of Botany, LeMaout and Ducaisne. (Translated by Mrs. Hooker, 1873).
Southeastern Drug Journal, Vols. 20-30, 1945-1956.
Taylor, Frances Long, *Crawford W. Long and the Discovery of Ether Anaesthesia.* New York: Paul Hoeber, 1928.
Telamon Cuyler Collection, University of Georgia Library, Athens.
Tennet, John, *The Poor Planter's Physician or Every Man His Own Doctor.* Philadelphia, 1734.
Turnbow, Grover, and P. H. Tracey, and Andrew Rafetto, *The Ice Cream Industry* (2nd edition). New York: J. Wiley & Sons, Inc., 1947.
Urdang, George, *Pharmacy's Part in Society.* Madison, Wisconsin: American Institute of the History of Pharmacy, 1946.
U. S. D. A. Agricultural Marketing Service, Statistical Bulletin, No. 136, 1953: No. 169, 1954; No. 199, 1956.
U. S. Dispensatory (19th edition), Wood, Remington, and Sadtler.
Wesley, John, *Primitive Physic or An Easy Way to Treat Most Ordinary Diseases* (32 editions). Philadelphia, 1747.
White, George, *White's Historical Collections of Georgia.* New York: Pudney & Russell, 1854.
White's Statistics of Georgia. Savannah, Georgia: W. Thorne Williams, 1849.
Woolley, Samuel Walter, and G. P. Forrester, *Pharmaceutical Formulas* (10th edition), Vol. 1. London: Chemist and Druggist, 1929.
Wootten, A. C., *Chronicles of Pharmacy,* 2 Vols. London: Macmillan Co., 1910.
Youngken, Heber W., "Drugs of the North American Indians," *American Journal of Pharmacy,* Vol. 95: 329, 1923; Vol. 96: 485, 1924; Vol. 97: 158 and 257, 1925.

www.ingramcontent.com/pod-product-compliance
Lightning Source LLC
Chambersburg PA
CBHW072129220426
43664CB00013B/2186